Explorations
in Child
Psychiatry

CONTRIBUTORS

E. James Anthony

L. Eugene Arnold

Lauretta Bender

Gaston E. Blom

Hilde Bruch

Justin D. Call

Dennis P. Cantwell

Stella Chess

Donald J. Cohen

Leon Cytryn

Joseph Fischhoff

Edward H. Futterman

M. W. Laufer

Reginald S. Lourie

Ake Mattsson

Louis W. Sander

Theodore Shapiro

Explorations in Child Psychiatry

EDITED BY

E. James Anthony

William Greenleaf Eliot Division of Child Psychiatry
Washington University School of Medicine
St. Louis, Missouri

WITH A FOREWORD BY

Jean Piaget

PLENUM PRESS • NEW YORK AND LONDON

Library of Congress Cataloging in Publication Data

Anthony, Elwyn James.
  Explorations in child psychiatry.

  Includes bibliographies and index.
  1. Child psychiatry. 2. Psychiatric research. I. Title. [DNLM: 1. Child
psychiatry. 2. Child psychology. WS350 A628p]
RJ499.A58   618.9'28'9   75-2308
ISBN 0-306-30819-3

© 1975 Plenum Press, New York
A Division of Plenum Publishing Corporation
227 West 17th Street, New York, N.Y. 10011

United Kingdom edition published by Plenum Press, London
A Division of Plenum Publishing Company, Ltd.
Davis House (4th Floor), 8 Scrubs Lane, Harlesden, London, NW10 6SE, England

Printed in the United States of America

To "Le Patron"

PROFESSOR JEAN PIAGET

Who taught us how to talk to children,
to understand them, and to learn from them.

FOREWORD

It is a great pleasure for me to write a foreword to this fine work by many different collaborators under the aegis of my friend and one-time colleague in Geneva, Dr. E. James Anthony, because it represents a collective effort toward a goal that today seems very necessary yet difficult to attain. This goal is the synthesis of developmental psychology with all the other aspects of child psychology into *a science of ontogenetic development* from birth to maturity encompassing three points of view—the biological, the behavioral, and the internalization of the behavioral into mental life.

This synthesis is indeed necessary since it is not possible to understand a disorder or a developmental arrest without having a sufficient knowledge of the ensemble[1] of elements that has brought it about. At each level of development, the personality of the subject attempts to integrate a multiplex system of factors in varying proportion, and without carefully and fully considering this interdigitating whole, it is not easy to disentangle the mechanisms involved in any particular functional disintegration. Similarly, the fact that child psychiatry is largely based on the principle of "syndromes" demands, as a matter of course, the inclusion of an "analytic" approach to the problem being studied, not only with regard to the specific psychogenesis but also with respect to the pathogenic processes making up the interdependent, interrelated system, since the elements of disorder share a conjoint responsibility for the functioning of the system as a whole. However, since there are those who remain normal in situations where others become variously disturbed, the meaning of the disorder to be remedied can be extremely diverse, and in order to grasp it, it is necessary to immerse oneself in the ensemble at the different developmental stages, the order of which is by no means fortuitous but resembles the orderly sequence of stages observed in em-

---

[1] This is a most important word in Piaget's psychological system but very difficult to translate precisely. It has a Gestalt sense that implies a total organized and coordinated whole—a well-orchestrated functional unit. (Editor)

bryogenesis. Thus, for example, when the psychiatrist is confronted clinically with a learning disability, he should not content himself merely with the signs and symptoms or with measures of intelligence and emotionality; what he must discover is the level at which the cognitive process has foundered and must, therefore, examine the patient as to his stage of operational thinking (logical, arithmetical, spatial, temporal, causal, etc.) and integrate these data with others derived from the more clinical inquiry.

However, this procedure is difficult to carry out for all sorts of reasons, the two main ones being the following:

1. Since an integrated diagnosis of development is, by its very nature, interdisciplinary, it is essential, in order to effect a synthesis, to evolve and to use a *common language*. It is not enough simply to put together thick dossiers juxtaposing findings relating to physical growth, electroencephalography, family conflict, social environment and intellectual performance. What is needed to coordinate all these different aspects is a linguistic medium that is sufficiently "general." However, an integration of this sort is by no means easy, especially in relation to the complex interaction between cognition and feeling, and I do not, in any way, consider that my particular language and my particular cognitive approach is adequate for this task.[2] However, I am hoping

---

[2] Readers might like to be reminded that at an interdisciplinary symposium in 1958 Professor Piaget spoke tentatively to the international group about the prospect of a common language and attempted to illustrate his point by "translating" the dynamic concepts of psychoanalysis into the language of equilibrium. In this new language, the oedipus stage represented a certain form of affective equilibrium "characterized by a maximization of the 'gains' expected from the mother and by a minimization of the 'losses' expected from the father". Piaget pondered as to whether the equilibrium point corresponded to a Bayes strategy, the criterion of which would be a simple maximum of "gain minus loss" or whether it corresponded to a "minimax" strategy, with a search for the minimum or the maximum loss which the subject supposes that a hostile environment is trying to inflict on him. He felt that the solution depended on the overall environmental conditions of each child. His "common language," as described at the time, consisted of modern applications of probabilistic language (information and games theory) coupled with the language of equilibrium. (*Discussions On Child Development,* Volume 4, pg. 8. Editors: J. M. Tanner & B. Inhelder. New York: International Universities Press, 1960.) Earlier, in 1942, he attempted to translate certain parts of psychoanalytic theory into the language of schema. Thus, when an individual rebelled against his father (the "father complex") and subsequently adopted the same rebellious attitude to other authority figures, it did not follow, he said, "that he was unconsciously identifying each of these persons with the image of his father." In the language of schemas the child acquired a primary affective schema with respect to his father and generalized this in later situations that were subjectively analogous. If, following a rebellious encounter, the individual dreamed of his antagonist in a childhood setting, this simply signified that the affective schemas were less susceptible to generalization and abstraction than the cognitive schemas. Piaget, of course, is doing more here than mainly translating into his own language; he is reconceptualizing the psychoanalytic belief in a conservation of affect in the unconscious behind a repression barrier. (*Play, Dreams, and Imitation in Childhood,* p. 189. London: Heinemann, 1951) (Editor)

that it is child psychiatry that will enlarge our frame of reference and achieve these crucial syntheses, the most essential being the *preservation of the dynamic and psychogenetic outlook* that has guided so much of my own work.

2. The second difficulty lies in the necessity of using an *experimental approach* to clinical problems. Clinicians are always tempted to overstate the value of the individual "case" and to construct theories on isolated and exceptional instances. If psychopathology is ever to be a completely scientific discipline, it requires an effort and an attitude of mind that approximates more nearly that of the physiologist or biologist than that of the practitioner. On the other hand, the cooperation between the "case" study and the general processes at work can also make a most informative contribution, and we can, therefore, look forward very much to the child psychiatry that develops out of this.

To put it briefly, developmental psychologists (including myself, here honored by having this work dedicated to me) are looking forward with great expectation to the emergence of *developmental psychopathology* as a new discipline still struggling to organize its own relevant field of knowledge. They are hoping especially that in spite of all the obstacles in the way and the huge amount of creative effort required for the purpose that this science will constitute itself on an interdisciplinary basis as wide as possible and on a common language that helps to unify what is precise and generalizable. The present collective study already represents a good beginning, activated as it is by the dynamism and conviction of Dr. Anthony. I am happy to express to him here, in the name of the School of Geneva, our warmest wishes for the pursuit and success of this endeavor.

JEAN PIAGET

École de Psychologie et des Sciences de l'Education
Université de Genève
Switzerland
December, 1974

PREFACE

One can suppose that the reason why *Tristram Shandy* appeals so much to child researchers (as evident from Dr. Lourie and the editor, who both quote him) is because he is "so developmental" that, when he traces his history, he does so *ab ovo*. He begins with the intrauterine life of the "little Gentleman," the homunculus, wrapped in "his melancholy dreams and fancies" until he was brought forth on the fifth day of November, 1718, after "as near nine calendar months as any husband could in reason have expected" into "this scurvy and disastrous world." He is even able to fix the time of his begetting (from a memorandum in his father's pocketbook) to the night "betwixt the first Sunday and the first Monday in the month of March" because his father was away between March and May in London.

> "But pray, Sir, What was your father doing all December, January, and February?"
> "Why, Madam, he was all that time afflicted with a Sciatica."

The ability to take a careful and precise developmental history is a prerequisite for the child researcher!

Every good child psychiatrist knows quite well that a child needs a certain amount of genetic, developmental, and environmental luck if he is to progress reasonably well through life. As things are fashioned, there are good and bad places in which to be born, good and bad families to be born into, and good and bad times at which to arrive. On opening his eyes the neonatal Shandy could only wish, without inconveniencing his father and mother unduly, that his begetting had been postponed some 20 or 25 years, when circumstances would have been more propitious. As a subdiscipline child psychiatry was begotten (and then promptly forgotten) on a convivial night of an international congress sometime between 1930 and 1935, when it received its present name. Its birth had been preceded by several miscarriages and more than one illegitimate movement. For a long time after its birth it was not quite clear who its parents were, and it has since been fostered by a wide variety of disciplines, which have never been quite sure what to do about it. With the hindsight now available it might have been better for it to have been born more respectably within a university medical center surrounded by helpful and friendly departments about 20 or 25 years later. One suspects that its whole scientific path might have been much smoother.

As a good developmental investigator Tristram Shandy is at pains not to bias the protocols with his own reactions. "My way," he says, "is ever to point out to the curious *different tracts of investigation*," and to indicate how it is "by slow steps of casual increase, that our knowledge—physical–physiological–technical, biographical–chemical, and obstetrical—has gradually been creeping upwards toward that acme of their perfections from which, if we may form a conjecture from the advances of these last seven years, we cannot possibly be far off."

Like him, we want, in this book, to call attention to the "different tracts of investigation," and to indicate the growth of knowledge over the past few decades in a whole range of areas pertaining to our discipline—the genetic, the chemical, the physiological, the developmental, the psychosomatic, the clinical, the naturalistic, and the experimental. We do not, for even a wild moment, propose that we are even within 100 years of an acme of knowledge within this field. We are only beginning; we are late starters; and we have been much distracted by the demands of our art, as suggested in the epilogue to this book.

We had many thoughts about this book during the process of inception, and many hopes for its future. Like Shandy we were anxious lest it should become, to quote Montaigne, "a book for a parlour window." We are hopeful that it will be taken seriously by our colleagues in child psychiatry and all our colleagues in the field of mental health and disease. We would like it to be read by others in order to make them more aware of ourselves, and we would like it to be read by our colleagues in order to make us more aware of ourselves: what we are trying to accomplish and where we are trying to go. We believe that the book will have a useful purpose not only in delineating our own field of endeavor but in setting a fashion for other disciplines to follow in which the researcher, as a person, and his research, as part of his personal achievement, are seen together in the same perspective. For this reason we would like to commend this book to as wide a scientific public as possible. The learned Bishop Hall, in the seventeenth century, had this to say in his book on the divine art of meditation, "that it is an abominable thing for a man to commend himself," let alone a group of men and women.

Shandy adds, "And I really think it is so."

"And yet," he goes on, "when a thing is executed in a masterly kind of fashion, which thing is not likely to be found out;—I think it is full as abominable, that a man should lose the honor of it, and go out of the world with the conceit of it rotting in his head."

This is precisely our situation. This was a book that needed to be written by the authors who contributed so enthusiastically to it, because it is seldom that the researcher, in any field, gets the opportunity to bring his heart and his head together in the same paper. Generally he is able to confide only to his closest friends what it cost him emotionally to carry out a particular investigation.

There is a further point to commend this volume. It is concerned with the doing of research. Child psychiatry needs to do research and to encourage its members to do research because without research it may flourish as an art form but is doomed as a scientific discipline. This is the editor's Hobby-Horse, and this is what Tristram Shandy, Gentleman, has to say about the subject: "A man and his Hobby-Horse, tho' I cannot say that they act and react exactly after the same manner in which the soul and body do upon each other: Yet doubtless there is a communication between them of some kind; and my opinion rather is, that there is something in it more of the manner of electrified bodies,—so that if you are able to give but a clear description of the nature of the one, you may form a pretty exact notion of the genius and character of the other."

It is not only the editor who has his Hobby-Horse. Every contributor to this book has one, and by getting to know and recognize the various types, one begins to learn something about the authors, since each chapter is as "full of Hobby-Horsical material as it can hold." There is nothing wrong with the possession of a Hobby-Horse, provided, as Shandy puts it, you can get on its back and ride it about as far as it will go, "leaving the world to determine the point as it thought fit."

E. JAMES ANTHONY

St. Louis
February, 1975

ACKNOWLEDGMENTS

I wish to record, firstly, my deep appreciation of my sixteen child psychiatric colleagues who responded so emphatically to the central idea of this book—the bridging of the gap between research as formally reported and research as informally lived and experienced, so as to provide a more authentic portrayal of the process of investigation as it actually exists.

My second debt of gratitude is to Mrs. Martha Kniepkamp and Miss Carol Cordes who have stage-managed the production at its different stages of development, and without whose help it might have languished indefinitely as scribbles on an editorial pad.

Thirdly, my thanks are due to the Administrative Assistant of the Division, Miss Doris Diephouse, who has for fifteen years so lightened my administrative load as to render the making of books feasible within a very active clinical, educational, and investigative life.

My final acknowledgment, as always, is to my family, who jointly provided me with my basic education in child psychology.

E. J. A.

CONTENTS

Developmental Research

Psychosomatic Research

Clinically Oriented Research

GENERAL
INTRODUCTION

INTRODUCTION

A GENERAL PERSPECTIVE OF
RESEARCH AND RESEARCHERS

E. JAMES ANTHONY

The purpose of this book is to be encouraging. It is largely addressed to those many clinicians in the field of child mental health who have often been tempted to explore a problem that interested them but have felt some diffidence about doing so because of a lack of research knowledge and training. Now it is true that research, like any other academic pursuit, benefits from training in methodology, but what becomes apparent on the reading of the different contributions to this volume is the self-made quality of the investigators. They have all carried out research not because they were trained to do research but because something within them that one can only nebulously term an attitude of mind compelled them to this activity. Technical proficiency can be acquired on the job and competence tends to increase with experience. The research attitude, however, is more difficult to acquire in its absence since its origins are often lost in the earliest years of life. It undoubtedly begins in wonder at the nature of things and with the wish to discover how they work. Anyone who has watched a year-old infant at work investigating the world around him will appreciate the zest and persistence with which it is done. Piaget (1952) has painted a vivid developmental portrait of the stage-5 baby during the sensorimotor period "discovering new means through active experimentation," and one can glimpse the once and future researcher in the making if the environment proves to be facilitating:

> *Observation 1 for 2.*—At 0; Laurent examines a watch chain hanging from his index finger. At first he touches it very lightly simply "exploring" it without grasping it. He then starts it swinging a little and at once continues this thus rediscovering a "derived secondary reaction." But instead of stopping there, he grasps the chain with his right hand and swings it with his left while trying some new combinations (here the "tertiary reaction" begins); in particular he slides it along the back of his left hand and sees it fall off when it reaches the end. Then he holds the end of the chain (with his right index finger and thumb) and lets it slide slowly

E. JAMES ANTHONY, The Harry Edison Child Development Research Center, Washington University School of Medicine, St. Louis.

between the fingers of his left hand (the chain is now horizontal and no longer oblique as before). He studies it carefully at the moment when the chain falls from his left hand and repeats this ten times. Afterward, still holding the end of the chain in his right hand, he shakes it violently which makes it describe a series of varied trajectories in the air. He then shows these movements in order to see how the chain slides along the quilt when he merely pulls it. Finally he drops it from different heights and so rediscovers the schema acquired in the preceding observation. From his twelfth month Laurent repeated these kinds of experiments with everything that his hand came upon. He entertains himself either by making them slide or fall or by letting them go in different positions and from different heights in order to study their trajectory [p. 269].

As if to demonstrate that infantile research was not sex-linked, his sister Jacqueline at about the same age also engaged industriously in the same series of investigations, making of her bassinet a veritable laboratory:

Observation 1 for 6.—At 1; 2 Jacqueline holds in her hands an object which is new to her: a round, flat box which she turns all over, shakes, rubs against the bassinet, etc. She lets it go and tries to pick it up. But she only succeeds in touching it with her index finger, without grasping it. She, nevertheless, makes an attempt and presses on the edge. The box then tilts up and falls again. Jacqueline, very much interested in this fortuitous result, immediately applies herself to studying it. . . . Afterward she puts her finger on the box and presses it. But as she places her finger on the center of the box she simply displaces it and makes it slide instead of tilting it up. She amuses herself with this game and keeps it up for several minutes. She finally again places her finger on the edge of the box which tilts it up. She repeats this many times varying the conditions but keeping track of her discovery.

Here one can observe all the basic elements of research: the persistence in spite of failure, the repetition under varying conditions, the need for replication, and, above all, the open-mindedness that goes along with what Piaget refers to as "experimenting in order to see." The drive to investigate is clearly very powerful and gradually lays bare the workings of the world to the infant. What happens to it eventually? Unfortunately, this active reaching out into the unknown soon becomes blunted by habit and routine, and assigned tasks gradually take the place of self-generated explorations. Bit by bit, the drive to investigate is snuffed out along the course of development, and potential researchers are lost to the world. Neither Laurent nor Jacqueline went on to become adult investigators. Yet they had an interested parent who aided and abetted them in their infantile researches and was manifestly well disposed to their continuation. We do not know the reason, but it may be that competition with an inordinately successful researching parent may have finally spelled failure to the child in this particular occupation.

Psychoanalysis has attempted to link the research interest to vicissitudes of the psychosexual drives. The original sexual interests and curiosities are sometimes no more than displaced into less blatantly sexual fields, but more often the sublimations seem far removed from the original drives with the gratifications hardly detectable on the surface. The scoptophilic who glues his eyes to the microscope may not be aware at all of the forces that keep him looking so persistently. On the other hand, there is a well-documented case of the toddler with intense anal conflicts who grew up to become one of the most inventive sanitary engineers, whose intricate and complicated plumbing designs became the pride of many cities.

According to Klein (1948), honest and frank answers to all the questions proposed by little children ensure the inner freedom to develop epistemophilic drives unhampered by repression. She described different types of researchers who developed as a result of different degrees of injury to their instinct for knowledge. Within the framework of psychoanalytic theory, she classified subsequent researchers into three main groups according to the way in which their childhood curiosities regarding both natural phenomena and forbidden knowledge were handled. The categorization was based on the extent to which the "injury" affected the dimensions of surface, depth, or breadth:

> In the *type 1 investigator* all impulses to investigate deeper questions become inhibited and there is a marked distaste for "penetration downward," although the breadth of research is unaffected. These researchers are adaptable, clever, and practical, able to appreciate the surface realities but curiously blind to any deeper connections. This avoidance of penetration represented a "repression in the depth dimension." This type 1 investigator generally constricts his studies to epidemiology, survey, and follow-up.
>
> In the *type 2 investigator* the quantity of the "investigating impulse" is "bound" in the dimension of breadth, suggesting that the child had overcome a phase of inhibition in his earlier researches and had returned to active investigation, but with an aversion to attacking new questions. As an adult researcher, he is inclined to direct his remaining unfettered energy to a few problems which he tackles, from surface to depth, with intense concentration. In the extreme case, he may be attracted by a single problem, such as maternal deprivation, and devote the labor of a lifetime to it without developing any interest outside this sphere. This is particularly true of some psychoanalytic investigators.
>
> In the *type 3 investigator* penetration is deep and broad so that new knowledge and new insights over a range of problems can be obtained, but there may be a complete lack of appreciation of the surface realities of daily life so that the work done seems to lack any practical or tangible significance. This type of researcher fails because of methodological ineptitude. He seems unable to turn his attention to anything simple and immediately at hand. Klein considers this ineptitude as being due to a concomitant inhibition of other repudiated primitive things surmised at that early time to be real. Thus, after overcoming a certain period of inhibition, the researcher tends to plunge into the depths and to stay there, becoming, in the process, utterly impractical.

Klein postulated a further limitation on all three types of researchers: permanent submission to the authority principle, stemming from intellectual dependency on parent figures. Some of these researchers are able to oppose established ideas and carry out entirely original researches, while others can move only along lines of authority or when backed by authority. It is hard enough for the adult, let alone the child, to strike a balanced viewpoint between the authoritative contributions of eminent precursors and the authoritarian dicta that have become traditionally incorporated into the discipline and that represent so many barriers to the freedom of thought. The resolution of the parental complex determines the proportion of critical acceptance, intellectual surrender, or oppositional cynicism that is brought to "the review of the literature."

It would be pleasing to the editor of this book to assume that the original impulse to investigate is lying latent in many adults, awaiting some unleashing experience, such as the efforts of others like them, to reemerge. When an occasion for research arrives, it may be seized upon with the early enthusiasm or once again suppressed on the grounds of lack of time, knowledge, or experience. Those who feel deficient in knowledge or experience stand to gain most from the message implicit throughout this book: that there is really no worthwhile excuse for the potential researcher not to do research and that both internal and external obstacles are the common experience of all who set out to explore. The principal difference between this and other research accounts is that this one has been written entirely by child psychiatrists who, in the midst of their busy clinical lives, have pursued some compelling idea to its conclusion. This is not to say that any of them could afford to follow Skinner (1956) in his relentlessness: "When you run into something interesting, drop everything else and study it." A clinical researcher, because of his responsibilities to his patients, cannot sacrifice all his time and effort to investigation, but there is no doubt that he can convert a substantial proportion of his daily clinical work into research without jeopardizing the needs of his patients.

Another dissuading factor is the stereotype developed by many clinicians about research. They often regard it, and the people who do it in contrast to their humane selves, as cold, hard, mechanistic, tough, exacting, and joyless, and it is apparent that they cull these ideas from formal textbooks and journals on research in which the finished products are presented so parsimoniously that nothing but established facts and figures are revealed. Bachrach (1962) has attempted to explode some of this mythology, pointing out that people simply do not do research in the way that people who write books about research say that people do research! He complained that it is often forbiddingly represented as a matter of "white ties and tails," whereas it is much more an affair of "blue jeans" and full of "fun and frustration." In his view it is also a pity that research is frequently equated with statistics, which are, in reality, no more than useful tools for handling some but not all research data. This is especially important for clinicians to realize, since they are often intimidated by the thought that before they can legitimately enter the field of research, they must take a course in advanced mathematics. Since they see themselves as possessing nonmathematical minds, this apparent qualification puts research out of court. Bachrach admitted that in the final presented version scientific studies are logical, consistent, coherent, orderly, and organized; while they are in process, however, they are frequently great big muddles with the researcher himself equally muddled. Another prominent investigator, Young (1951), said that the researcher "may hardly know himself what law he is trying to prove. He is constantly observing, but his work is a feeling out into the dark, as it were. When pressed to say what he is doing he may present a picture of uncertainty or doubt, even of actual confusion."

The research world is, therefore, not a bureaucratic world of in-trays and out-trays, and of time schedules and precisely anticipated aims and objects, although proposals for research grants are expected to give this impression. Chronological developments of the investigation, in three-monthly and six-monthly intervals, are often included in applications, but the genuine research mind is not fashioned to evolve programmatically. What can one say about the research mind apart from the fact that it is often confused and uncertain? It has, apart from built-in inquisitiveness, enough openness and flexibility to move in the direction of maximal scientific reward. There are certain contradictions about it. As Bachrach said, it is both careful and casual, relaxed and alert. In its quintessence, it is constantly "prepared," ready to be deflected by an unexpected finding and to regard it as a fortunate rather than a disturbing occurrence.

The route from question to answer can be a circuitous one, reaching out into many byways, by-products, and diversionary activities on the way. The initial aims may give place to amended or even quite different ones. A classical example was provided by Fox (1958) in her fascinating saga of the floppy-eared rabbits:

> A medical investigator, Thomas, was exploring the possibility that the vascular lesions induced by hypersensitivity to certain substances might be due to a release of proteolytic enzymes. Since he happened to have some papain in the laboratory, he injected this and, low and behold, in a rather bizarre and funny manner the ears just flopped. Being a good research scientist, he did not let it drop at that. "I chased it like crazy, but I didn't do the right thing—I did the expected things." He cut sections and stained them but could find nothing the matter. He did take a casual look at the cartilage but dismissed the idea that the dramatic collapse of the ears could be associated with cartilaginous dangers since, like everyone else, he believed this substance to be relatively inert. At this point, he abandoned the investigation, partly because he had used up his supply of rabbits but more because he was preoccupied with another problem. About two years later, he was once again working on the use of proteolytic enzymes to deplete fibrinogen and once again injected papain intravenously and "the same damned thing happened again." He demonstrated the spectacular effect to a student class, explaining that he had no idea what caused it, but this time he cut sections of the ears before and after the injection of papain.

"This is the part of the story I am most ashamed of. It still makes me writhe to think of it. There was no damage to the tissue in the sense of a lesion, but what had taken place was a quantitative change in the matrix of the cartilage." In a terse report to the *Journal of Experimental Medicine,* he reported the changes in the cartilage omitting any reference to the years of bewilderment and exasperation that had preceded the discovery.

This research tale not only illustrates the ups and downs of life in the laboratory but also the dangers of so-called "hypothesis myopia," a condition in which preconceptions make it impossible to see what is actually in front of one's eyes. This is particularly apt to happen in clinical psychiatric research, since psychiatry is top-heavy with theory, which often acts as a deadweight on research. People perceive what they have been brought up to perceive, what they have been trained to perceive, and what they expect to perceive; they fail to perceive facts that are opposed to their predilections and suppositions.

Should the researcher, therefore, discard all his theories and work empirically? On a reading of this book, it will be observed how differently different investigators respond to this problem: some seem to prefer an overall systematic theory by which to judge their data; some prefer working models that have a built-in obsolescence and can be continually subjected to modification as the data accrue; but quite a few are pure empiricists who believe data to be the stuff of science and sedulous theorizing. Some insist that theoretical systems help one to see better and others that they prevent seeing at all. The history of science has reflected both the theoretical and the atheoretical approaches. Men like Bacon (1868) have berated the system builders who "with infinite agitation of wit spun out of a small quantity of matter those laborious webs," and have asked, "To what purpose are these brain-creations and idle plays of power?" There can be nothing but romantic chaos, certainly not science, if "everyone philosophizes out of the cells of his own imagination, as out of Plato's cave."

The Baconian attitude is perhaps too rigorous for a young, developing science to follow as an ideal; yet it would be hard for the great inductivist to dismiss any of the contributions in this volume as "brain-creations" or "idle plays of power," and some are more likely to have emerged out of a Freudian rather than a Platonic cave. The Baconian man of science carries out carefully measured observations and experiments in the area in which he hopes to make discoveries and gradually amasses a great deal of hard data. Sooner or later this collection of data begins to exhibit certain general features that suggest to him a lawlike hypothesis that explains all the individual facts and their interconnections. Having arrived at such a hypothesis, he seeks to verify it by finding evidence that conclusively proves it. If he is successful, the finding becomes a permanent addition to the body of certain knowledge, and he will have discovered another regularity of nature, another law that can be put to use wherever it applies. The most important feature of the method is held to be the way that general statements can be reached from observed instances, and the process, known as induction, is generally regarded as the very hallmark of science, the criterion of demarcation between what can count as science and what cannot. Thus any statements based on intuition or authority or argument from first principles are *ipso facto* excluded, and only statements of observable fact and statements validly induced from them have the right to be termed scientific, since only these are testable and provable facts.

The strictness of this approach is eminently suitable to the physical sciences, but it is less applicable to what Popper (1965) has termed the "historical" sciences, in which the fundamental activity lies less in testing universal hypotheses and predicting specific events than in exploring the past systematically and establishing continuities by means of meaningful connections (Jasper's *Verständliche Zusammenhange*). This approach allows a certain amount of latitude to the behavioral scientist but not a great deal, since Popper is, in many respects, just as hard as Bacon on pseudoscience, although he would be more likely to accept the earlier stages of scientific development that are more concerned with relevance than with rigor. However, in contrast to the inductive method, he has put the onus on disproof rather than proof and has made falsification the valid method of science. Statements can, therefore, be tested by systematic attempts to prove them wrong rather than to prove them right. This is somewhat nearer the clinical approach in which the tendency in general is to accept whatever is presented and then gradually to eliminate what is obviously false or redundant. This would seem to be a different way of arriving at the truth: superseding a theory that was once serviceable with a better one. In this approach, theories are accorded a more fundamental role since they precede the observations and experiments that are designed to test them. Knowledge is thus advanced by fruitful theorizing and not by inductive procedures, the claims of which, according to Popper, have been grossly overstated. Knowledge, he says, consists of theories, not of facts. Empirical investigators, who are sometimes scathing about the airy abstractions of theory, need to be reminded of Lewin's aphorism that "there is nothing so practical as a good theory."

After theory, the second major factor that differentiates investigators is language, which ranges in this book from the loosely anecdotal to the precise. With all reporters in the field of the behavioral sciences, the contributors to this book share the problem of the absence of a universal data language to which their observations can be related. The language difficulty is more than apparent in the use of operational definitions: frequently too much is taken for granted, and there is an uncritical assumption of mutual understanding. Clinicians, in general, are inclined to beg a great many questions and leave them loose-ended in their daily practice, and the same tendency overflows into their research. It will take a little time to sharpen our definitions and eradicate some of their current cloudiness and ambiguity. In time we should, like our colleagues in the "harder" disciplines, be able to say shortly, simply, and succinctly what we try to do, how we do it, and what we have done.

A third point of difference among investigators lies in the hardware that they use. Some have a penchant for apparatus and may naïvely indulge this addiction without stopping to consider its effect on the subject. They may have a similar scotoma for the influence of their own presence in the field of investigation. A preponderance of investigators in child psychiatry is clearly more at home sitting passively, looking at and listening to the subject rather than doing something with him or to him. The history of science records both types of activities: Descartes did all his work in bed, whereas Bacon is said to have died from a cold that he contracted while experimenting in a snowdrift.

A fourth difference is readily discernible throughout the book and relates to the way in which the individual investigator attempts to deal with the mind–body problem as he encounters it in research. Some prefer to deal with somatic aspects, giving only slight acknowledgment to the psyche, whereas others hardly mention the body at all but treat it as an embarrassing appendage to the mind. Even when they profess a psychobiological point of view, one or the other element of the dualism may obtain scant recognition. The difficulty stems from theoretical orientations that cannot cover both sides of the *psychesoma*, and this has led in recent years to various efforts at formulating a general scientific theory of human behavior. So-called general system theory has still to gain a firm footing in psychiatric research, and although the needs for such a comprehensive unified approach are obvious, it will be some time before researchers in child psychiatry develop sufficient sophistication in the field of methodology to handle such multidimensional problems.

Child psychiatrists are becoming active investigators in this decade. As a result, ethical problems of research are becoming increasingly salient, and powerful restrictions are being placed on the use of human subjects, especially children. The child researcher is particularly sensitive to this issue, since his training in clinical work has tended to accentuate the natural protectiveness that most adults feel toward children. It is well-nigh impossible for him to regard them as Ss anonymously occupying cells within research design, and for this reason a great many biases may creep into the investigation. Nevertheless, many child researchers are learning to discipline their softer feelings and to comply with the requirements of "blindness" in their studies.

Perhaps to a greater extent than their nonclinical colleagues, clinical researchers are sensitive to the confidentiality of research documents and registers, to the use of very explicit consent forms, to the dangers of "deficit" research, to deceptions practiced on subjects in psychosocial experiments, to invasions of family privacy, to intrusions into the educational environment of the child and into his records, and, above all, to the possible exploitation of the child as a research subject. The ethical issue is discussed at some length elsewhere in the book, but it is clear that the fundamental humanism of the child psychiatrist, his knowledge and liking of children, and his intensive therapeutic training all provide an essential safeguard to abuse. This considerate and concerned approach is summarized by Anna in Margaret Landon's well-known book *Anna and the King of Siam*, when she says; "Understanding children and conducting research on them is largely a matter of getting to know them, getting to like them, when you are with them getting to know what to say, seeing it their way as well as putting it your way, but nicely." One can do a great deal with children in research if one does it "nicely."

The range of research activities represented in this volume may come as a surprise to many who have so far tended to regard child psychiatrists as little more than clinical practitioners limited to almost a single approach and a single set of theories. The various studies indicate that as far as research is concerned, this is far from being the case. The various contributors are clearly under no obligation to limit their thinking, and this augurs well for the future scientific growth of this particular discipline. Freedom is of great importance to the investigator if he is bent on opening up new ways and not simply following well-trodden paths; but he also has a responsibility when doing this. In this context, Flournoy once enunciated two scientific principles approvingly quoted by Piaget (1944): the first is the Hamlet principle that all things under heaven and on earth are possible, and the second is the Laplace principle that the weight of evidence must be proportional to the strangeness of the facts. These two considerations certainly give the investigator a lot of leeway in conducting his research.

References

BACHRACH, A. J. *Psychological research*. New York: Random House, 1962.

BACON, F. Of the proficience and advancement of learning. In J. Spedding, R. L. Ellis, and D. D. Heath (Eds:), *The works of Francis Bacon*. London: Longmans, 1868.

BARBER, B., & FOX, R. C. The case of the floppy-eared rabbits: An instance of serendipity gained and serendipity lost. *American Journal of Sociology*, 1958, **54,** 2.

KLEIN, M. *Contributions to psychoanalysis*. London: Hogarth, 1948.

LANDON, M. *Anna and the King of Siam*.

PIAGET, J. Presidential address. *Revue Suisse de Psychologie*, 1944.

PIAGET, J. *The origins of intelligence in children*. New York: International Universities Press, Inc., 1952.

POPPER, K. R. *Conjectures and refutations: the growth of scientific knowledge*. New York: Basic Books, 1965.

SKINNER, B. F. A case history in scientific method. In *Cumulative record*. New York: Macmillan, 1956.

YOUNG, J. Z. *Doubt and certainty in science*. Oxford: Clarendon Press, 1951.

RESEARCH AS AN ACADEMIC FUNCTION OF CHILD PSYCHIATRY[1]

E. JAMES ANTHONY

The longer I live and the more tolerant I grow, the more convinced I become that the universe I live in is a pluralistic one and that it takes all types and conditions to make a world, particularly a scientific world. Nevertheless, I cannot claim that I have completely outgrown every bit of my infantile egocentrism, and the models I use to conduct my daily professional business—whether of teaching, treating, or investigating—tend to be idiomatic and pervaded with personal attributes and feelings. What I have to say about research, therefore, will bear the mark of my bias. I would like this consideration to be kept in mind during the reading of these comments when any seemingly inconsistent ideas make their appearance.

One's attitude toward research is closely linked with his hopes and expectations for his discipline. Depending on the quality of these hopes and expectations, the undertaking can be romantic and colorful or humdrum and pedestrian. It can be a mission or a job. Joel Elkes (1966) made the distinction elegantly when he wrote, "We all have our private image of the growth of science. A rising curve, a tree, a many-roomed mansion inhabited by a society of friends. My image, I am afraid, is more prosaic. To me, science is a sort of creature that, like Napoleon's army, marches on its stomach. It subsists on facts and does not care where it finds them."

Whereas Elkes lives on facts like a good empirical researcher, I myself have an inordinate appetite for ideas, even in the form of useful fictions like myths, but, like him, I am ready to look for these wherever I can find them.

My heterogeneous collection of ideas began to accumulate in the lumber room of my mind during my heterogeneous training in London. The aim of the Institute of Psychiatry there was to expose the residents to a maximum

[1] Read before the annual meeting of the Society of Professors of Child Psychiatry, Gainesville, Florida (1968), and published in the Archives of General Psychiatry, October 1969, Volume 21.

E. JAMES ANTHONY. The Harry Edison Child Development Research Center, Washington University School of Medicine, St. Louis.

number of experiences, ranging from the very concrete in the way of brain specimens to the most abstract and fantastic elements in our art-science. When I came to the United States, I was at once struck by the formal, homogeneous training offered in most psychiatric centers, especially in centers for child psychiatry. It was as different as Stilton cheese is from good American processed cheese. Stilton, you may remember, is rather acrid, crumbly, and moldy, with a variegated coloring, whereas the American cheese is smooth, hard, and solid; it is more dependable and lasts longer. It is also a much more predictable cheese and offers little surprises to the taste. What I am trying to insinuate by means of this cumbersome analogy is that the average training received currently in the United States is very likely to turn out a first-rate practitioner but one devoid of any research interests or urges. I am inclined to believe, biased by my own experience, that a heterogeneous training, with a great deal of self-teaching opportunity available to the resident, is altogether more liable to spawn future investigators. An environment in which incompatible and conflicting ideas and techniques live cheek by jowl is an uncomfortable but stimulating setting in which to work. It is not necessarily a happy place to be in and the hedonistic culture of America may prefer to do without it, but, as Redlich (1961) once remarked on the emotional climate of research settings, "I have observed too many happy ships bobbing up and down at the moorings without going anywhere."

We have to recognize that in the world of medicine, psychiatry has a poor reputation with regard to research, while child psychiatry, about which I am here concerned, has as yet no reputation at all. Until we begin to develop systematic research, our academic image will remain negative and we will continue to feel, as we have felt for some time, that we are not acceptable in our schools of medicine. In order to survive at all, we have to do research. Research in our field, according to Brosin (1955), is not a luxury but a vital necessity.

An important GAP report (1959), put out more than a decade ago, underlined most of these comments:

> In comparison with other fields, psychiatry does not have a strong research tradition oriented to systematic empirical investigation of important problems. At the same time, we do have a great need for immediately applicable working formulations which offer sure guides to treatment. These conditions favor quick and often premature closure on many basic questions. Any information vacuum tends to be quickly filled with plausible hypotheses revived by respected authorities. In time, it may easily be forgotten that they are unverified hypotheses and may come to be treated as established fact. It is, however, as true in psychiatry as in other scientific fields that authority is no substitute for evidence.

I would say that in child psychiatry we are especially prone to take in and shelter for indefinite periods of time a free, workable, and apparently worthwhile idea, especially if a hallowed name has become attached to it. In addition, there is not enough research in child psychiatry to challenge such ideas or generate new ones, so that the content of our programs remains relatively unchanging. Of course, we do not have to change for the sake of change, but in the words of Hamburg (1961), "science is not a monolithic body of knowledge, settled now and for all time. It is a continuing, evolving, developing process in which yesterday's answers become today's questions." For us, yesterday's answers are still today's answers and, sad to say, we do not confront ourselves with many questions.

I want now to deal with three separate issues in the field of research: (1) the fostering of a propitious atmosphere; (2) the stimulation of research as a continuous, matter-of-fact process in child psychiatric facilities; and (3) the setting up of training facilities to encourage research interests and activities in residents and staff.

Fostering a Research Atmosphere

It is difficult to define or describe atmosphere. It clearly has as much to do with people as with buildings, equipment, or funds, but it is often confused with these latter elements. The atmosphere can be regarded as an emanation from special people whose very presence is an incitement to investigation, people who not only create excitement and interest by their own drive for discovery but also ensure the proper conditions for research by their open-mindedness and lack of dogmatic traditionalism. They also serve as models to be imitated and identified with. Here they must be especially powerful and stimulating, since they are in competition with other models in the form of teachers, administrators, and private practitioners.

The dearth of investigation in any particular setting can most often be ascribed to an absence of adequate research models, to the presence of many practitioner models, and to a lack of genuine interest in research on the part of the director of the facility. It is not enough for him simply to pay lip service to the importance of research, or to support it in order to be "in" with the medical school, or to preach it because it is becoming respectable and fashionable. He has to believe in research with a faith that can override the many impediments in a clinical unit that hinder research developments. Best of all, he should be a researcher himself, actively engaged in research and not simply talking about it, telling others to do it, or writing grant proposals.

The director of a facility should also be able to counteract the antiresearch atmosphere prevalent in many clinical settings. There are many clinicians whose experience of grants from the National Institute of Mental Health have been such that they are ready to condemn all contemporary research in the field of psychiatry (especially that done by nonpsychiatrists) as trivial and given to "methodolatry." They warn residents against engaging in research before they have acquired adequate clinical background and experience. They sneer at findings that are no more than long and elephantine glimpses into the obvious. Clinicians are understandably sensitive about the relevance of research to theory and practice. They are not, as a rule, impressed by technological tricks or by a complex but corrupt analysis of the data. It is also well for the researcher to remember (and, in fact, fatal for him to forget) that for many clinicians there is something vaguely threatening about research. They may see it as intrusive, intimidating, dehumanizing, and fixated on numbers. Perhaps its greatest crime in their eyes is approaching children in a nontherapeutic way and perceiving them in terms of means and not ends. Such an approach implies an absence of alliance, of working through defenses, and of respect for defenses. The patient loses his identity and becomes a figure among other figures, and following the statistical analysis he is no longer considered to exist. There is no responsibility for him and no concern about his future except in follow-up studies.

This distorted picture of clinical research is as false as many of the other stereotypes associated with psychiatry. I mention it as a reminder that there is a great deal of rational and irrational resistance to the development of systematic research in child psychiatry.

In spite of many of these unpropitious attitudes, a certain amount of research activity still continues in our field, but it is done by a disproportionately small number of investigators who are, for the most part, nonpsychiatrists. It is important to ask ourselves how much longer we can afford to have our research gardens cultivated by investigators from other disciplines with whom our younger members are unable to identify.

Research has yet another adverse aspect that may disenchant the clinician: it can and does affect the "happy" working conditions in a clinic. Alan Gregg (194) conceded that research people frequently appear very disagreeable, and Redlich (1961) concurred with this impression, depicting the typical researcher as vain, arrogant, irritable, narcissistic, possessive about his ideas, jealous of others with similar ideas, and paranoid about having ideas stolen. "To keep a department of such personalities together," he went on to say, "is no small task." It is not surprising that clinicians, with their sensitivity to morbid personality and behavior, prefer to keep a distance from individuals described in such unpalatable terms.

On their side, researchers working in a clinical division tend to become unhappy with the antiresearch atmosphere. If they are irritable, it is often because they have experienced many frustrations and snubs in attempting to collect their samples. Clinicians deal with them guardedly and suspiciously and are as possessive of their patients as researchers are of their projects. It is obvious that there is room for a great deal of misunderstanding and failure to communicate. These barriers are by no means insuperable if the two parties involved make some effort to penetrate each other's worlds and see psychiatry from the same side. As Plato might have said, when clinicians become researchers and researchers clinicians, then is the time when a good scientific republic will be established.

Establishing a Research Program

In a symposium on the future of psychiatry, one of the participants (Rothman, 1962) remarked that unless our philosophy of science became "more critical, experimental, more deductive, and inventive," we would remain in the renaissance period of medical history, awaiting some Harvey to catapult us into the seventeenth century. We are certainly waiting for something to happen in child psychiatry, and I feel that unless something happens in the way of productive basic and clinical research in the next few years, we may very well become extinct as a medical discipline. and get ourselves transplanted into the school of social work.

The first thing we have to remember about the undertaking of research is that it is a serious, time-consuming, and energy-sapping business that requires concentrated attention and technical knowledge and competence. It is surprising how many clinicians run away with the idea that it takes no special training and that "clinical experience and mature reflection" are quite sufficient. In many respects, and in different ways, it is as complicated as carrying out intensive psychotherapy, and it takes as much dedication, insight, ability, and experience. People of similar capacities may move into research or into therapy and we must get away from the old idea, to paraphrase Shaw, that those who can, treat, and those who cannot, do research. As I see it, the good clinical investigator needs many of the qualities that the good therapist also requires. He needs his intuitions, his empathy, his understanding, and his background of knowledge. He needs to form a good research alliance with his subjects and to be concerned with what happens to them once the investigation is over. I always remember a motto once proclaimed at the Tavistock Clinic in London: "No therapy without research and no research without therapy." It is not always possible to follow up and offer the investigated subject treatment should he require it, but this might well become one of the goals of applied research, about which we are beginning to hear more. The treatment-oriented child psychiatrist might well be won over to research by such built-in policies.

The development of research in any child psychiatry division must proceed in stages. Most importantly, it should not attempt to grow overnight into a huge research center, nor should it start with bricks and mortar before the necessity for research has clearly been established. Creating the right atmosphere, winning over the clinicians, encouraging the residents, and creating a competent research staff are all important steps, none of which should be overlooked if the foundation is to be solid.

Research is often presented to clinicians in a somewhat narrow way, and it is often necessary to point out the obvious fact that the research spectrum is a wide one and that there is a place along it for most competent clinicians, whatever their point of view. At one end of the spectrum lies brain research and at the other mind research, and at the points between the two there is the possibility of various types of brain–mind investigation. On the organic side, there is the prospect of exciting work on the correlation of localized cerebral activity and behavior or on the action of chemical substances on neural areas. On the other side, one can have psychoanalytic research associated with the observation of infants and toddlers, family studies, and therapeutic evaluations. And between these two sides there are the now-thriving areas of epidemiology, learning theory, and psychophysiological development. In addition, the exciting idea of a developmental psychopathology involving a consideration of critical periods and vulnerability is now moving to the center of the research stage and demanding research space, time, and attention. There is, therefore, a niche for everyone and no excuse for anyone on the grounds of limited interests. It is merely a question of developing the habit of research and a knowledge of what good investigation entails. In time, research can become a way of life. One of our few, pioneer researchers, David Levy (1959), as made this point very well:

> Physicians frequently make clinical inferences on the basis of their experiences. . . . They particularly are encouraged to test their inferences by systematic accumulation of data. The value of doing so, aside from the possibility of making a scientific contribution, lies in gaining the habit of thinking in terms of the observations that are needed and can be collected in order to answer the question. Sometimes the observations that are needed are at hand and require very little extra time.

Therefore, the time given to research can be small or large, but time itself should not be allowed to become a barrier to all research, although admittedly, service time, as Sir Thomas Lewis once said, can become a "crippling routine which the care of numbers of patients renders inevitable."

Training for Research in Child Psychiatry

One of the reasons for the little research in child psychiatry is the lack of research training during residency. Individuals who are attracted to research are often among the best students, and they may well be discouraged from entering the field at all because of the lack of research opportunities. Alan Gregg

(1941) declared that psychiatry does not attract the best minds among medical students (although this is becoming less true), and it could be added that child psychiatry does not attract the best among psychiatric residents.

Of course, irrespective of their capacities, not all residents should be expected to do research. In Redlich's (1961) experience, compelling residents to do research has produced poor results, and he concludes that staff investigators should stimulate but not force research. He feels that there are subtle ways of encouraging interest, such as selectively rewarding such activity or letting the trainee know that "good clinical work is all right but not enough." This may seem a little hard on the less research-minded resident, but a division has to think of its own total program as well as of the individual student. A system of academic priorities is always implicit in the functioning of any department, and trainees usually get the message. On the other hand, it is not always the staff or students who are culpable. In a personal communication to Redlich (1961), Nurnberger wrote that "there is something woefully wrong with the program or with the criteria of selection if no resident will engage in scientific or scholarly work," which puts the onus where it chiefly belongs. It is too easy to blame the resident for one's own ineptness.

Lack of encouragement to do research may be matched by discouragement from doing research. In certain dedicated service settings residents are asked to justify their research interest, which may be regarded by their seniors as some form of maladjustment.

How can we recognize a good potential researcher among the residents who come to us? It is by no means easy, since the investigative drive may be swamped in such a heavy load of commitments that it goes unrecognized. After many years in the field of clinical research, I have reached the conclusion that most researchers can be classified along the lines of the Shakespearean statement about greatness: some are born researchers; some achieve research by dint of hard work; and some have research thrust upon them under conditions that are unavoidable and often painful. It is usually impossible to mistake the person in the first category: his curiosity, drive, and persistence will seek out research opportunities without much help from his seniors. These born researchers show themselves fairly early in life, so that they have a reputation for scientific interest almost by the time they get into grade school. James Clark Maxwell is a beautiful illustration. When he was a very small boy in Scotland he constantly plagued people around him with the kinds of questions likely to drive even a child-centered adult to distraction. "What's the go of it?" he would repeatedly ask when confronted with anything new, and when people tried to explain, in the generalizing way of adults condescending to small children, he would stamp his foot and demand: "Yes, but what's the *particular* go of it?" We want not only residents who are curious about "the particular go" but also senior staff who can give specific answers because they too are interested in the "particular go." Unfortunately, we know as yet so little of the "go" in child psychiatry, and virtually nothing of the "particular go," that the senior is often pushed to give solid answers that make the whole problem seem more completely delineated and understood than it actually is.

Clearly those of us engaged in postgraduate education are obligated to recognize and further whatever talent for research our students possess. Even for those who possess very little it should be possible to find a small area, "even if only 2 mm in diameter," as Aubrey Lewis (1967) used to say. It would not be kind, according to him, "to encourage competent clinicians to attempt scientific investigations beyond their powers"; on the other hand, it would be "an ominous situation if the special training of psychiatrists did little to promote their activity in suitable research." The ratio should be determined by the trainee with the help of a little encouraging prodding by the director. The research carrot should not be hung tantalizingly and unattainably in front of the resident but should form an integral part of his staple professional diet.

The weekly research seminar has been used by many, including myself, to familiarize the resident with research problems, research techniques, and ongoing research work. An important part of this seminar is the practice of evaluating research in terms of its aims, its procedures, and its value to the field. Using this type of approach, Hamburg (1961) found "a striking increase in research interest and awareness among the residents" at the end of a year. He also remarked on the importance of staff respect for the seminar which signifies to the resident from the outset that research is highly valued in the institution and is viewed by the faculty as an integral part of the training.

The resident who manifests strong research interests and inclinations while attending the seminars should receive further encouragement and perhaps more formal instruction in scientific method and should carry out some research under supervision. He should become a participant in the division's ongoing research, which, at worse, might mean no more than carrying out routine procedures and, at best, might include an active role in planning a research strategy that might orient him toward a research career. As an alternative, he might be guided in the design and execution of a manageable investigation that he himself has chosen and that could lead to a small dissertation or a scientific paper. It is important as part of the general policy of encouragement not to load the resident with administration, with insatiable demands of service, or with excessive "nose-wiping, spoon-feeding, toilet-training" teaching and training activities. All of these may exercise a malignant effect on research drive.

I would very much like to see the development of a career-teaching and research-fellowship program that would add a third and fourth year to the academic training. Such a program would help to create well-rounded academic child psychiatrists who would pass these two years in a well-organized program, devoting one third of their time to research, one third of their time to teaching, and one third to clinical practice. Each of these three thirds would feed into a common reservoir of academic experience essential for the evolution of the academic mind. I have tried to keep these three thirds operating in my own professional life, although I have been compelled to add a fourth third (!) of administration, which to me signifies not merely routine paper work but the planning and provision of research opportunities for the resident and the junior staff member.

Conclusion

Every discipline grows and develops through research, and where there is a lack of research the discipline is stunted. In child psychiatry the responsibility for carrying out systematic or even sporadic research has not been settled, and so the practitioner goes about his daily business of diagnosis and treatment without being aware of, or even caring, who is laying the foundations of the house in which he lives; he himself is too busy metaphorically minding the baby, paying the rates and taxes, and finding enough money to live on. Someone, however, has to do the basic work, and those who devote themselves to this work need training, recognition, and acceptance by the rest of the faculty. To create a research division demands a great deal of effort (apart from money) and a director who has a passion for investigation and who is also ready to sacrifice himself in the service of research carried out by others. He must be able to convince the resistant group of practitioners that research is indispensable to the life of the clinic and to the future of the discipline; often a "selling job" must be done before research can be made an integral part of the life of the division. Only directors can do this job and we have an obligation both to our division and to our discipline to do it. I like to think that we can, by so doing, sway the course of child psychiatry in this country and direct it toward more scientific goals. To some extent, we are still locked up in the old system of child guidance and unable to get away from the ritualized method of looking at things. I am not sure whether we can change our direction, but if we cannot, we should make room for those who can. How indispensable are we to the forward movement of our discipline? The great surgeon Bilroth once said to his medical colleagues in Germany: "I do not doubt that if we professors were all to die at once today, we should be replaced immediately and so ably that the development of science would not be halted for a moment." Who knows, as Lewis (1967) remarked, it might even be hastened!

References

BROSIN, H. W. On discovery and experiment in psychiatry. *American Journal of Psychiatry,* *1955,* **111,** 561–575.

ELKES, J. Psychoactive drugs: Some problems and approaches. In P. Soloman (Ed.) *Psychiatric drugs.* New York: Grune & Stratton, 1966.

REPORT. *Some observations on controls in psychiatric research,* Report No. 42, May 1959.

GREGG, A. *The furtherance of medical research.* New Haven: Yale University Press, 1941.

HAMBURG, D. Recent trends in psychiatric research training. *Archives of General Psychiatry,* *1961,* **4,** 215–224.

LEVY, D. *The demonstration clinic.* Springfield, Ill.: Charles C Thomas, 1959.

LEWIS, A. *Essays and addresses.* Vol. 1: *State of Psychiatry.* New York: Science House, 1967.

REDLICH, F. C. Research atmospheres in departments of psychiatry. *Archives of General Psychiatry, 1961,* **4,** 225–236.

ROTHMAN, R. Future of genetic development and organic approaches. In P. Hoch and J. Zubin (Eds.), *The future of psychiatry.* London: Grune & Stratton, 1962.

BRIDGING TWO WORLDS OF RESEARCH

A QUESTION OF COMPLEMENTARITY[1]

E. James Anthony[2]

> *The future belongs to interdisciplinary research, yet because of reciprocal and often systematic ignorance, this is in fact frequently difficult to organize.*
>
> —*Towards a Theory of Knowledge, Jean Piaget*

The Two Worlds of Research

Behavioral research today has become too complex for the skills of a single discipline, especially in the area of clinical investigation. In this area a moderate-to large-sized project is commonly parceled out among different groups of specialists. The task of collaboration is strained by differences in language, in theory, and in method. Attitudes toward the collecting and processing of data can be almost antithetical. One might envisage a "soft" and a "hard" side in terms of data and a "tender" and "tough" side (to use William James's categories) in terms of personnel. For all practical purposes there is a gap between the two, perhaps more apparent than real and certainly more felt than reasoned. (See Fig. 1.) It is by no means easy to bridge this gap, even when one is strongly motivated to do so, but in order to carry out a coherent and comprehensive program of research, one must talk to the other side. Therefore he may have to learn a new language, expand or contract a theoretical framework, and tolerate a radical transformation of his most precious ideas. The incompatibilities may appear insurmountable, the approach on the soft side being subjective, impressionistic, uncontrolled, "unblinkered," qualitative, and nonnumerical, and, on the hard side, objective, instrumental, controlled, "blind," quantitative, and statistical. The "tender-minded" behavioral

[1]The Cameron Memorial Lecture, Institute of Psychiatry, Maudsley Hospital, London, July 1971
[2]Supported by U.S.P.H.S. Research Grants MH12043, MH14052, and MH23441

E. JAMES ANTHONY, The Harry Edison Child Development Research Center, Washington University School of Medicine, St. Louis.

DATA		DATA
"Soft"		"Hard"
Subjective		Objective
Impressionistic	?	Instrumental
Uncontrolled	Bridging	Controlled
Unblinkered	Concepts	Blind
PERSONNEL		PERSONNEL
"Tender-minded"	?	"Tough-minded"
Anthropologists	Bridging	Anthropometrists
Social workers	Procedures	Psychophysiologists
Psychiatrists		Experimentalists
Projective Psychologists		Psychometric Psychologists

FIG. 1.   The two worlds of research (in terms of a semantic differential).

scientists include anthropologists, social workers, dynamically oriented psychiatrists, and projective psychologists, while the "tough-minded" behavioral scientists include psychometric psychologists, experimentalists, psychophysiologists, and anthropometrists.

There is much to be said for and against both sides. Those on the soft side have been characterized by those on the opposite end as "pseudoscientific" because of their supposed propensity for treating tenuous impressions as unassailable dogmas that cannot be tested, repeated, or refuted. Clark Maxwell (1948), on the other hand, was surprisingly positive about the soft approach and had this to say about the two sides:

> In the statistical method of investigating social questions . . . (persons) are grouped according to some characteristic, and the number of persons forming the group is set down under the characteristic. Other students of human nature proceed on a different plan. They observe individual men, ascertain their history, analyze their motives, and compare their expectation of what they will do with their actual conduct. This may be called the dynamical method of study as applied to man. *However imperfect the dynamical study of man may be in practice, it is evidently the only perfect method in principle.* . . . If we would take ourselves to the statistical method, we do so confessing that we are unable to follow the details of each individual case . . .

Unfortunately, the "only perfect method in principle" does not always work out well in practice, and this represents the dilemma "between the significant and the exact," to quote Merton Gill (1968). To put it differently, is it possible to be relevant and meaningful as well as quantitative and exact? Loevinger (1963) rightly maintains that no one-sided resolution of this issue should be sought; in her words, "The function of the research is to look for what is objective, behavioristic, and quantifiable without losing the sense of the problem. The function of the clinician is to preserve the depth and complexity of the problem without putting it beyond the reach of objective and quantifiable realization. As in the battle of the sexes so in the clinical research dialogue, if either side wins, the cause is lost."

The gap is not only a conceptual and methodological one; there is also a gulf created by language. According to Abraham Kaplan (1964), the language of inquiry is so completely different on the two sides that communication across the gap is constantly garbled. Investigators on the "soft" side tend to use what he terms the "literary" style with an emphasis on people, places, and events, whereas those on the hard side employ what he calls an "eristic" style characterized by deduction and experimentation and, in its more advanced forms, by rigorous and logical conceptualization accompanied by explicit rules for deriving propositions and testing them by equally rigorous mathematical proof.

If one maintains the position that there are good things on both sides and that it is essential to establish a dialogue across the gap, it becomes necessary to search for bridging concepts and procedures that will permit the process of research to cross uninterruptedly from one side to the other.

A Bridging Concept

A useful bridging concept is that of complementarity put forward by Niels Bohr (1958) with regard to physical phenomena. According to Bohr's concept different and mutually exclusive but equally truthful statements can be made on one and the same occurrence. Blackburn (1971), a theoretical chemist, has carried the matter of complementarity further. His term for the soft approach is "sensuous." He points out that an experience is not a number and that both sensuous and quantitative information are projections of nature into disjunctive mental spaces. Thus sensuous information is not independent of quantitative knowledge, since both have their referent in the same system of nature. However, both may be true and both may lead by a continuous process of self-correction to reliable models of nature. Neither is complete in itself, each representing an undernourished view because each lacks the information available through the other approach. Blackburn recognizes that the mind sets of the two classes of investigators are so different that rarely, in the history of science, have they been able to tackle a task conjointly. A mechanism of contempt, detracting from the assets of each side, operates from both ends. The hard scientist, as Whitehead (1956) remarked 40 years ago, must be prepared to relinquish his lopsided, one-eyed view of the world and to recognize that there are other ways of knowing besides reading the pointer on a scale. Today the soft procedures are being looked at with increasing interest and wonder. It is obvious that the human mind and body can process information with staggering sophistication and sensitivity by the direct sensuous experience of their surroundings; they therefore must be included in, not excluded from, the field of research. Blackburn feels that "hard" scientists must school themselves to come into direct and open confrontation with phenomena and to train their bodies, by "trusting and cherishing" them (strange terms from a physical scientist), to respond sensitively to the natural and human environment. Since the self and its environment are interlinked inextricably, he says, it follows that *one can best understand one's surroundings by one's own sensitive reactions to them.*

The crucial question is whether a combination of soft and hard knowledge can be used to provide a complete and complementary description of phenomena. Such a result would require that certain conditions be satisfied. First, although the results from the two approaches may seem conflicting, each should strive to be consistent and repeatable in itself. Second, the bridging concepts and procedures must be given some time to work, since the complementary vision can become the natural viewpoint only after fairly long periods of total immersion in the mutual problem. Third, workers from both sides must be trained in "cross-over" techniques, the tender investigator learning to perceive order in a welter of numerical data and the tough investigator learning how to intuit the complex behavioral system as an organic whole. Finally, since we cannot hope to inject "relevance" and meaning into what both sides regard as essentially trivial projects, it is important to find a significant area of concern in which to attempt the complementary modes of approach.

Bridging Procedures

There are three procedures in the management of data, either soft or hard, that might be used in bridging the gap. These can be summarized as follows:

1. Reshaping data, that is, "hardening" or quantifying soft data, or "softening" hard data or making them anecdotal.
2. Admixing data, that is, blending soft and hard data within a common descriptive or theoretical frame of reference.
3. Redeploying data, that is, using soft data strategically to generate testable hypotheses in hard studies, and using hard data to direct the observer in naturalistic studies.

All these maneuvers demand a certain amount of respect for data generated from "the other side," together with some knowledge and understanding of the methods by which they were obtained. Respect for the data clearly implies respect for the collector of the data and the point of view that dictated his choice of procedures. The gap is unlikely to be bridged as long as either side continues to indulge in abrasive and polemical exchanges. The members of an interdisciplinary research team must do more than just tolerate each other's presence in the project if they hope to carry out something more than routine, pedestrian investigations. To appreciate the problems connected with a particular research role, they need to have played the role itself. Such reciprocity can prove invaluable in overcoming scientific egocentrism, but the undertaking of ego-alien roles can prove uncomfortable and can sometimes increase rather than diminish resistances to opposing points of view.

In the field of the behavioral sciences, the soft and hard polarities are less far apart than in many other disciplines, and the distinction is between telling stories and measuring differences between individuals or groups. The approach to family studies by an interdisciplinary team affords a good illustration of the ways in which bridges can be set up to span adjoining areas that project toward each other in a kind of cantilever system.

To demonstrate how this is done, examples are taken from a current multidisciplinary research project in which the eruption of psychosis within a family has been the main target of investigation. A large number of families have been studied by a multiple, overlapping approach, but in this presentation a single family is used to illustrate the method, to demonstrate what a rich portrayal of family life is obtained, and to exemplify how data can be manipulated to enhance the understanding of the field from which the data are drawn.

The P. Family

The P. Family is constituted as follows:

Nuclear Group	*Extended Group*
Father—business executive	Paternal grandfather
Mother—chronic schizophrenic (noninvolving type)	Paternal grandmother
John—thirteen years	Maternal grandfather
Susan—ten years (being seen in guidance clinic)	Maternal grandmother
Robert—eight years	Paternal aunt and husband
	Maternal uncle and wife

The battery used to investigate the functioning of the family included "softer" (nonnumerical) and "harder" (numerical) procedures, as follows:

Softer procedures	Harder procedures
Home visit	Behrens-Goldfarb Family Interaction Scale
Living-in with the family	
"Focal" interviewing of nuclear and extended members	Bene-Anthony Family Relations Test
	Identification test
	Rating of nonpsychotic spouse
	Like–unlike score profiles on standard psychological tests

Reshaping Data: Soft into Hard

The living-in procedure with families containing a psychotic parent was theoretically designed to provide a naturalistic account of the trivia of everyday living and not a diagnostic picture highlighting the psychopathology.[3] A female observer attempted to record both her objective and subjective impressions of family life as she experienced it in the home. The extract is taken from one of the daily protocols that the observer tape-recorded each evening.

> As a special treat for me, Mr. P. had brought home TV dinners, which only required heating up. "Now for goodness sake, don't go and burn them," he said to his wife. "I know you're going to forget all about them as soon as I turn my back." Mrs. P. didn't say anything but I noticed that her head seemed to tremble. John came in and said that he had some work to prepare and would be late coming down to dinner. Susan and Robert stuck close to me and constantly touched me or stroked my face or played with my hair or made comments on my dress. Susan said, "You look sad today. Why are you sad?" Then she said, "It makes me feel sad when you are sad like that." Although she was talking to me, she kept looking at her mother from time to time. Mr. P. asked both children not to pester me and said it was rude to say unpleasant things to people about their appearance. Mrs. P. had said nothing so I asked her if she liked ready-made dinners. She began to titter in a silly way, which made Susan also laugh quite hysterically, I thought. Mr. P. shouted at Susan to stop. Then he said to Mrs. P., "You are not looking so good today, have you forgotten to take your pills?" Mrs. P. mumbled something like, "Please don't." Everyone looked at her and she said, "We've all got to be good—we'll all go to heaven one day." Robert came over to her and put his hand on her shoulder and said, "Please don't talk like that, Mom—I don't want you to die—I don't want you to go away." Mrs. P. began rubbing her hands together and Susan began to rub her knee. Then they turned away from her and seemed to vie for my attention. If Robert would hold my hand, Susan would snatch it away from him, or if Robert asked me a question, Susan would ask a question as well. Mrs. P. was now bent over, rocking slightly and smiling in a sly manner. Susan said to me, "You're looking sad again—why don't you look happy? Everybody must be happy—everybody must sing and be happy." I said to her, "Even when they're feeling sad?" She

[3] See "Naturalistic Studies of Disturbed Families" by E. James Anthony in this volume.

said immediately, "'Specially when they're feeling sad." (She had diagnosed my mood correctly. I was beginning to feel quite miserable about what was happening.) Mr. P. now said, "Why don't you leave our guest alone? She's not sad— she's just mad at you for the way you're pestering her—you'll drive her crazy before the end of the week." As he said "crazy," both kids looked startled and Susan said, "But she likes us—she likes us to be with her." Mr. P. seemed quite angry and said, "But I'm telling you how she really feels, and I'm telling you that she's not going to stand it if you both don't stop." (No one bothered to ask me how I thought that I felt.) Robert covered his eyes with the backs of his hands and said, "You never want us to have a nice time." Mr. P. said to him very sharply, "When you talk to me, look at me directly. People who can't look at you are heading for the mental hospital." Robert buried his head in his hands. Mrs. P. made no effort to defend him. John now came in and he and Mr. P. immediately started talking about a school test that John had taken in which he scored an A— and Mr. P. wondered where he had slipped up. John looked across the table at his mother and brother and said loudly, "What's gone wrong with those two people?" Mr. P. said, "We're not feeling too well today—we don't think we took our pills." John said somewhat rudely to his mother, "How do you expect to get better if you don't do the right thing?" Susan said, "She's my mother and you leave her alone." There was an uncomfortable silence for a while and I broke it and said, "I think it's going to be a sunny day tomorrow, so Susan, Robert, and I can go and play in the park." Susan said, "I think it's going to be a horrid day with lots and lots of rain." And Robert said, "There's going to be a big storm. You'll see." John laughed and said, "Shows how much you both know about the weather forecast. It says it's going to be warm and sunny and so it's going to be warm and sunny." Mr. P. looked up from his paper and said, "That's the first rational remark I've heard the whole evening."

In this family, the mother's psychosis is essentially a withdrawing or noninvolving type, so that the children must initiate most of the approaches to her. The degree of involvement of the child with the psychotic parent is a function of the parent's involvement with the child, of the child's involvement with the parent, of the psychosis involving the child (for example, in making the child part of a delusional or hallucinatory system), and of the child's involvement in the psychosis (as evident in his curiosity about, interest in, and knowledge of the psychotic phenomena). In the noninvolving psychoses, this observer is better able to assume an objective posture and to observe events objectively and dispassionately, but with the involving psychoses she almost invariably feels herself caught up in a maelstrom of seething emotions beneath which she may feel submerged.

A striking fact about the content of the session is the way in which everyday events are distorted through conflict and confusion. This does not happen all the time but is triggered by a situation that then snowballs into increasing abnormality. A number of different features stand out: Mr. P. seems almost adamant about pushing his wife further into her craziness by constantly reminding her of her inadequacies, deficiencies, and abnormalities, as if driven by a "psychosis wish"; Susan and Robert manifest marked "affect

TABLE 1
Analysis of 100 Sequential Responses in Living-in Protocols

Variable observed	Noninvolving psychosis (the P. family) Raw score	Involving psychosis (the M. family) Raw score	Chi-square[a]	Sig. level[b]
Interaction of children with sick parent	19	52	23.78	.001
Interaction of children with well parent	32	26	.87	ns
Interaction of children with observer	28	15	5.01	.025
Hostile projections	9	11	.22	ns
Incongruous affects	13	4	5.21	.025
Conflicting communications	6	8	.31	ns
Magical thinking	29	22	1.29	ns

[a] Result gained from 2×2 chi-square.
[b] Significance level associated with a two-tailed test.

hunger" in competition for the observer, and Susan, especially, is hypersensitive to the flow of affects; her identification with her mother on the motoric level is also very evident; she is especially aware of how elation is often used to mask unhappiness; Mr. P. makes use of his wife's psychosis to threaten or reproach the children and to make them feel afraid and guilty; the coalitions within the family show father and John drawn together so that John shows the same impatience with his mother, but the ego boundaries of the younger children and their mother are so tenuous that the coalition between them is not at all firmly established; finally, the "contagiousness" of the situation is such that the observer is already manifesting symptoms.

The research psychologist, on the quantitative side, was fascinated by but dissatisfied with the "anthropological" account of the "culture of psychosis" and set to work to carry out a "blind" analysis of a hundred sequential responses from the living-in protocols. The results are shown in Table 1.

The significant differences between the two types of psychotic subcultures were found in the interaction of the children with the sick parent, in the interaction of the children with the observer, and in the occurrence of incongruous affects in the children in response to the noninvolving psychosis in the parent. Three other variables also showed up strongly in most protocols and these had to do with hostile projections on the part of the children, conflicting or confusing communications in the family, and interactions of the children with the "well" parent.

Reshaping Data: Hard into Soft

Although not hard in the sense of the physical sciences, and reckoned to be softer today than in the past, psychometric testing can still be placed on the harder side of the behavioral science research spectrum. The P. family were all given a battery of psychological tests that included both intelligence and projective procedures. The ratings of certain sensitive variables extracted from the raw scores were carried out blindly on each member of the family. When these, together with the intelligence scores, were put together, a comprehensive picture of family functioning emerged, within which certain patterns and groupings could be detected. When the children's scores are compared with those of the parents, a child may be like the sick parent, predominantly like the "well" parent, or mixed.

In the case of the P. family (see Table 2), John's scores are very much like his father's and Robert's like his mother's, whereas Susan's scores reflect both parents', although she is somewhat nearer to her mother in most of the ratings. On the basis of these findings it could be predicted that Mr. P. and John would approach problems with a similar cognitive style, which is charac-

TABLE 2

Family Profile as Manifested by Individual Responses on Intelligence Test and by Ratings[a] Based on Responses to Battery of Psychological Tests

	The P. family				
	Mr. P.	Mrs. P.	John	Susan	Robert
Test IQ V/P:F	$\frac{133}{113}$: 125	$\frac{97}{117}$: 107	$\frac{143}{124}$: 134	$\frac{103}{120}$: 112	$\frac{85}{107}$: 95
V-P	+20	−20	+19	−17	−22
Ratings					
Reality testing	1	4	1	2	3
Concreteness	1	3	1	2	3
Relationships	3	4	2	3	3
Aggressivity	3	4	2	3	3
Coping	1	4	1	3	3
Content pathology	2	4	2	2	3
Overall severity	3	4	2	3	3
Emotionality	2	4	2	4	3
Means	2.00	3.88	1.63	2.75	3.00

[a] Ratings are from 0, denoting absence of indications of disturbance for that variable, to 4, denoting incapacitating disturbance, too much, or too little. The ratings were made blind by two independent raters, and the interrater reliability ranged between .76 to .81.

teristically convergent with high scores on intelligence tests and low scores on open-ended tests, and which is generally accurate, consistent, realistic, logical, and action-oriented. The cognitive styles of Robert and Susan would tend to be divergent, like their mother's, with low scores on intelligence tests and high scores on open-ended ones, and with generally amorphous, unrealistic, inaccurate, and nonpersistent characteristics.

It was therefore expected that in an interactional situation in which the family was set to work on a problem the two subgroups would handle the situation quite differently and reach radically different solutions. The following protocol has been taken from a session in which the parents and the children were asked to reach a joint conclusion on the meaning of the proverb, "A rolling stone gathers no moss."

> The father immediately took command of the situation and discoursed fully and confidently on the subject. He said that in order to get on in life and not stagnate in a menial job you have to keep on the move. People who got places were dynamic, lively people who refused to stay put. The rest of the family listened impassively without interruption and there was some silence after he had concluded. When the interviewer turned to the mother, she attempted a vague, disjointed statement, to which her husband listened with obvious impatience. For a while, what she seemed to be saying appeared tangential to the problem, but, in a somewhat roundabout way, it gradually began to make a little sense. What she said was: "Moss is soft and lovely—I've always loved moss—gave mossy baskets for presents with little pebbles in it—like to lie on moss—soft like a cushion—cool—kind—doesn't worry you—not like stones, they hurt—can't lie on stones—too hard—go away, horrible stones—nice moss." The father's impatience communicated itself to the 13-year-old John, who broke out irritably, "You're absolutely wrong, Mom, moss is just dirt. It does you no good. You can't use it for anything. You can't make cars and vacuum cleaners and freezers out of it. It's just garbage. It dirties your clothes and that's all. Dad's right, if you want to get to the top you've got to keep going. I'll be class president next year. If I just sat at my desk and did nothing, they wouldn't elect me president. I tell you I'm not going to stay in one place all my life. I'm going to go places like Dad. That's how Dad got all his money." The two younger children looked shy and withdrawn, but after a while, with a little prompting, the younger boy, Robert, in a quiet, self-contained manner, but quite lucidly, said, "I don't like shifting about too much. Whenever we've changed houses I've had a bad time. When you move about you lose your friends and the good teachers who know you. I liked my bed in the old house. It was just right for me. When we came here, we bought a new one and I can't get used to it. I can't sleep for a long time when I get to bed. I think you're happy when you stay in one place and make lots of friends. You only lose things when you move. I lost my fishing tackle when we moved." Susan's eyes filled with tears as the interviewer looked in her direction. The interviewer told Susan that she didn't have to talk but that she was here with her family and families were good to talk with. She looked first at her father and then at her mother and slowly began. "I think dad's right because you get left behind unless you take part in a lot of things and go to different clubs and try everything even if people don't like you and they are mean to you. You can become president like John if you are popular and good at games and take the class register and

everything." She now looked at her mother and saw that her head was bent and her eyes closed, and she hurriedly changed her direction. "I think Mom's right because it's so nice to be quiet and still and stay in one place and just look at the same trees. You can never tell with new things, they always seem to go wrong. I once had one of those new dolls that talked and all the talking went wrong and it just screeched and said the same thing over and over again and I hated her. You never knew what was going to happen next. It was just horrible."

This vignette illustrates how helpful it can be to juxtapose the quantitative with the qualitative. The harder data give new meaning to the softer material of the session and enable one both to anticipate and to understand the interactional process. The psychometric results come to life and acquire a new richness when transposed to the family group setting.

Admixing Data

The family procedures in this research were selected on the basis of the battery principle, according to which a conglomerate of tests are put together to cover different aspects of a total problem preconceived within a particular theoretical framework. A different type of bridging procedure has been put forward by Glaser and Strauss (1967), based on what they call "grounded theory." According to their view, the behavioral scientist should generate his own theory relevant to the research on which he is engaged and not simply fall back on using the research field to test old and well-established constructs. This means that the concepts are not extrapolated from psychoanalysis, learning theory, field theory, etc., but are "grounded" in the investigation. One therefore discovers theory as one goes along, and, like any deduced theory, it must be assessed in terms of logical consistency, clarity, parsimony, density, scope, integration, fitness, and workability. It also follows that neither qualitative nor quantitative approaches have any special advantage, since both can be relevant to the verification and generation of new theory.

In this approach, the investigator's task is to develop a theory that accounts for much of the relevant behavior and that can be presented either as a well-codified set of propositions or as a running theoretical discussion using conceptual categories and their properties. The advantage of this method of commentary is that it puts emphasis on theory as process, that is, as an ever-developing entity, and not as a perfected end product. Since the investigator is discovering theory, it is important for him to enter the field of investigation without a loading of preconception. This approach is thus a form of theoretical sampling that looks at the field of investigation from different vantage points through the use of different techniques of data collection, and provides slices of different data about the same phenomenon.

Although the approach has been criticized by laboratory investigators, it

TABLE 3

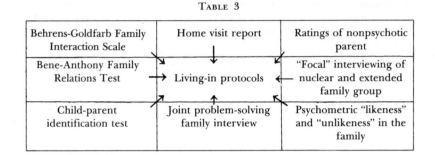

Behrens-Goldfarb Family Interaction Scale	Home visit report	Ratings of nonpsychotic parent
Bene-Anthony Family Relations Test	Living-in protocols	"Focal" interviewing of nuclear and extended family group
Child-parent identification test	Joint problem-solving family interview	Psychometric "likeness" and "unlikeness" in the family

has evoked a sympathetic response from clinicians interested in using primary field data because it respects the richness of clinical material, involves a low level of abstraction, treats qualitative and quantitative material equally, and offers excellent opportunities for searching out large and striking regularities. It permits one to enter an unknown culture, rather as an anthropologist does, without the expressed purpose of proving or disproving some presupposition.

If the repertoire of family studies is considered as an opportunity for finding grounded theory, each test in the battery begins to assume a different aspect than the other tests and than the battery as a whole, and gradually a coherent theoretical framework begins to take shape (Table 3).

The nuclear "theoretical commentary" is provided by the living-in experience,[4] since in this "anthropological" setting, the grounded theory of *involvement* appears to obtain its fullest expression.

In the Behrens-Goldfarb Family Interaction Scale, Mr. P. and John were rated as being in close contact and communication. There was also minimal interaction between the parents and between the father and the two younger children. The nonverbal impact of the mother on the two younger children was appreciable, and it was not surprising that the two younger ones were also rated independently as the more disturbed. The Family Relations Test disclosed a marked preoccupation of John with his father and of Robert with his mother, with Susan showing an ambivalent involvement with both parents. During the home visit the mother reported, somewhat incoherently, that she had brought up her oldest child "by the book" and had done everything right but that later she began to get tired and lose interest in everyone and everything so that the two younger children had brought themselves up as best they could. She was constantly confused about the child-rearing data pertaining to Susan and Robert and mixed them up. Her account of family life was equally nebulous and confused. She said that she liked to have her husband around because he always knew exactly what to do no matter what the

[4] See "Naturalistic Studies of Disturbed Families" by E. James Anthony in this volume.

problem was, but she felt so far away at times from the children that she hoped that their father could do things for them. When the father was invited to give his perspective of family life, he immediately began to interview the interviewer and make careful notes of his responses. The father remarked dispassionately that his wife no longer really existed, but he felt that it was important for the sake of the children and for his own career that they should stick together as a family. He had high hopes that his older son would be very successful but did not place much store on the abilities of the two younger ones, both of whom, he said, had been "brainwashed" by their mother. At no time did he express any compassion for or understanding of the illness of his wife. His main concern was to isolate her in the family and insulate her from the outside world. For the sake of the children, he said, he was striving to mitigate her influence in the family and reduce her to a nonentity. In the focal interviews, John discussed his mother's illness with remarkable objectivity and detachment. "I feel sorry for her but she has only herself to blame for letting herself go. I have tried to help her but she doesn't seem to have any interests in doing better. She's just not motivated." (*Motivation* was his father's favorite word.) Susan admitted to being mystified by her mother's behavior. "When she got sick last time, she just seemed to forget all about me. I cried every night in bed and could not go to sleep. I know she cares, but she doesn't seem to care. I wish Daddy would be nicer to her. She might get better." Robert said that he sometimes dreamed that his mother was laughing and talking with them and that she was "like an ordinary lady." He really would like her to come and watch him play baseball, he said, but she never wanted to do anything. Sometimes he got angry and hated her, but then he was sad and loved her.

In the identification test, the children were confronted with a series of questions asking them which parent they felt they were more like with respect to a number of physical, social, and psychological attributes. Robert showed a strong, unwavering identification with his mother, to the point of renouncing his gender identity; Susan was also closely identified with her mother but showed a surprising number of likenesses to her father; John was wholly identified with his father in every respect. (It was noted that even the intonation of his voice was hard to distinguish from that of his father.) Identification not only signifies a certain degree of involvement but also generates further involvement.

The rating of the nonpsychotic spouse constitutes a good prognostic index, since he or she is frequently the only barrier against the forces of unreality and irrationalism emanating from the psychotic parent. Mr. P. scored poorly on all counts: his attitudes were rated harmful, particularly for the two younger and more vulnerable children. His disengagement from them and his readiness to link them to his wife's disorder had the effect of driving them into greater involvement with their noninvolved mother and therefore a constant re-experiencing of the trauma of psychological abandonment. Having no one to turn to, they would frequently reach out indiscriminately to strangers and build up false hopes from every transient relationship.

The battery of tests could now be viewed as a gestalt that combined the salient features of each test in a comprehensive picture of involvement or noninvolvement. The observer in the household was able to experience at first hand the central, convergent process as it influenced her during the course of her stay (Table 3).

The central theme of involvement is thus seen in the separate context of the parents' involvement with the child, in the child's involvement with the parent, in the child's involvement with the illness, in the psychosis involving the child, in the well spouse disinvolving the sick parent, in the sick parent's differentiated or nondifferentiated response to the children, and in the barrier to the process of involvement set up by an amorphous cognitive style.

Redeploying Data

The use of soft data to generate testable hypotheses in hard experimental studies is illustrated elsewhere in this volume.[5] In Table 1, the sequential analysis of the living-in protocols isolates a number of responses in the children that could be classified under four headings:

1. Hostile projections: actions, reactions, or interactions in which the children interpreted experiences in their environment in malevolent rather than benign terms.
2. Incongruous affects: in which the children appeared not to recognize the affects of others, to misinterpret them grossly, or to give an inappropriate affective response to situations.
3. Conflicting communications: in which there were indications of not understanding, misunderstanding, and perplexity occasioned by communications from others.
4. Magical thinking: in which nonnatural or supernatural explanations were furnished by adults and children as an explanation of events.

These observations from the living-in experience became hypotheses, which were put to the test in experimental situations that were so devised as to simulate the natural conditions under which the observations had been made in the household.

---

[5]See "The Use of the 'Serious' Experiment in Child Psychiatric Research" by E. James Anthony in this volume.

The reverse of this process was then carried out: hard data were used to direct the observer in naturalistic studies of the family. In the method of "focal" interviewing, each member of the family group, both nuclear and extended, was interviewed solely in the context of their reaction to the psychotic disorder manifested by Mrs. P., special attention being placed on the extent to which their lives had been altered, positively or negatively, by the predicament that had descended on the family. The ratings of the responses were then carried out blindly by two independent raters unacquainted with the project. In Table 4 the influences of the psychotic member on the different members of the P. family are juxtaposed so that one can appreciate at a single glance the impact on the individual as well as an inferred influence on the group as a whole.

Table 4 creates expectations for anyone entering the family for the first time as an observer. It would alert him to the existence or potential development of the following phenomena in the P. family:

1. The family as a whole is fairly sharply bifurcated for and against the psychotic member. Those in sympathy tend to regard her in the context of being victimized by mysterious external forces, while those opposed to her hold her responsible for the downfall of the family and regard her as mischievously disposed toward it.

2. The sympathizers tend to be tainted with the same pathology, whereas the opposition manifests reverse pathology at the other extreme.

3. The family is in constant conflict as these two contrary elements within it attempt to pull it in different directions, and the younger members are most inclined to reflect the agony induced by these pressures.

4. A particularly vulnerable member is apt to attempt ineffectually to straddle both attitudes and to end up with the external conflict internalized, with the ambivalence expressing itself symptomatically in indecision.

5. The stronger forces, in opposition, are apt to strive to isolate and insulate the psychotic one from the general life of the family and to succeed in doing so, thus driving the patient into increasing withdrawal and regression.

6. The extended family group shows a [similar] division in siding with either the paternal subgroup, reflecting the paternal point of view and all its positivism, or the maternal subgroup, curiously amorphous and unsure of itself, mirroring the mother's negativism.

TABLE 4

"Focal" Interviewing of Nuclear and Extended Family Group Members on the Impact of the Psychosis on Them[a]

The P. family

Variable	Mr. P.	John	Susan	Robert	MGF[b]	MGM[c]	PGF[d]	PGM[e]
Progress (bettering/worsening)	5	4	3	1	2	1	5	4
Prognosis (good/bad)	5	4	3	1	3	2	5	5
Responsibility (ours/hers)	4	3	2	2	3	4	5	4
Stigma (little/lot)	4	4	3	2	2	2	5	4
Feelings (love/hate)	4	3	2	1	3	2	4	3
Upsetting (min./max.)	2	1	3	4	3	4	2	3
Extrusion (in/out)	4	3	2	1	2	1	5	4
Means	4.00	3.14	2.57	1.71	2.71	2.85	4.43	3.86

[a] Ratings were made "blindly" by independent raters for the protocols, ranging from 1 to 5, 1 denoting *for* the patient and 5 *against* the patient.
[b] MGF = maternal grandfather.
[c] MGM = maternal grandmother.
[d] PGF = paternal grandfather.
[e] PGM = paternal grandmother.

Armed with this information, the observer entered the household and sub-sequently emerged with much richer and fuller protocols that, on sequential analysis, provided a whole new set of hypotheses to be tested experimentally.

It was found that this type of interplay between the soft and the hard ap-proaches increased the instrumental power of both in almost a dialectical man-ner. It was not the traditional mode of doing research, but it appeared to add a mechanism of enrichment, facilitating the continuous emergence of new ideas and new data.

Conclusion: The Benefits of Complementarity

The hard approach creates models within laboratories that serve as blue-prints of reality. It should be acknowledged that, useful though these are, their purpose is to simplify complex systems by projecting them into a simpler space that has a smaller number of dimensions than are required for a complete description of the original system. The experimenter thus relocates pluralistic phenomena in an underdimensioned space, where he feels both less involved in and more in control of the situation. This amount of control is not possible on the soft side, and the hard-nosed researcher will do his best to avoid direct contact with the soft side. However, it is important for him to experience it in its fully nebulous state so that he can have no illusions about what he himself can accomplish alone.

This presentation can be understood as a plea for some form of scientific synthesis that can comprehend complex systems with a minimum of abstrac-tions, so that these systems can be really apprehended as an organic whole through an active, trained intuition in the same way that the good experi-menter is able to find order in a large mass of numerical data. The soft re-searcher, bearing in mind Clark Maxwell's (1948) comment that "however imperfect the dynamical study of man may be in practice, it is evidently the only perfect method in principle," should not be too apologetic about his type of data but should try to regard them as complementary to data obtained under more controlled conditions and to work continuously toward a reconci-liation of the two approaches. Brewster Smith (1970) reflected this catholicity of the sources of knowledge when he wrote, "One may glean insights and hypotheses from many sources, including common human experience and its refinement in the arts, later to be tested by firmer criteria. I am convinced that there is no royal road to Truth, not even that of the experimentalist. Truth is elusive, and we do best to converge upon it from multiple perspectives." This summarizes, briefly and succinctly, the theme of this presentation.

References

BLACKBURN, T. R. Sensuous-intellectual complementarity in science. *Science,* 1971, **172,** 1003–1007.

BOHR, N. *Atomic physics and human knowledge.* London: Chapman and Hall, 1958.

GILL, M. et al., Studies in audio-recorded psychoanalysis, I, General Considerations, *Journal of the American Psychoanalytic Association,* 1968, **16,** 230–244.

GLASER, G. B., & Strauss, E. *The discovery of grounded theory: Strategies for qualitative research.* Chicago: Aldine, 1967.

KAPLAN, A. *The conduct of inquiry.* San Francisco: Chandler, 1964.

LOEVINGER, J. Conflict of commitment in clinical research. *American Psychologist* 1963, **18,** 241–251.

MAXWELL, C. Quoted by K. H. Wolff in The unique and the general: Toward a philosophy of sociology, *Journal of Philosophical Sciences,* 1948, **153,** 192–210.

SMITH, M. B. *Social psychology and human values.* New York: Basic Books, 1970.

WHITEHEAD, A. *Sciences and the modern world.* London: Penguin, 1956.

THE CHILD AS A RESEARCH SUBJECT

E. James Anthony

Like many eminent child psychologists such as Binet, Piaget, Stern, and others, Valentine (1942) used his own children as subjects in his studies on child development. One of them, in later years, was asked whether he resented his father's professional approach toward him when he was small and answered that, on the contrary, he remembered his childhood as a most pleasing and fascinating experience. Not many individuals, he thought, could claim to have had the undivided attention and boundless interest of a parent during their entire development. He recalled endless hours of play with delightful and challenging materials. It was no concern of his at the time whether his father's rapt circumspection had affectional or academic sources, but he suspected, looking back, that there was a good deal of both.

We have heard children at our research center in St. Louis express in more naïve terms sentiments that were similar to these, and it could be that our intense absorption with questions, which could be answered only by our subjects, provided the basis for what we have termed the "research alliance." Like the therapeutic alliance, this is cultivated by facilitating conscious and unconscious factors in both child and investigator, and it is therefore prominent in some research settings and negligible in others. It is particularly apt to occur in clinical investigations conducted by clinicians habitually in contact with patients. Therapeutic attitudes engendered by such investigations are likely to overflow into the contact with subjects, so that at least some part of the research alliance may be therapeutically derived. Clinicians have a tendency to transform most situations into clinical ones, and the more therapeutically oriented the researcher is, the more therapeutically infused his research is likely to be. This type of contamination is an advantage in naturalistic exploration but interferes with the more rigorous forms of investigation. Yet it can, with the imposition of certain safeguards, be used with profit even in highly controlled experimentation.

It is a surprising fact that textbooks dealing with research methodologies

E. JAMES ANTHONY, The Harry Edison Child Development Research Center, Washington University School of Medicine, St. Louis.

41

may cover every aspect of technique from design to the analysis of data
inherent but omit or take for granted the considerable set of problems inherent
in the investigation of children: how to make contact with the child, how to
engage his cooperation, how to maintain his interest, and how to prevent being
bamboozled by him. Child subjects, like child patients, have almost infinite
resources for leading the unsuspecting researcher up the garden path.

The Nature of the Child Subject

One must remember that an average sample of children drawn from any
source can run the gamut from negativism to complete acquiescence, so that a
standard approach, rigidly enforced, may alienate or antagonize a significant
proportion of the research group. With clinical subjects one must exercise even
greater flexibility if the responses are to count for anything. Research
obsessiveness, like clinical compulsivity, often defeats its own purpose: the
administration provokes all degrees of resistance from the subjects and hence
many degrees of unresponsiveness. Instructions, meticulously enunciated or
even taped, can be completely misunderstood or misinterpreted, depending on
the first impressions created by the researcher. The subject may go no further
than his immediate subjective reaction to the objectivity. This is what makes it
well-nigh impossible to replicate a human project.

A certain number of generally acceptable statements can be made about
the child subject, bearing on the quality of his participation in research
(Anderson, 1954):

1. The child is a growing, differentiating organism who becomes
   increasingly complex with each step in development.
2. He is an organized whole who functions as such within every
   situation in which he is placed. "Since neither the child nor his
   behavior can be broken up and reassembled in the literal sense,
   difficulties arise in scientific child study."
3. He lives in a context that is neither simple nor unitary and that
   continuously affects his behavior and development. He perceives
   the environment in certain ways and selects parts to which he
   responds. "At all times there is a reciprocal relation between the
   human being and this biosocial context."
4. He is engaged in a continuous process of development that is not
   reversible, and therefore he does not step into the same research
   stream twice. On the second occasion, he is in all respects a different child.

The interplay between the child and the research environment is also
complicated. He affects his environment and is in turn affected by his envi-

ronment. He can be regarded at any moment as a highly organized energy system within a field of forces. There are no simple or single interactions between him and his environment. They are all composed of multiple factors, reciprocal relations, progressive recessions of causes, and continuous cumulations of effects. When this complexity is misunderstood, erroneous conclusions are often drawn from individual to environment, from individual to group, and, in Lewin's (1939) terminology, from genotype to phenotype and *vice versa*. In doing research one must keep in mind the differences between the individual and the group. Generalizations may be possible about the group that are not equally true of the individual, and *vice versa*.

With projects involving visual or auditory displays, it is important to remember that a wide variation of acuity exists and that within a given group some may see and hear much more than others. Class and ethnic experiences may accentuate such differences even further.

Children during development may also vary a great deal in terms of language capacity, in the ability to recall, in being able to reflect or introspect, and in taking up an objective and dispassionate attitude toward the research task confronting them.

The setting may also influence a child's reactions. So-called "habitat" research is thought to elicit more "natural" responses than laboratory situations. Whether the latter appear "unnatural" to the child is a moot point. Most child researchers are aware that the majority of their subjects continue to manifest interest and motivation under even the most artificially contrived conditions, taking the unusual very much in their stride.

What one might call the "psychopathology of everyday research" may cause some of the variability not accounted for by the factors previously mentioned. The time of the day, the time of the year, the state of his bowels, the time of his last meal, or an incipient cold may transform an otherwise reliable respondent into a very haphazard one. If he is tired, hungry, or bored, his research behavior can deteriorate into a stubborn silence or a playful confabulation, and it is then questionable whether one can take his responses seriously. He may clown, play the fool, "romance," or guess with little concern for his responsibility as a subject. The younger the child, the more suggestible he is and the more likely he is to reflect the researcher's expectations.[1]

In addition, not only is the child's research behavior different in different research situations or with different researchers, but there have also been different conceptualizations of child subjects by different theorists who have investigated them.

[1]This is discussed more fully in "The Use of the 'Serious' Experiment in Child Psychiatric Research" by E. James Anthony in this volume.

Lewin and the Child Subject

According to Lewin (1939), the child subject brings certain qualities to the research situation that may allow him to feel more at home in it than his adult counterpart. Lewin is talking here of his own very special conception of the research environment. First of all, he sees it as a "life-behaving system," but different from real life in being more controlled and more contrived. To adults it appears essentially artificial but to the child, who has been elaborating miniature life situations since infancy, it represents a reasonable facsimile of life to be taken as seriously as any play situation.

Secondly, Lewin restricts his research attention to the "here and now," and this approach fits the nature of the child like a glove. His time perspective is less extensive than that of the adult, and he is essentially a creature of the present (*"Das Kleinkind ist wesentlich jetzt"*). He is accustomed to adapting himself to what is current, and his field of action can be comfortably confined to what Erikson terms the "microsphere." His units of action are smaller in scope and duration than the adult's, and the past and future play less part in determining the events of his psychological environment (or so Lewin prefers to think because this is in keeping with his experimental approach).

It is not only easier to contain the child psychologically within the experimental life space, but it is also easier to persuade him to accept the rules and regulations that govern life within the space as established by the investigation. As Piaget (1932) demonstrated, children assimilate the "morality" of a given situation quite uncritically and will assume that the edicts in existence have been handed down from eternity. The child therefore understands that rules are necessary before games can be played and that certain arbitrary conditions are needed before an experiment can be carried out. It is possible that he regards the research task as the adult's game and therefore graciously concedes that he can conduct it in his own fashion. (This view of research may not be entirely foreign to the truth.[2])

It was Lewin who first encouraged researchers to take a close look at the research situation as a whole and at the research subject as a totality far transcending the narrowness of the epithet *subject*. To understand the behavior of the child in a particular research context, Lewin (1939) asked us to remember the following:

1. There is a distinction between the situation as constructed and perceived by the researcher and the situation as experienced by the child; the researcher needs to know something of the child's life space experiences, such as fears, affections, aspirations,

[2]See "The Use of the 'Serious' Experiment in Child Psychiatric Research" by E. James Anthony in this volume.

dreams, and realities as they are interpolated into the experimental situation.

2. These psychosocial aspects are as essential to the researcher's understanding of the situation as the physical factors involved in the setting.

3. The atmosphere generated reciprocally by the researcher and his subject may sometimes contain too much tension, suspicion, fearfulness, and antagonism for the research process to work at all.

The emotionally disturbed child has many of the characteristics of the normal research subject but in somewhat exaggerated form. Lewin discussed these exaggerations in considering the so-called "marginal" child, whose unsureness and uncertainty emanate from an in-between status with respect to definite groups. In this sense all clinical subjects can be regarded as "marginal" and may manifest such characteristics of marginality as excessive tensions, undue fluctuations between attack and timidity, strong aggressive reactions to frustrations, rapid alternations among values, and overwhelming feelings of rejection. Research responses might therefore be expected to be less stable, less confident, and more likely to terminate in such seemingly nonsolutions as unresolvable conflict, withdrawal, heightened emotionality, increased psychomotor activity, disorganized behavior, and transient regressions involving dedifferentiation, derealization, and loss of motivation. In short, the clinical subject may, and often does, respond to the research demand clinically. This response can be kept within acceptable levels of deviation by the exercise of a more therapeutic approach.[3]

Marginal behavior can take two forms: it can be more rigid, more concrete, and more differentiated on the one side; or more plastic, more unrealistic, and more undifferentiated and regressed on the other. The marginal child may also show too little or too much of many normal characteristics, and therefore in intergroup investigations the extreme responses may cancel each other out and get lost in the analysis.

There is a further feature considered by Lewin that is especially relevant to clinical research with children. The child, to a far greater extent than the adult, reacts to situations as a dynamic unity; he tends to put all of himself into the response and learns only gradually through the process of development to give more selective and partial answers. Because of this, he fatigues rapidly from the impact of the extensive and intensive research batteries to which some investigators inconsiderately expose him. He is easily tired by too much experimenting and may fall back on random or nonsensical

---

[3] See "The Use of the 'Serious' Experiment in Child Psychiatric Research" by E. James Anthony in this volume.

replies. It is important to keep this psychophysiological limitation in mind and to maintain a reasonable tempo of presentation and some opportunity to relax between exposures. Social class and ethnic affiliation seem to be important factors in determining the level of tolerance to research, but before they come into play the stranger reaction can sometimes produce a general paralysis of the research drive. These "tropisms" are not all in-bred; life experiences of a negative kind help to generate negative tropisms in the laboratory, and the sensitive researcher must beware of replicating life's mistakes and inculcating a "negative research reaction" analogous to the "negative therapeutic reaction" of psychoanalysis.

The Child Research Subject as Perceived by Piaget

In their studies of child behavior, Gesell and his colleagues made use of a method that involved making highly refined observations on subjects placed in certain experimental situations. By this means they were able to work out norms of development and to delineate "behavior patterns" at various stages of growth. This external, descriptive approach was carried a step further by Piaget (1931), who began to explore an in-between area of unconsciousness. He adopted a "clinical" method that was at first largely an interrogation but that later included the concurrent manipulation of test material. By this means he was able to open up to research this intermediate area, where thought is largely preoperational and intuitive and is bounded on the "darker" side by unconscious fantasies and feelings not ordinarily available to consciousness. These levels of observation and communication have been discussed in some detail by the author in two previous papers (1964, 1968). Piaget was well aware that the verbal approach to the child contains many pitfalls. He noted how suggestible the child is to adult influence and how earnestly he tries to please grown-ups by living up to their expectations. He also noted how rapidly the child shifts from the level of seriousness and task orientation to playfulness and "romancing," but he felt sure that in proper hands the "clinical method" diminishes the likelihood of such pseudoresponses by allowing the child to take the lead in the inquiry and that if the researcher keeps psychologically behind the child, the element of suggestion can be greatly reduced. He suggested that an additional means of ensuring the eliciting of normative responses is the inclusion of as many children as possible at the same level of development.

The Child as a Research Subject as Seen by Griffiths

The importance of Griffiths (1935) lies in the fact that she is one of the few child researchers who has thought deeply about the nature of children as research subjects. She is exquisitely sensitive to the defense structure and the way to approach it with tact and consideration. She warned against direct questioning as inevitably tending to promote evasion, confusion, and unconscious rationalization. The younger child may find himself completely blocked and unable to respond. She also cautioned against betraying too much interest in any particular point, since this is likely to cause the suppression of the very facts that are being sought. She counseled a policy of waiting and of being content with scattered fragments of information, which, like the pieces of a jigsaw puzzle, will eventually come together to provide a complete picture. The child's thought develops in bits and pieces and to ask for more than he produces at any given time is to demand what he does not yet possess: "There would seem to be something almost of impertinence in an impatient forcing of a child's thought by continual questioning." Griffiths reminds us that the essence of the scientific method lies in the observer's refraining from influencing the phenomena that he is observing. Research, she declared, *begins with respect for the child*.

This gradualism is best described in her own account of the research situation. She is seated in a large room, not too comfortable and not too well lighted; the austerity and comparative gloom are favorable elements since they afford less distraction for her purpose, which is to explore the child's capacity for imagination. She is careful, therefore, to remove all distracting influences and to maintain a fairly quiet environment. The child is slowly accustomed to the situation until he is no longer engaged with its external aspects.

She went on to discuss the "research alliance," pointing out that however desirable it is to eliminate the influence of the experimenter, in most instances it is actually impossible.

> A very delicate relationship grows up between the experimenter and each subject, and this situation needs careful handling. We owe to psychoanalysis the recognition of the importance of "transference," and it is not only in an analytic situation that this phenomenon is at work. On every occasion that a child comes under the influence of an adult other than his parents, this parent-child relationship is reproduced.

The experimenter must at all times be aware of his influence on the subjects and take this into consideration when dealing with the results. In research work with children he must preserve "a good, positive relationship" with them; this is not usually difficult. The experimenter must exercise "a quiet, restrained, although sympathetic manner." When he does, the children respond "with astonishing rapidity" and seem to enjoy the situation.

Gradualism is the key to Griffith's approach. The child must be gently but thoroughly habituated both to the personality of the experimenter and to the new environment: "There is no work to which the dictum 'hasten slowly' can be applied with greater advantage than to psychological work with little children."

The Child as a Research Subject as Seen by Murphy

Murphy's (1956) eclectic approach borrows a little from everybody and infuses it all into "a positive approach." As she studies the child, she is reminded (presumably at different times) of Bergson's *élan vital*, Freud's unconscious conflict, Rorschach's experience balance, her husband's biosocial view of the organism in society, Lewin's notion of life space, Frank's idiosyncratic patterning of development, and Anna Freud's sensitivity to childhood feelings and experience. Surprisingly, the only name missing from this pantheon is Piaget, although she is well aware of his work and makes several references to him.

This "positive" approach would be expected in turn to elicit positive approaches from the children, and this is what happens.

> It is impossible to have the experience of playing with hundreds of small children with miniature Life Toy Material without feeling considerable awe for the creative and integrative capacities of these young minds. Like the poets, they often distill what have been repeated sequences of life, experienced in large segments, into the simplest patterns which could convey these sequences.

This rather romantic view of childhood produces a very humanistic approach to the child as a research subject. The need for flexibility is stressed in preference to a fixed experimental plan. The essential factor is "to make each child feel as completely at ease as possible," and in order to do this the researcher must vary his attitude, being fairly aloof with one child, affectionate with another, and humorous with a third.

Murphy, like Griffiths, made a point of the importance of having a familiar setting with simple furnishings that can be quickly explored and then forgotten. The researcher, likewise, must be "a friendly, familiar and unthreatening person."

Murphy pointed out that not only do children respond differently to differently structured research situations, but they respond differently to investigators of different sexes, different ethnic origins, different classes, and so on, being productive with one and negativistic with another. As she put it:

> A child may vary from hour to hour, day to day, week to week, tester to tester, or test to test. This is one reason why a battery of tests over a period of time is the only way to get an adaquate basis for evaluation of the range within which this variation occurs, the ceilings or limits which distinguish one child from another, and the predominant patterns of persistence and change.

What is difficult to gauge is the persistent or transient significance of a child's response, whether it is related to phase or personality, local or general conditions, and the extent to which life in the research situation and life at home approximate one another. Children often behave differently at home than at school. They may be inhibited at school and very expressive in the home, or quiet and unobtrusive when at a neighbor's house and noisy and exuberant within the family circle. The "nearness to life" or the "lifelikeness" of the research situation may be a strong force in determining the type of reaction. The situation may be categorized according to its similarity or dissimilarity to previous situations experienced by the child: Is it like home? like school? like visiting friends? like staying at a hotel?

Murphy is of the opinion that the child's feeling about the adult researcher "profoundly affects" his behavior in the research session, but she does not go quite as far as Griffiths in linking this feeling to psychoanalytic transference. One thing is sure, if transference is presumed to enter the research situation, control becomes well-nigh impossible. It is complicated enough that the child may displace his current home experiences to the laboratory without throwing his difficult past into the situation as well. If the researcher analyzes the child's sequential responses, it is possible to disentangle various aspects of the researcher's influence as it is reflected in the child's compliance, in his imitation, in his defiance, in his seductiveness, or in his independence and autonomy. The laboratory reaction, like the therapeutic reaction, may tell us something of what goes on in the world outside.

Miniature Life Play

Most of the researchers mentioned are clearly aware of the variability of the child subject in relation to the nature of the experiment, the conditions of the experiment, and the behavior and expectations of the experimenter. They assume that this is an inevitable facet of the research situation with the child, and they therefore do very little to correct it or to enforce rigidly standardized conditions. A good example of the flexibility and even permissiveness with which research procedures are often handled with children is provided by miniature life play.

Miniature life play is one of the commonest research instruments used in the investigation of children. As a method for the study of personality development, it was first tried at the Iowa Child Welfare Research Station about 30 years ago and has been in extensive use since then, perhaps because it seems so much the most natural research situation to set up for children. It is the child's psychological laboratory, but what can the outsider glean from it? Herron and Sutton-Smith (1971) suggested that the best way to learn how to do a good doll-play study still seems to be to collect the "lore" from someone with experience in the area, since it is difficult to pick up the nuances involved from an examination of the literature. It is true that the child is better able to talk through the doll than more directly, but his responses may vary considerably, depending on how the research questions are constructed: Are

they too emotionally loaded? Is the subject asked to verbalize the feelings of a
child doll rather than an adult doll? Is he invited to tell what the doll would do
rather than what it would say? There is evidence to suggest that a doll family
that duplicates the child's own family tends to produce more identifications
than does the use of a standard family, and that indoor settings for the dolls
produce more stereotyped behavior than outdoor settings.

In keeping with evidence previously furnished in this chapter, it has been
found that high interaction in the miniature life play between experimenter
and child tends to produce more fantasy material, more thematic changes,
more aggressiveness, and an earlier onset of aggressive play than does a low
interaction level; and that subjects show more aggression in the presence of an
experimenter of the same sex. There have unfortunately been relatively few
studies of consistency during miniature play, and those that exist have mostly
to do with aggression, in which split-half reliabilities were fairly high (.77 in
one study).

A much more serious problem, one that is shared with other objective
techniques, has to do with validity. Does miniature life play reflect real life or
wish fulfillment? The advocates of miniature life play have claimed that three-
quarters of the child's free play is replicative, which is surprising, since it had
been assumed that play generally attempts to compensate for real life and that
the inhibited child takes advantage of the free conditions to indulge in fantasied
aggression. There does not seem to be any consistent direct or inverse relationship between reality and fantasy, which may be another way of saying that the
child's perception of the miniature life situation is highly variable.

It also cannot be taken for granted that the child will identify with a doll
child and express himself through it. In many clinical subjects there is a
tendency toward "metamorphosis," in which the subject speaks and acts
through the authority figure of an adult doll. When the doll children are
severely punished or when aggressive play is unbounded, there is a fairly
predictable association with punitive parents.

In summing up, one could say that miniature play is a useful research de-
vice but that its assets and limitations should be clearly understood. The play
of the child is as complex as any human activity and as difficult to unravel into
its component details. Children are said to play in order to rehearse; to gain
emotional release; to mitigate, deny, or temporarily resolve a conflict; to recapture an earlier omnipotence; to repeat and gradually assimilate a traumatic
experience; to overcome a specific fear; to conceptualize vague ideas; and to
experiment with possible modes of thought and action. It is the first aid station
to which the child goes to heal his wounds, to discharge his feelings, to
reassure himself about the future, and, in general, to feel better about himself.
One has also to remember that it is also a place where he goes to have a bit of
fun (*Funktionslust*). The main thing is the exercise of control. The drama of
the child's life can unfold on this stage *under his direction and management*,

and when this important element is taken over by the adult (be it parent, teacher, or researcher), the play at once begins to reproduce the qualities of the particular relationship. For children under five, the play is less a drama than a dream, with all the dream's tendencies to condensation and symbolism.

Conclusion

Children are elusive creatures. They slip through one's investigative fingers like eels; when we think we have them pinned down as research specimens, they suddenly evade us in gales of nonsense and laughter that ruffle our adult egos and cause our best-laid research plans to go far agley. We can come closest to finding out about them by pretending to be casual onlookers in search of trivia, although our sights are directed to profounder matters. This was Piaget's stratagem: the uninformed, somewhat simpleminded adult who wants to learn about the way the game of marbles is played (but who is really delving into the universal problem of morality). But he is aware of the pitfalls.

> We are more conscious than anybody of the defects as of the advantages of the method we have used. The great danger . . . is that of making the child say whatever one wants him to say. *There is no infallible remedy for this*; neither the good faith of the questioner nor the precautionary methods we have laid stress upon are sufficient. The only safeguard lies in the collaboration of other investigators [Piaget, 1932].

We seem to be caught here between a researcher's Scylla and Charybdis. If the research situation is rigorously controlled, what emerges seems sterile; if it is allowed to develop loosely in a play relationship, the richness of the product may be a function of the relationship.

It is the poet who is nearest the child in this respect but still at a distance away. One of them, Walter De la Mare (1935), had this morsel of comfort to offer all child researchers:

> I believe that those who can win nearest to childhood and be wholly at peace, at liberty, and at ease in its company, would be the first to acknowledge that they can never get nearer than very near, never actually there.

As will be seen through the rest of this book, the researcher can often get "very near," but he would be among the first to confess that he is "never actually there."

References

Anderson, J. E. Methods of child psychology. In L. Carmichael (Ed.), *Manual of child psychology*. New York: Wiley, 1954.

Anthony, E. J. Communicating therapeutically with the child. *Journal of the American Academy of Child Psychiatry*, 1964, **3**, 106.

ANTHONY, E. J. On observing children. In E. Miller (Ed.), *Foundations of child psychiatry*. Oxford: Pergamon Press, 1968.

GRIFFITHS, R. *A study of imagination in early childhood*. London: Routledge, 1935.

HERRON, R. E., & SUTTON-SMITH, B. *Child's play*. New York: Wiley, 1971.

LEWIN, K. Environmental forces. In C. Murchison (Ed.), *A handbook of child psychology*. Worcester, Mass.: Clark University Press, 1933.

LEWIN, K. Field theory and experiment in social psychology: Concepts and methods. *American Journal of Sociology,* 1939, **44,** 868.

MARE, DE LA, W. J. *Early one morning in the spring: Chapters on children and on childhood as it is revealed in particular in early memories and in early writings*. New York: Macmillan, 1935.

MURPHY, L. *Personality in young children*. Vol. 1: *Methods for the study of personality*. New York: Basic Books, 1956.

PIAGET, J. *The child's conception of the world*. London: Routledge, 1931.

PIAGET, J. *The moral judgment of the child*. London: Routledge, 1932.

VALENTINE, C. W. *The psychology of early childhood: A study of mental development in the first years of life*. Chicago: University of Chicago Press, 1942, Chap. XX.

ORGANICALLY
BASED RESEARCH

INTRODUCTION

What is striking about the presentations in this section is the clarity of concept, the general economy of language (especially striking in the two younger researchers), and the single-mindedness with which the research goal is pursued. In each chapter the hyperkinetic syndrome is looked at and studied in somewhat different ways, depending on the main focus of investigation.

Cantwell is lucid not only with regard to his philosophy of science but also with regard to the influences that have played upon him during his research career. He examines the hyperkinetic syndrome within the framework of a medical model, as a disease entity different from other disease entities and capable of being classified in relation to other disease entities. He explodes some of the mythology that others, antagonistic to this approach, have built up around the medical model. It does not, he feels, entail a cold-blooded labeling of subjects along organic lines with little or no respect for their personal qualities. The real objective, as in all scientific work, is to add one's own quote to the establishment of a "common language" that can be shared by workers in the same field. The "six steps" seem ideally suited to this approach and follow the classical outline that medical investigators have used so profitably for so long. It is, as Cantwell says, a "tough-minded" approach, but tough-mindedness is necessary to counteract the ever-present specter of subjectivity that haunts the psychiatric and psychological fields.

Arnold examines his neurochemical research in terms of its philosophy, its ethics, and its humanism, and he seems prepared to live with a foot in both the subjective and the objective worlds. He can allow himself to be introspective or experimental as the situation demands, and he is of the opinion that child psychiatrists should cultivate the attribute of "humanistic willingness" and apply it to all aspects of their work, including research. His ideology is suitably rigorous and his experimental design impeccable. Once the controlled study is over, he allows himself to "gossip" about its meaning and application. More than any other investigator in this volume, he examines the "morality" of his research and considers several important issues that come up in the investigation of children; one should not harm, nor withhold good treatment when this is required. As he says, he is primarily a clinician who has "backed into research," and it is to his clinical bent that he attributes his humanistic approach to research.

Laufer's chapter offers more personal background to the neurophysiological work he has carried out over many years. If he is not as single-minded as Cantwell and Arnold, it is not only because he belongs to an older generation but also because of his more dynamic orientation. There is no doubt that one's experience "on the couch" is inclined to have a long-range effect on one's activities in the laboratory and conflict in one's personality. In this instance, one of the investigator's feet was in neurophysiology and the other in psychoanalysis, and the inevitable result was a feeling of isolation. He found it difficult to talk to others. In his investigation of hyperkinesis he became increasingly preoccupied with the diencephalon as well as with the emotional aspects, and he tried to keep a dual perspective on malfunctioning *in utero* on one hand and rigid, impoverished mothering in the extrauterine world on the other.

These three investigators give us not only a considerable insight into the hyperkinetic syndrome from three different angles, but they also furnish us with a good deal of additional understanding of why their research outlook carried them in these three different directions.

A MODEL FOR THE INVESTIGATION OF PSYCHIATRIC DISORDERS OF CHILDHOOD

ITS APPLICATION IN GENETIC STUDIES OF THE HYPERKINETIC SYNDROME

DENNIS P. CANTWELL

Introduction

Although child psychiatry has had officially approved subspecialty training programs in the United States for over 10 years, many leaders in the field have decried the nearly negligible amount of research training occurring in these programs (Finch, 1973) and have emphasized the need for active, ongoing research if child psychiatry is to develop the body of scientific theory necessary for it to remain a viable discipline (Anthony, 1969a, 1973; Fish, 1969). However, if more clinical investigation in child psychiatry is to occur in the future, more medical students must be recruited into the field, and those who are recruited must be encouraged to undertake investigative work while they are in training.

At the present time, I find myself just embarking on a dual career—that of a clinical investigator and that of director of a fellowship training program in child psychiatry. In my latter role, it will be my task to persuade at least some of my trainees to follow the path that I have taken.

As my contribution to this volume, I thought it might be valuable for me to trace this path—to describe my own training briefly and to summarize the

DENNIS P. CANTWELL, Director of Residence Training in Child Psychiatry, University of California, Los Angeles.

influences that led me to choose a career in academic research in a comparatively young discipline. After summarizing the key influences in my training years, I will outline the model I have developed for the investigation of the psychiatric disorders of childhood. Finally, I will describe the application of this model to my own studies of children with the hyperkinetic syndrome.

The Making of a Clinical Investigator

My medical-school years and part of my adult psychiatric residency were spent at Washington University in St. Louis, Missouri. During these years, I worked as a research fellow for Dr. Samuel B. Guze and was also strongly influenced by people like Eli Robins and George Winokur. Following this training, I spent two years as a military psychiatrist at a base in Southern California. Fortunately, during these two years I began collaborating on a research project with Dr. James H. Satterfield, studying children with the hyperkinetic syndrome. This work continued during my years at UCLA, first as a trainee and now as a faculty member.

From the people named above, I learned certain principles that helped me to formulate my own research model. The most important of these principles can be summarized as follows (Guze, 1972; Robins and Guze, 1970):

1. Psychiatry is a branch of medicine and thus a "medical model" is entirely appropriate for the investigation of psychiatric disorders.
2. The medical model requires a primary focus on the *condition* that a patient presents, whether this condition is called a *disease*, a disorder, an illness, a sickness, or by some other term.
3. A corollary of this focus on a patient's disorder is the notion that patients may present many types of disorders that differ in their symptomatology, natural history, etiology, pathogenesis, and response to treatment.
4. A valid classification of the various psychiatric disorders is a necessary and essential step in the advancement of the field.
5. Precisely because psychological processes and phenomena are more subjective, more difficult to measure and quantify, a "tough-minded" approach is necessary in psychiatric research. More, rather than less, should be demanded in the way of systematically obtained data.

Based on these principles, the Washington University group has developed a five-phase system for establishing diagnostic validity in psychiatric disorders of adulthood. The application of this five-phase system has led to the establishment of specific diagnostic criteria for 14 adult psychiatric disorders

(Feighner *et al.*, 1972). Working within the context of this five-phase system during my years at Washington University, I took part in follow-up studies and family studies (Guze and Cantwell 1964, 1965; Guze *et al.*, 1967, 1968), developing a research approach and learning techniques for the evaluation of patients and the collection of data that have stood me in good stead throughout my career.

The major drawback of my training at Washington University was the almost total lack of exposure to child psychiatry. Despite the presence of a well-established division of child psychiatry at Washington University, there was little study of child psychiatry in the medical school curriculum and none in the adult psychiatric residency. It was not until I actually had an opportunity to collaborate with Jim Satterfield in an ongoing investigation of children with the hyperkinetic syndrome that I felt confident that child psychiatry was the speciality that I wished to pursue. Therefore, I entered fellowship training at UCLA. During my two years as a trainee at UCLA, I learned a good deal about observing children, talking to children, and working with children and their parents in a therapeutic way. However, I received little in the way of research training and felt that no effort was made to encourage me to pursue investigative efforts. I was able to continue my investigative work with hyperkinetic children, but only in addition to and outside of my fellowship program. Therefore, I chose to spend one year as a special research fellow with Professor Michael L. Rutter at the Institute of Psychiatry, Maudsley Hospital, in London, England.

I chose this course because his published works indicated that Professor Rutter's philosophy seemed to be similar to my own, particularly his emphasis on the necessity for the development of a valid classification system for the psychiatric disorders of childhood (Rutter, 1965; Rutter *et al.*, 1969). During this year in England, I learned new techniques for evaluating children and their families, and I developed a framework for applying the principles derived from my training at Washington University to the field of child psychiatry.

Each of these separate experiences—my years in St. Louis, my years at UCLA, my investigative work with Jim Satterfield, and my year in London—added something unique to my training that I would have missed had I spent all of my training years in any one of these places. The model that I have developed for the investigation of psychiatric disorders of childhood is an amalgam of all these influences.

The model assumes that an investigator begins with an index population of children and carries out studies that can be grouped under six "stages" of investigation. These six stages are as follows:

1. *Clinical description*: A careful clinical description of the behavior problem the child presents is the starting point for investigative work in this model. Obtaining this description requires

detailed, systematic, yet flexible questioning of the parents; obtaining reliable information from the school; and performing a reliable and valid diagnostic interview with the child. It also requires taking into account the age-appropriateness of behaviors, the sex of the child, his race, his social class, and other factors that may affect the clinical picture.

2. *Physical and neurologic factors*: A systematic physical and pediatric neurological examination should be performed and the results recorded in a standardized fashion. Special attention should be given to the evaluation of neurodevelopmental abnormalities. It is important to inquire systematically about events in the history suggesting possible CNS involvement.

3. *Laboratory studies*: Included here are the results of all types of laboratory investigations: blood, urine, spinal fluid, EEG, neurophysiological, etc. Valid, reliable psychometric studies can also be considered as laboratory investigations in this context.

4. *Family studies*: Included in this stage are two different types of investigations: (a) studies of the prevalence and types of psychiatric disorders in the close relatives of a clinically defined index group of child patients; and (b) studies of the relationships and interactions occurring between the members of a family.

5. *Natural history studies:* Prospective and retrospective follow-up studies of an index population of children to trace the course and outcome of their disorder help determine whether the original group formed a homogeneous diagnostic category. These studies also provide a standard against which to judge the effectiveness of various forms of treatment.

6. *Treatment studies:* At our present level of knowledge, marked differences, such as complete recovery and marked deterioration, in response to adequate trials of the same treatment can be considered as evidence that the original group of children did not form a homogeneous group. Thus differential response to treatment can also be used to subdivide the original index population of patients.

The application of this model in clinical research will be illustrated by a description of several studies of the hyperkinetic syndrome.

This syndrome was first described by the German physician Heinrich Hoffmann over 100 years ago (Hoffmann, 1845). Since Hoffmann's original description several authors have outlined a syndrome that begins early in life, is more common in boys, and is manifested by a symptom pattern of hyperactivity, impulsivity, distractibility, and excitability (O'Malley and

Eisenberg, 1973; Stewart et al., 1966; Werry, 1968). Aggressive and antisocial behavior, specific learning problems, and emotional liability are often considered part of the syndrome. Terms like *minimal brain damage* and *minimal brain dysfunction* used to describe this syndrome reflect the assumption of many clinicians that the etiology of this condition is some type of brain damage. However, it is now quite clear that while *some* hyperkinetic children may suffer from frank brain damage, the majority do not (Werry, 1972). Similarly, *most* brain-damaged children do *not* present the hyperkinetic syndrome (Rutter et al., 1970).

It was my clinical impression, gained from several years' experience in dealing with hyperkinetic children in two different clinical settings, that many of the parents of hyperkinetic children are psychiatrically ill as adults and had been hyperkinetic themselves as children. This conclusion suggested possible familial and/or genetic etiological factors.

Psychiatric Study of the Biological Parents of Hyperkinetic Children

The first study undertaken was a comparison of the psychiatric state of the biological parents of a group of hyperkinetic children and the parents of a matched comparison group of normal children. This study was designed to answer two questions: (1) Do the parents of hyperkinetic children have higher prevalence rates for psychiatric illness? (2) Is there anything specific about the nature of their psychiatric illness?

Selection of the Probands

The first problem to be faced was the selection of the hyperkinetic probands. Present evidence suggests that the term *hyperkinetic syndrome* describes a heterogeneous group of children with a behavioral syndrome that may be due to a number of different etiologies (Cantwell, 1973; Fish, 1971). The syndrome is known to be common in children with low IQ (Pond, 1961), with frank brain damage (Ingram, 1956), and with epilepsy (Ounsted, 1955). However, the syndrome also occurs in children in whom there is no discernible evidence of a neurological or other abnormality. At the moment the question is unanswered whether the hyperkinetic syndrome occurring in children with a low IQ, evidence of frank brain damage, or epilepsy is a different condition than the hyperkinetic syndrome occurring in children with no evidence of other abnormality. However, it was felt that as homogeneous a proband group as possible would have to be selected if meaningful family data were to be obtained (Winokur et al., 1969). In the absence of a specific laboratory test for the hyperkinetic syndrome, this plan of procedure meant selecting patients by strict clinical diagnostic criteria.

In order to be accepted as a hyperkinetic proband for the family study, each child had to meet all of the following inclusion criteria: (1) white boy between five and nine years of age; (2) currently attending school; (3) normal vision and hearing; (4) full-scale IQ of 80 or above on the Wechsler Intelligence Scale for Children; (5) free of any evidence of gross neurological disease; (6) living in an intact family with both biological parents in the home; and (7) manifesting a chronic symptom pattern of hyperactivity, distractibility, excitability, and impulsivity in both the home and the school settings.

The basic work-up of each hyperkinetic proband consisted of: (1) a structured interview with the parents; (2) a diagnostic interview with the child; (3) a teacher's behavior-rating scale; and (4) a parents' behavior-rating scale.

The structured interview with the parents covered the following areas: identifying data, present behavior and symptoms, developmental history, past medical history, school history, parental home experience, and family history of psychiatric disorder.

The diagnostic interview with the child was a modified version of one described by Rutter and Graham (1968) and consisted of both unstructured and semistructured parts. The aim of this interview was to determine the *nature* and *extent* of any abnormalities of emotions, behavior, or relationships shown by the child. At the end of this interview, ratings of specific items of behavior were made exclusively on the basis of *direct observation* during the interview. Another set of items was rated on the basis of the child's *verbal account* during the interview. All items were rated on a four-point scale: "absent," "mild," "moderate," or "severe."

The teacher's behavior-rating scale consisted of 36 items of classroom behavior arranged in checklist form so that the teacher could check off whether each individual item of behavior was exhibited by the child: "not at all," "just a little," "pretty much," or "very much." These individual items were given numerical scores of 0, 1, 2, and 3, respectively. These scales have been demonstrated to distinguish validly between hyperkinetic and normal children and to have high test–retest reliability (Satterfield *et al.*, 1973). The teacher's scale also contained an open-ended invitation for the teacher to make any comments he would like about the child. If the child had been seen by the school psychologist, results of intellectual and achievement testing were requested.

The parents' behavior-rating scale consisted of 45 items arranged in checklist form similar to the teacher's scale. Both the form for teachers and the form for parents had the checklist questions phrased so that a positive answer described undesirable behavior.

The information from all sources—the interview with the parents, the interview with the child, the teacher rating scale, and the parent rating scale— was used to make a judgment as to whether the child was or was not suffering from the hyperkinetic syndrome.

Fifty hyperkinetic probands were selected in this manner, and were matched to 50 normal comparison children for age, sex, race, and social class. The comparison children were screened by a pediatrician to ensure that there were no hyperkinetic children in their families and that they came from intact families with both biological parents living in the home.

Psychiatric Examination of the Parents

A somewhat similar diagnostic procedure was used in the evaluation of the psychiatric state of the parents of both groups of children. Each parent was interviewed separately in a systematic, structured psychiatric interview such as has been described in previous publications (Guze *et al.*, 1962). The interview included a history of current and past illnesses and injuries, a description of all hospitalizations and operations, and a detailed inventory of symptoms designed to elicit the manifestations of anxiety neurosis, hysteria, obsessional neurosis, phobic neurosis, schizophrenia, affective disorder, organic brain syndrome, sociopathy, alcoholism, drug abuse, homosexuality, transsexualism, anorexia nervosa, and mental retardation. In addition, a detailed family history of psychiatric difficulties and a detailed history of the parental home experience were obtained. The interview also included sections dealing with school history, job history, marital history, military experiences, and legal difficulties. Specific inquiry was also made about suicide attempts. A mental status examination concluded the interview.

The clinical picture presented by each parent was categorized in terms of syndromes that have been systematically described and validated by the validation criteria of Robins and Guze (Feighner *et al.*, 1972). A category of "undiagnosed psychiatric illness" was reserved for those parents who were felt to be psychiatrically ill but whose symptoms did not meet the specific diagnostic criteria for any psychiatric diagnosis. In addition, an attempt was made to characterize a parent as having manifested the hyperkinetic syndrome as a child if he or she had demonstrated symptoms in both of the following areas during childhood: (1) learning difficulties, short attention span, distractibility, and poor concentration; and (2) hyperactivity, impulsivity, recklessness, and aggressive outbursts.

In addition to specific criteria's being necessary for each psychiatric diagnosis, one of the following specific criteria had to be met for an individual symptom to be scored as positive: (1) the symptom required some type of medical consultation; (2) the patient's usual routine was disrupted by the symptom; (3) the patient took some type of medication on more than one occasion to relieve the symptom; or (4) the symptom was so clinically significant that the examiner felt that it should be scored as positive even though none of the above criteria were met (e.g., a period of unexplained paralysis lasting for more than a few moments). With the exception of cases of organic brain syndrome, no symptom was scored as positive if it could be explained by a known medical illness of the patient (Feighner et al., 1972).

As part of the family history elicited from the interviewed parents, information was obtained about first-degree relatives of the person being interviewed. This information was concerned primarily with hyperkinesis, alcoholism, sociopathy, affective disorder, schizophrenia, suicide attempts, successful suicides, and psychiatric hospitalizations. The only psychiatric diagnoses attempted for a noninterviewed relative based on the family history obtained from the interviewed parents were hyperkinesis, hysteria, alcoholism, schizophrenia, affective disorder, organic brain syndrome, and sociopathy. These were global diagnoses using the same general criteria as were used for the diagnoses for the interviewed parents.

Results

The psychiatric diagnoses and other clinical data for the interviewed parents are presented in Table 1. The data indicate that most of the inter-

TABLE 1

Individual Psychiatric Diagnoses and Other Clinical Data (Interviewed Parents)

	Subjects		Controls	
	Females ($N=50$)	Males ($N=50$)	Females ($N=50$)	Males ($N=50$)
Alcoholism	4 [a]	15	0	7
Sociopathy	0	8 [a]	0	2
Hysteria	6 [b]	0	0	0
Probable hysteria	2	0	1	0
Primary affective disorder:				
Unipolar type	4	2	4	2
Bipolar type	1	0	1	0
Undiagnosed	1	2	0	1
Total psychiatrically ill	18 [c]	27 [c]	6	12
Outpatient psychiatric care	15	20	4	8
Psychiatric hospitalization	2	2	0	1
Attempted suicide	2	1	0	0

Statistical analyusis by χ^2 (subject males vs. control males and subject females vs. control females):

[a] $= p < .05$
[b] $= p < .025$
[c] $= p < .005$

TABLE 2
Individual Psychiatric Diagnoses and Other Clinical Data (Noninterviewed Relatives)[a]

	Subjects				Controls			
	Males (N= 251)		Females (N= 263)		Males (N= 256)		Females (N= 245)	
	N	%	N	%	N	%	N	%
Alcoholism	50 [d]	20	5 [b]	2	13	5	0	0
Sociopathy	30 [d]	12	0	0	1	<1	0	0
Hysteria	0	0	21 [d]	8	0	0	0	0
Primary affective disorder:								
Unipolar type	1	<1	0	0	0	0	2	<1
Bipolar type	0	0	0	0	0	0	0	0
Organic brain syndrome	1	<1	0	0	0	0	1	<1
Psychiatric hospitalization	10 [c]	1	2	<1	2	<1	0	0
Attempted suicide	1	<	1	<1	0	0	0	0

[a] Includes grandparents, aunts, and uncles of the index patients and controls.

Statistical analysis by χ^2 (subject males vs. control males and subject females vs. control females):
[b] $= p < .05$
[c] $= p < .010$
[d] $= p < .001$

viewed parents in the control group were free of any psychiatric illness, whereas nearly half of the parents of the hyperkinetic children had some psychiatric diagnosis ($p < .005$). The fathers in both groups tended to be ill more than the mothers. The specific differences between the groups were in the greater prevalence of alcoholism, sociopathy, hysteria, and probable hysteria in the parents of hyperkinetic children. Suicide attempts and psychiatric care ($p < .001$) were also more frequent in the parents of the subject group.

The undiagnosed group contained two fathers of hyperkinetic children who were heavy drinkers but who did not meet the specific criteria for alcoholism, and one mother of a hyperkinetic child and one father of a control child who had histories of episodes suggestive of mild depression but did not meet the specific criteria for a diagnosis of primary affective disorder. The clinical diagnoses and other clinical data concerning the noninterviewed relatives are summarized in Table 2. These findings from the family histories of the interviewed parents were very similar to the comparable ones from the personal interviews. In particular, they confirmed the high prevalence of alcoholism, sociopathy, and hysteria among the relatives of the hyperkinetic children.

The data concerning hyperkinetic relatives are presented in Table 3, and the psychiatric diagnoses of the interviewed, previously hyperkinetic parents are summarized in Table 4. Most striking is the finding that six of the eight fathers in the previously hyperkinetic patient group were alcoholics and that one fell into the undiagnosed group but was also a heavy drinker who did not meet the specific criteria for alcoholism. The one father in the control group who was previously hyperkinetic was also alcoholic. The two mothers in the previously hyperkinetic patient group were diagnosed as hysterical and probably hysterical as adults.

These data suggested that a significant percentage of the biological parents of hyperkinetic children are psychiatrically ill. Systematic psychiatric examination of these parents revealed high prevalence rates for alcoholism, sociopathy, and hysteria. Family history data elicited from the interviewed parents confirmed the high prevalence of alcoholism, sociopathy, and hysteria among the relatives of hyperkinetic children. In addition, it was also noted that the hyperkinetic syndrome occurred more often in the biological first- and second-degree relatives of the hyperkinetic children than in the relatives of the comparison group of normal children. Moreover, a significant number of these "grown-up" hyperkinetic children were given diagnoses of alcoholism, sociopathy, and hysteria as adults.

TABLE 3
Relatives Diagnosed as Hyperactive

	Subjects			Controls		
	Total number	Hyperactive		Total number	Hyperactive	
		N	%		N	%
Mothers	50	2	4	50	0	0.0
Fathers	50	8 [a]	16	50	1	2.0
Aunts	163	0	0	145	0	0.0
Uncles	151	15 [c]	10	156	0	0.0
First cousins:						
Women	301	6 [c]	2	282	0	0.0
Men	251	30 [a]	12	248	5	2.0
Total relatives	966	61 [d]	63	931	6	0.6

Statistical analysis by χ^2 (subject relatives vs. control relatives):
[a] $= p < .010$
[b] $= p < .001$
[c] $= p < .025$
[d] $= p < .05$

TABLE 4
Psychiatric Diagnoses of Parents Previously Hyperactive

	Subjects		Controls
	Males (N= 8)	Females (N= 2)	Males (N= 1)
Alcoholism	6	0	1
Sociopathy	1	0	0
Undiagnosed	1	0	0
Hysteria	0	1	0
Probable hysteria	0	1	0

These data suggested two hypotheses: (1) there is a familial relationship between the hyperkinetic syndrome and three adult psychiatric disorders: alcoholism, sociopathy, and hysteria; and (2) the hyperkinetic syndrome is a familial disorder that is transmitted from generation to generation. These data did not explain, however, whether the familial relationship is a genetic or an environmental one, nor whether the mechanism of transmission is genetic or environmental.

Psychiatric Study of Nonbiological Parents of Adopted Hyperkinetic Children

To test the hypothesis that the relationship between the hyperkinetic syndrome and the three adult psychiatric disorders is a genetic one and the hypothesis that the hyperkinetic syndrome is genetically transmitted, a systematic psychiatric examination of the nonbiological parents of adopted hyperkinetic children was carried out. If the nonbiological parents and their extended families were found not to show the same increased prevalence rates for hyperkinesis and other psychiatric disorders found in the biological parents and their relatives, then an argument could be made for a genetic component operating in the hyperkinetic syndrome.

Selection of the Adopted Hyperkinetic Probands

The 39 adopted hyperkinetic probands included a group referred to the author and a group garnered from the private practice of several physicians in the Southern California area who specialize in the treatment of hyperkinetic children. They met the same inclusion criteria listed above as the biological probands, with the exception of criterion number 6. The criterion substituted for the adopted group was that they have had no contact with their biological parents after one month of age and live in an intact family with both *adopting* parents living in the home. The same basic diagnostic work-up as described above was carried out with each adopted proband prior to his inclusion in the study.

Psychiatric Examination of the Adopting Parents

Each adopting parent was interviewed separately in the same structured interview as described above. The psychiatric diagnoses for the interviewed parents of all three groups of children are presented in Table 5, and the clinical diagnoses of the noninterviewed relatives are summarized in Table 6. The high prevalence rates for alcoholism, sociopathy, and hysteria found in the biological first- and second-degree relatives of hyperkinetic children were not found in the nonbiological first- and second-degree relatives of the adopted hyperkinetic children.

The data concerning hyperkinetic relatives are presented in Table 7. Of

TABLE 5
Individual Psychiatric Diagnoses of Interviewed Parents (in Percentages)

	Biological		Adopted		Control	
	Mothers (N = 50)	Fathers (N = 50)	Mothers (N = 39)	Fathers (N = 39)	Mothers (N = 50)	Fathers (N = 50)
Alcoholism	8[d]	30[c]	0	5	0	14
Sociopathy	0	16[b,d]	0	0	0	4
Hysteria	12[a,e]	0	0	0	0	0
Probable hysteria	4	0	3	0	2	0
Primary affective disorder:						
Unipolar type	8	4	5	5	8	4
Bipolar type	2	0	3	0	2	0
Undiagnosed	2	4	5	5	0	2
Total psychiatrically ill	36[a,f]	54[c,f]	15	15	12	24

[a] = $p < .05$ Biologic vs. adopted   [d] = $p < .05$ Biologic vs. controls
[b] = $p < .025$ Biologic vs. adopted   [e] = $p < .025$ Biologic vs. controls
[c] = $p < .005$ Biologic vs. adopted   [f] = $p < .005$ Biologic vs. controls

TABLE 6
Individual Psychiatric Diagnoses of Noninterviewed Relatives (in Percentages)

	Biological		Adopted		Controls	
	Females $(N = 263)$	Males $(N = 251)$	Females $(N = 176)$	Males $(N = 218)$	Females $(N = 245)$	Males $(N = 256)$
Alcoholism	2^d	$20^{c,f}$	0	3	0	5
Sociopathy	0	$12^{c,f}$	0	1	0	1
Hysteria	$8^{c,f}$	0	1	0	0	0
Primary affective disorder:						
Unipolar type	0	1	1	1	1	0
Bipolar type	0	0	0	0	0	0
Organic brain syndrome	0	1	0	0	1	0

$^a = p < .05$ Biologic vs. adopted $^d = p < .05$ Biologic vs. controls
$^b = p < .025$ Biologic vs. adopted $^e = p < .025$ Biologic vs. controls
$^c = p < .005$ Biologic vs. adopted $^f = p < .005$ Biologic vs. controls

TABLE 7
Relatives Diagnosed as Hyperactive

	Biological		Adopted		Controls	
	Total number	Percentage hyperactive	Total number	Percentage hyperactive	Total number	Percentage hyperactive
Mothers	50	4	39	0	50	0
Fathers	50	$16^{a,e}$	39	3	50	2
Aunts	163	0	98	0	145	0
Uncles	151	$15^{c,f}$	140	.7	156	0
First cousins:						
Female	307	$2^{a,e}$	211	0	282	0
Male	251	$12^{c,f}$	267	1	248	2
Total male relatives	452	$12^{c,f}$	446	1	454	1
Total relatives	966	$6.3^{c,f}$	794	.6	931	.6

$^a = p < .05$ Biologic vs. adopted $^d = p < .05$ Biologic vs. controls
$^b = p < .025$ Biologic vs. adopted $^e = p < .025$ Biologic vs. controls
$^c = p < .005$ Biologic vs. adopted $^f = p < .005$ Biologic vs. controls

note is the relatively low incidence of the hyperkinetic syndrome in the nonbiological relatives of the adopted hyperkinetic children compared to the rather high incidence of hyperkinesis in the biological male relatives (fathers, uncles, and first cousins) of the hyperkinetic children.

Comment

The familial association of alcoholism, sociopathy, and hysteria has been noted by a number of investigators (Forest, 1973; Guze *et al.*, 1962, 1967, 1968; Robins, 1966). The data from the first of the two studies described above suggest a familial relationship between these same three adult psychiatric disorders—alcoholism, sociopathy, and hysteria—and the hyperkinetic syndrome. Several environmental mechanisms could explain this association. Parental mental illness might produce psychiatric disorder in children through involvement of the child in the parents' symptoms (Anthony, 1969*b*) or through some nonspecific environmental influence (Rutter, 1966). Learning theorists might go further and argue that a parent could "teach" his child to be hyperkinetic through selective reinforcement of certain behaviors or through modeling. A direction of effect from child to parent could also be hypothesized. That is, parents demonstrate psychopathology as a result of living with a deviant child.

However, the data from the second study described above strongly suggest that the familial relationship between the hyperkinetic syndrome and alcoholism, sociopathy, and hysteria is a genetic one. The relative absence of psychopathology in the parents of the adopted hyperkinetic group does not lend support to a purely environmental explanation for this association.

The data from the second study provide even stronger evidence for the hypothesis that there is a genetic transmission of the hyperkinetic syndrome from generation to generation. Table 7 clearly shows that the hyperkinetic syndrome was found to a much greater degree in the biological first- and second-degree relatives of hyperkinetic children than in the adopted relatives. The prevalence rate for the syndrome found in the adopted relatives is no greater than that found for the relatives in the comparison group and is less than the prevalence rate for the syndrome in the general population (O'Malley and Eisenberg, 1973). These data clearly favor a genetic mechanism operating in the transmission of the syndrome.

Directions for Future Research

In the first stage (clinical description) of the six-stage model proposed above, a group of behaviorally defined hyperkinetic children were selected by strict diagnostic criteria. When the biological families were studied in the fourth stage of the model, it was discovered that the index population of hyperkinetic children could be divided into two groups: (1) those whose parents gave histories of hyperkinesis in childhood and had increased prevalence rates for psychiatric illness as adults (the "positive family history group": FH+); and (2) those whose parents were free of any such history (the "negative family history group": FH−).

Since 1968, I have been collaborating with Jim Satterfield on a longitudinal study of hyperkinetic children. This group of children has been intensively investigated from behavioral, neurological, neurophysiological, psychological, familial, and therapeutic perspectives. They form an ideal population to investigate the FH+ and FH− groups in the other four stages of the model to see if these two groups differ in ways *other* than familial patterns of illness. Relevant findings from our own work and the work of other investigators are listed below along with possible lines of investigation in each stage of the model.

Stage 2: Physical and Neurological Factors

Although the physical examination is usually completely normal in hyperkinetic children, one group of investigators (Waldrop and Goering, 1971) has reported a high incidence of minor physical anomalies, such as epicanthus, widely spaced eyes, curved fifth finger, adherent earlobes, etc. This finding is being followed up in our population to see if these anomalies occur more frequently in the FH+ group. This would add weight to the idea of a genetically determined subgroup of hyperkinetic children.

We have found that about one-half of our group of behaviorally defined hyperkinetic children have an excess of minor neurological abnormalities indicative of sensorimotor incoordination (Satterfield et al., 1973), usually described as "soft signs" in the neurological literature. This finding is consistent with those of other investigators (Millichap, 1973; Werry et al., 1972). There is some evidence that those with such signs are distinguished from those with no such neurological signs by a greater likelihood of response to stimulant drug treatment (Satterfield et al., 1973), suggesting that this may be a meaningful subgroup.

Stage 3: Laboratory Studies

Laboratory findings are generally more reliable, precise, and reproducible than are clinical descriptions. If some measure could be found that was consistently associated with the hyperkinetic syndrome, it would simplify diagnosis and permit subdivision of the syndrome. At present, there is no such measure. However, neurophysiological studies from our laboratory and the laboratories of other investigators (Calloway, 1973; Knopp *et al.*, 1972; Satterfield *et al.*, 1972, 1973) suggest that a significant number of hyperkinetic children have lower levels of basal resting physiological activation than age-matched normals. That this group of "low-arousal" hyperkinetic children is a meaningful subgroup is suggested by the fact that they show the best response to stimulant drug treatment.

Studies in our laboratory have also revealed that approximately 20 percent of behaviorally defined hyperkinetic children have a definitely abnormal EEG. Forty percent of those with abnormal EEGs have epileptiform abnormalities and 60 percent have slow-wave abnormalities. Those with abnormal EEGs show a better response to stimulant medication than those with normal EEGs (Satterfield *et al.*, 1973). Differences have also been found between the epileptiform and slow-wave groups on tests of cognitive performance and academic achievement (Satterfield *et al.*, 1974). Thus the EEG also seems to select meaningful subgroups of the index population of children.

Stage 5: Natural History Studies

Both retrospective and prospective studies indicate that antisocial behavior is prevalent in "grown-up" hyperkinetic children (Mendelson *et al.*, 1971; Menkes *et al.*, 1967; Minde *et al.*, 1971, 1972; Weiss *et al.*, 1971). The finding that 10 percent of the biological parents of hyperkinetic children gave histories suggestive of hyperkinesis in childhood and that a significant number were alcoholic and sociopathic as adults also suggests that the hyperkinetic syndrome in childhood may be a precursor to the development of antisocial behavior in later life.

The mechanism of the association between hyperkinesis in childhood and antisocial behavior in later life is unknown at present. Since the percentage of hyperkinetic children who develop significant antisocial symptomatology increases with the age of the children, it could be hypothesized that the antisocial behavior develops as a reaction to the primary symptoms that define the syndrome. Children who are unable to succeed in an academic setting, who are unable to develop satisfactory peer relationships, and who find rejection at home and at school are likely prospects to act out and rebel against the values of society.

However, the family studies described above, which suggest a genetic relationship between sociopathy and hyperkinesis, support another hypothesis: That is, that "antisocial hyperkinetic" children form an etiologically distinct subgroup of the hyperkinetic syndrome. There are other lines of evidence that tend to support such a view. Recent research on waking autonomic functions and EEG patterns in sociopathic adults suggests that many have the same underlying neurophysiological abnormality that has been discovered in hyperkinetic children: lower levels of basal resting physiological activation than age-matched normals (Dela Pena, 1973). Were this "low-arousal" group of hyperkinetic children found also to be the FH+ group, this would be even stronger evidence that "antisocial hyperkinetic" children are a meaningful subgroup. It would also suggest that in this group there may be a genetically transmitted neurophysiological abnormality that leads to hyperkinesis in childhood and sociopathy in adulthood. There is also indirect evidence that among hyperkinetic children, antisocial, aggressive behaviors may be mediated by Dopamine, while the symptoms of hyperactivity may be mediated by norepinephrine (Arnold et al., 1973). This evidence tends to indicate a possible biochemical difference between "antisocial hyperkinetic" children and those without antisocial behavior.

Since antisocial disorders in childhood are difficult to treat and so often portend serious psychiatric and social pathology in adulthood (Robins, 1966), the unraveling of the mechanism of the association between hyperkinesis and sociopathy is an important research task. Our longitudinal study of hyperkinetic children and their families should help us to answer some important questions about the mechanism of this association: Is it the hyperkinetic children with evidence of low CNS arousal who are most likely to develop antisocial behavior? Is antisocial behavior in hyperkinetic children mediated through educational retardation? Are the hyperkinetic children whose parents are antisocial more likely to develop antisocial behavior themselves? Do adopted hyperkinetic children (whose biological parents may have been antisocial) growing up with nonantisocial adopting parents, have the same incidence of sociopathy as children being raised by their antisocial biological parents?

Stage 6: Treatment Studies

The notion that there is *one* hyperkinetic child who requires only one treatment—stimulant drugs—has clearly been shown to be a "scientific myth" (Fish, 1971). However, there is general agreement in the literature that *some* hyperkinetic children do have a dramatic, positive, short-term response to dextroamphetamine or methylphenidate treatment. In our own population some 70 percent have shown a favorable response to methylphenidate, while approximately 20 percent deteriorated following stimulant treatment (Satterfield et al., 1973). We have shown that those children who are most likely to respond to stimulant treatment are neurophysiologically and neurologically different from those with a poor response (Satterfield et al., 1972, 1973). At our present level of knowledge it is reasonable to assume that these two groups of children may have different conditions with similar clinical pictures. If this is so, one could expect these two groups to differ in familial patterns of psychiatric illness.

It is apparent from the above discussion that these six stages interact with one another. New findings in one stage may lead to changes in one or more of the other stages.

For example, beginning with a population of children with the clinical picture of the hyperkinetic syndrome, we find that one group shows a positive response to stimulant medication while another group shows a negative response. When we compare these two groups—the "responders" and the "nonresponders"—we find they differ in a number of other parameters. The responders show laboratory evidence of low CNS arousal, more abnormal EEGs, and a greater number of minor abnormalities on neurological examination. Thus this group begins to look as if they have their disorder on a neurodevelopmental basis. One might then go back and take a closer look at the clinical picture of the two groups, using techniques such as cluster analysis to see if differences can be found in the behavioral picture. A family study of the two groups may yield different familial patterns of illness. Follow-up studies should reveal a different natural history for the two groups, if they do in fact have different disorders.

Or, beginning with the same population of children, we find one group with a positive family history and one with a negative family history, as in the studies described above. We might then compare the behavioral picture of the two groups or look at a variety of laboratory measures. Since the family studies offer tentative evidence for a possible genetically determined subgroup of hyperkinetic children, it is reasonable to assume that one might find metabolic, biochemical, or chromosomal differences between the FH+ and FH− groups.

Thus the continued application of this model to the same index population leads to increasingly refined diagnostic criteria, and ultimately to more homogeneous subgroups of the original index patient population. These homogeneous patient populations provide the best starting point for studies of etiology and treatment. The role of dynamic factors, family relationships, sociological factors, genetic factors, etc., in the etiology of any condition is more easily elucidated when the patient population under study is as diagnostically "pure" as possible. Likewise, response to any treatment modality, be it psychotherapy, pharmacotherapy, behavior therapy, or some other modality, is best evaluated in a homogeneous patient population.

The Clinical Investigator as Clinician

In discussing this research model in my everyday teaching activities, I have found there are certain misconceptions that arise when one mentions the term *medical model* in a psychiatric setting. I would like to outline and comment on some of these misconceptions.

Misconception 1: "The medical model implies the existence of 'organic disease entities' and therefore organic modes of treatment."

This model does not assume that psychiatric disorders are disease entities, nor does it assume any etiology *a priori* or that any one type of therapeutic intervention is better than another. It assumes only that a patient who presents *disorder A* may have a different condition than a patient who presents *disorder B*. Furthermore, if disorder A is truly different than disorder B, then it should be possible to characterize and differentiate the two conditions from each other in a number of ways.

Misconception 2: "The focus on the patient's *disorder* minimizes the importance of the patient as an *individual*."

The medical model does imply that the focus of scientific inquiry is *disorder A* or *disorder B* rather than the *patient* with disorder A or B. Important questions that must be answered include: What factors do cases of disorder A have in common? What factors do cases of disorder B have in common? What factors are present in disorder A that are not present in disorder B and *vice versa*? However, the focus of inquiry in no way diminishes the importance of the patient as an individual. Every patient is a unique human being, and this uniqueness must be taken into account in any doctor–patient relationship. This consideration is part of the art of medicine. However, excess emphasis on the unique aspects of each patient and lack of recognition of the common factors shared by patients who present a particular disorder will impede scientific study. For if patients share no common factors, then training and experience are valueless, and dealing with each new patient becomes a research project in itself.

Misconception 3: "The process of diagnosis is merely a form of labeling a child and is a meaningless exercise for clinical purposes."

Making a diagnosis does result in applying a label to the *psychiatric disorder* a child presents. It does not result in applying a label to a *child*. Just as a child may have measles at one age and pneumonia at another age, he may present one psychiatric disorder at one age and another psychiatric disorder at a different age. For clinical purposes, no one would state that it is a meaningless exercise to distinguish between measles and pneumonia. Therefore it is difficult to fathom why it should be a meaningless exercise to distinguish similarly between two psychiatric disorders.

For research purposes, a valid diagnostic classification scheme is a vital necessity (Rutter, 1965). If findings from various centers are to be compared, investigators with different theoretical backgrounds must have a "common language" in which they can communicate. A proper classification system serves this purpose. It should be recognized that a classification system emphasizes what a particular patient has in common with other patients. It is not to be confused with a diagnostic formulation—which emphasizes what a particular patient has that is different from other patients. Both are necessary and one cannot do the work of the other.

Misconception 4: "A disorder-oriented approach in investigative work is incompatible with a humanitarian approach in therapeutic work."

A tough-minded scientific approach in the study of psychiatric disorders is far from being incompatible with a warm, compassionate, humanitarian approach in therapeutic work. From my own personal standpoint I feel that the techniques of evaluating children and their families that I learned in my investigative work have made me a better clinician. From a more general standpoint it is difficult to see how *more* knowledge about a patient's *disorder* makes one *less* effective in dealing with the *patient* as an individual.

The effective use of knowledge about a child's psychiatric disorder to relieve the suffering of the child and his family caused by that disorder is humanitarian in the highest sense of the word. The psychiatrist who uses this knowledge can do so in a warm, compassionate way, or in a cold, unsympathetic way—quite independently of the model he uses in his investigative work (Guze, 1972).

Implications for Training

The end product of a fellowship training program in child psychiatry could theoretically be any one of three types of individuals: a pure artist, a pure scientist, or a scientifically minded artist. The pure artist would be able to use his clinical skills to apply currently recognized solutions, usually based on inadequate data, to currently recognized clinical situations. The pure scientist would not acquire or use clinical skills and in his pursuit of ultimate truth would not be prepared to take action on inadequate data. As a result, he would be a danger to patients, despite his ability to think scientifically. The third type—the scientifically minded artist—should be the only acceptable end product of any fellowship training program in child psychiatry. He will think scientifically and will acquire and use clinical skills effectively. He will accept the fact that at the same time as he is searching after ultimate truth in his investigative work, he must frequently take action on inadequate data in his therapeutic work.

The scientist-artist must acquire in his training years the dual personality necessary to reconcile the rather contradictory approaches of the clinician and of the scientist. As a clinician he must be a pragmatist. He must treat children and their families using information that he knows as a scientist is based on inadequate, incomplete data. Moreover, to be effective as a clinician he must deliver this treatment with therapeutic enthusiasm. Yet as a scientist he must be wary of accepting enthusiastic therapeutic claims. He must develop the capacity for critical evaluation of data and for making controlled observations in a clinical context. He must be able to appreciate and evaluate critically new knowledge as it appears. Finally, the scientist-artist must integrate what he learns in his investigative work with what he learns in clinical practice so that one contributes to the other.

If we endeavor to graduate such individuals from our training programs, both the art and the science of child psychiatry will flourish in the future. We can graduate such individuals only if we make research training an important and integrated part of our fellowship programs.

References

ANTHONY, E. J. Research as an academic function of child psychiatry. *Archives of General Psychiatry*, 1969, **12**, 385–391. (a)

ANTHONY, E. J. A clinical evaluation of children with psychotic parents. *Archives of General Psychiatry*, 1969, 177–184. (b)

ANTHONY, E. J. The state of the art and science in child psychiatry. *Archives of General Psychiatry*, 1973, **29**, 299–313.

ARNOLD, L. E., KIRILCUK, V., CORSON, S. A., & CORSON, E. O. Levaoamphetamine and dextroamphetamine: Differential effect on aggression and hyperkinesis in children and dogs. *The American Journal of Psychiatry*, 1973, **130**, 165–171.

CALLOWAY, E. Personal communication, 1973.

CANTWELL, D. P. The hyperkinetic syndrome. In M. Rutter and L. Hersov (Eds.), *Recent advances in child psychiatry*. London: Blackwell, 1973.

DELA PENA The habitually aggressive individual—progress report to the National Institute of Mental Health, 1973.

FEIGHNER, J. P., ROBINS, E., GUZE, S., WOODRUFF, R. A., WINOKUR, G., & MUNOZ, R. Diagnostic criteria for use in psychiatric research. *Archives of General Psychiatry*, 1972, **26**, 57–64.

FINCH, S. M. The current status of child psychiatry. *The American Journal of Psychiatry*, 1973, **130**, 799–801.

FISH, B. Discussion on "Research as an Academic Function of Child Psychiatry" by E. J. Anthony. *Academic Child Psychiatry* (Adams, Work & Cramer, eds) 91–95, Gainesville, Florida, 1969.

FISH, B. The "one child, one drug myth" of stimulants in hyperkinesis: Importance of diagnostic categories in evaluating treatment. *Archives of General Psychiatry*, 1971, **25**, 193–203.

FOREST, A. D. The differentiation of hysterical personality from hysterical psychopathy. *British Journal of Medical Psychology*, 1967, **40**, 65–78.

GUZE, S. B. Psychiatric disorders and the medical model. *Biological Psychiatry*, 1972, **5**, 221–224.

GUZE, S. B., & CANTWELL, D. P. The prognosis in organic brain syndromes. *American Journal of Psychiatry*, 1964, **120**, 878–881.

GUZE, S. B., & CANTWELL, D. P. Alcoholism, parole observations and criminal recidivism: A study of 116 parolees. *American Journal of Psychiatry*, 1965, **122**, 436–439.

GUZE, S. B., TUASON, V. B., GATFIELD, P. D., STEWART, M. A., & PICKEN, B. Psychiatric illness and crime with particular reference to alcoholism: A study of 223 criminals. *Journal of Nervous Mental Disorders*, 1962, **134**, 512–521.

GUZE, S. B., WOLFGRAM, E., MCKINNEY, J., & CANTWELL, D. P. Psychiatric illness in the families of convicted criminals: A study of 519 first-degree relatives. *Disorders of the Nervous System*, 1967, **28**, 651–659.

GUZE. S. B., WOLFGRAM, E., McKINNEY, J., & CANTWELL, D. P. Delinquency, social malad-justment and crime: The role of alcoholism. *Disorders of the Nervous System*, 1968, **29**, 243–289.

HOFFMANN, H. *Der Struwwelpeter: oder lustige Geschichten und drollige Bilder*. Leipzig: Insel Verlag, 1845.

INGRAM, R. A characteristic form of overactive behaviour in brain damaged children. *Journal of Mental Science*, 1956, **102**, 550–558.

KNOPP, W., ARNOLD, L. E., ANDRAS, R. Electronic pupilography: Predicting amphetamine benefit in hyperkinesis. Paper read at the 125th annual meeting of the American Psychiatric Association, Dallas, Texas, 1972.

MENDELSON, W., JOHNSON, J., & STEWART, M. A. Hyperactive children as teen-agers: A follow-up study. *Journal of Nervous Mental Disorders*, 1971, **153**, 273–279.

MENKES, M., ROWE, J., & MENKES, J. A twenty-five year follow-up study on the hyperkinetic child with minimal brain dysfunction. *Pediatrics*, 1967, **39**, 392–399.

MILLICHAP, J. G. Drugs in management of minimal brain dysfunction. *Annals of the New York Academy of Sciences: Minimal Brain Dysfunction*, 1973, 205.

MINDE, K., LEWIN, D., WEISS, G., LAVIGUEUR, H., DOUGLAS, V., & SYKES, E. The hyperactive child in elementary school: A five-year, controlled, follow-up. *Exceptional Child*, 1971, **38**, 215–221.

MINDE, K., WEISS, G., MENDELSON, M. A five-year follow-up study of 91 hyperactive school children. *Journal of the American Academy of Child Psychiatry*, 1972, **11**, 595–610.

O'MALLEY, J., & EISENBERG, L. The hyperkinetic syndrome. *Seminars in Psychiatry*, 1973, **5**, 95–103.

OUNSTED, C. The hyperkinetic syndrome in epileptic children. *Lancet*, 1955, **269**, 303–311.

POND, D. A. Psychiatric aspects of epileptic and brain-damaged children. *British Medical Journal*. Lectures I and II, 1961, 1377–1382, 1454–1457.

ROBINS, E., & GUZE, S. B. Establishment of diagnostic validity and psychiatric illness: Its application to schizophrenia. *American Journal of Psychiatry*, 1970, 983–987.

ROBINS, L. N. *Deviant children grown up*. Baltimore: Williams and Wilkins, 1966.

RUTTER, M. Classification and categorization in child psychiatry. *Journal of Child Psychology and Psychiatry*, 1965, **6**, 71–83.

RUTTER, M. *Children of sick parents: An environmental and psychiatric study*. London: Oxford University Press, 1966.

RUTTER, M., & GRAHAM, P. The reliability and validity of the psychiatric assessment of the child. I: Interview with the child. *British Journal of Psychiatry*, 1968, **114**, 563.

RUTTER, M., GRAHAM, P., & YULE, W. *A neuropsychiatric study in childhood*. Lavenham, Suffolk: The Lavenham Press Ltd, 1970.

RUTTER, M., LEBOVICI, S., EISENBERG, L., SNEZNEVSKIJ, A. V., SADOUN, R., BROOKE, D., & LIN, T. S. A tri-axial classification of mental disorders in childhood. *Journal of Child Psychology and Psychiatry*, 1969, **10**, 41–61.

SATTERFIELD, J. H., CANTWELL, D. P., LESSER, L. I., & PODOSIN, R. L. Physiological studies of the hyperkinetic child. I. *American Journal of Psychiatry*, 1972, **128**, 1418–1424.

SATTERFIELD, J. H., CANTWELL, D. P., SAUL, R. E., LESSER, L. I., & PODOSIN, R. L. Response to stimulant drug treatment in hyperactive children: Prediction from EEG and neurological findings. *Journal of Autism and Childhood Schizophrenia*, 1973, **3**, 36–48.

SATTERFIELD, J. H., SAUL, R. E., CANTWELL, D. P., & YUSIN, A. B. Intelligence, academic achievement and EEG abnormalities in hyperactive children. *American Journal of Psychiatry*, 1974, **131**, 391–395.

STEWART, M., PITTS, F., CRAIG, A., & DIERUF, A. The hyperactive child syndrome. *American Journal of Orthopsychiatry*, 1966, **36**, 861–867.

WALDROP, M. F., & GOERING, J. D. Hyperactivity and minor physical anomalies in elementary school children. *American Journal of Orthopsychiatry*, 1971, **41**, 602–607.

WEISS, G., MINDE, K., WERRY, J. S., DOUGLAS, V. I., & NEMETH, E. Studies on the hyperactive child. VIII: Five-year follow-up. *Archives of General Psychiatry*, 1971, **24**, 409–414.

WERRY, J. Studies on the hyperactive child. IV: An empirical analysis of the minimal brain dysfunction syndrome. *Archives of General Psychiatry*, 1968, **19**, 9–16.

WERRY, J. Organic factors in childhood psychopathology. In A. Quay and J. Werry (Eds.), *Psychopathological Disorders of Childhood*, 1972, 83–121.

WERRY, J. S., MINDE, K., GUZMAN, A., WEISS, G., DOGAN, K., & HOY, E. Studies on the hyperactive child. VII: Neurological status compared with neurotic and normal children. *American Journal of Orthopsychiatry*, 1972, **42**, 441–451.

WINOKUR, G., CLAYTON, P. J., & REICH, T. *Manic depressive illness.* St. Louis: The C. V. Mosby Company, 1969.

A HUMANISTIC APPROACH TO NEUROCHEMICAL RESEARCH IN CHILDREN

L. EUGENE ARNOLD

Introduction

In this discussion of the problems, philosophy, ethics, and techniques of neurochemical research with children, I will describe only enough of the research in which I have been involved to illustrate various points. Those who wish a more complete description may consult the references at the end of the chapter (Arnold *et al.*, 1972, 1973; Corson *et al.*, 1972; Knopp *et al.*, 1973).

In one sense I have not researched the topics that are the real focus of this chapter. I have done neurochemical research in children, but I have not methodically investigated the techniques, philosophy, ethics, and development of such research. Therefore most of the following discussion will necessarily be rather subjective, experiential, and even anecdotal, though hopefully also pragmatic and logical. Such an admission of subjectivity may sound strange coming from a neurochemical investigator. However, it is consistent with Popper's (1963) call for scientists to be zealous partisans who reveal their biases explicitly in order to clarify communication. It is also consistent with a humanistic willingness to learn from introspection, deduction, and empirical serendipity as well as from rigorously "scientific" experimentation. I believe that child psychiatrists, whether engaged in patient care, teaching, or research (hopefully all three), should be humanistic and that their research should tend toward the goals of Promethean humanism.

Prometheus, you may recall, was the mythical figure who stole fire from

L. EUGENE ARNOLD, Associate Professor of Psychiatry and Pediatrics, Ohio State University School of Medicine, Columbus.

81

the gods and gave it to the human race. He was punished severely for his transgressions, benefiting mankind at his own expense. The Promethean humanist, when engaged in research, attempts to "steal" the secrets of nature for the benefit of mankind even though the theft costs him personal inconvenience. He holds human values above the pure pursuit of knowledge. Although the pursuit of knowledge is itself a human value, there are times when other human values should supersede it.

Preparation and Initiation: "The Seduction"

Selecting the Research Area

This section could just as well have been titled "Being Selected by the Research Area." Besides graduate students who need a dissertation or thesis, there may be some far-sighted, well-organized individuals with hypertrophied frontal lobes who follow a logical sequence of deciding to do research and then choosing their areas of research. However, I suspect that many investigators are led into research the same way I was: I first became intrigued with the area of research and then decided to do research. As Paul Clements said in describing how he started his work, "It caught my attention."

During my child psychiatry residency, I was introduced to the problem of medicating hyperkinetic children. Among the recommended references was Laufer's 1967 article, which, like Bradley's previous article (Bradley, 1950), mentioned that some hyperkinetic children respond better to DL-amphetamine (the racemic mixture of amphetamine's optical isomers) than to pure dextroamphetamine, and *vice versa*. This "caught my attention"; I couldn't help wondering what the levoamphetamine in the racemic mixture was doing to make the difference. As I thought about it and discussed it with Paul Wender, one of my supervisors, I gradually convinced myself I had to investigate. I was at Johns Hopkins at the time, where Solomon Snyder *et al.* (1970) had just completed their laboratory work *in vitro* and in rats, suggesting that for dopaminergic actions the two isomers of amphetamine were approximately equal, though for norepinephrinergic actions dextroamphetamine was about 10 times as potent as levoamphetamine. He had naturally become curious about the differential effect of the two isomers in hyperkinetic children. It seemed natural to collaborate on a study (Arnold, Wender *et al.*, 1972). Thus I was seduced into my first neurochemical research without ever having really made a decision to "do research."

I soon discovered that neurochemical research was like eating Cracker Jacks. Each answer brings with it many new questions, which the investigator feels obliged to sink his teeth into. Any reluctance I felt toward further entanglement succumbed to my second seduction on joining the Ohio State University faculty. Irresistible overtures came through two of my new colleagues there. Walter Knopp (1973) was interested in pupillographic correlates of clinical improvement with drugs. He had already found in patients with Tourette's disease that deviant electropupillograms were normalized by the anticatecholaminergic haloperidol when it was clinically efficacious. He was eager to investigate pupillographic correlates of amphetamine-induced behavioral improvement in hyperkinetic children. This offered hope of developing a reliable predictor of currently unpredictable stimulant effect. Samuel Corson (Corson *et al.*, 1972, *Experimental Control* . . . ; Corson *et al.*, 1972, "Interactions . . .") had discovered naturally hyperkinetic, untrainable dogs that were "paradoxically" normalized by amphetamine in a manner similar to that of hyperkinetic children, and he was eager to collaborate on related experiments. The opportunity for worthwhile investigation was an irresistible temptation.

Thus both at Hopkins and at Ohio State I was seduced into research because of my clinical interest in an area in which knowledge gaps interfered with rational treatment. I feel very comfortable with this kind of clinical backing into research. Though some may disagree, I feel that at our present state of knowledge child psychiatry cannot afford specialized researchers, clinicians, and teachers. Rather, there should be child psychiatrists who are interested in various areas of expertise and who treat patients, do research, and teach within these areas of expertise. I feel that these three activities are complementary and synergistic. Research sharpens patient care and teaching; patient care helps delineate appropriate questions for research and keeps both teaching and research relevant; teaching keeps patient care updated and clarifies research questions and relevance.

Delineating the Questions

This section might just as well have been titled "Being Confronted by the Questions." Seduction into research through clinical concerns tends to open the gate for meaningful research questions to pounce on the unwary clinician-investigator and capture his imagination. Clinical concern also offers guidelines for assigning priorities among the many questions that emerge from a critical reading of the valiant scientific guesswork and sophisticated ignorance that abound in the literature. I do not mean to denigrate the contributions of those who have long labored in child psychiatric research, but rather to dramatize the ignorance that handicaps all who explore the frontiers of a discipline as new and undermanned as ours. Fortunately, clinical experience provides some rudimentary guidance, showing where we're starting from and suggesting where we would like to be and how we might get there.

1. *Where we're starting from*: In the area of medicating hyperkinetic children, some of the starting-point facts were these. Empirically, it seemed well established that the majority of hyperkinetic children respond favorably to stimulants, but there was no way of predicting confidently which children would benefit, which would be unaffected, and which would fall into the approximately 10 percent who would actually be made reversibly worse. (The contributions of Satterfield *et al.*, 1972, and Barcai, 1971, had not yet been published at that time.) Neither was there a good way of estimating ahead of time the optimum dose for a given child, which might vary 20-fold from child to child. Furthermore, some children respond best to one stimulant, others best to another. Again, there was no way of predicting which stimulant would be best for which child. Also, some children who do not respond well to a stimulant respond to a tranquilizer or diphenhydramine, again without apparent rhyme or reason. Thus there was a threefold predictive problem: qualitative, quantitative, and idiosyncratic. This situation naturally led to a trial-and-error approach to clinical management, with some children unfortunately not helped by any medication and some so plagued by side effects than an efficacious medicine had to be discontinued.

It appeared that the state of knowledge about the hyperkinetic syndrome was approximately the same as about "dropsy" before the elucidation of the different causes of edema. Once the basic knowledge was gained to allow clinical differentiation of cardiac, renal, hepatic, endocrine, and other causes of edema, the clinician could specifically treat each condition with the appropriate medication, or at least withhold inappropriate treatment. Prior to that time clinicians were forced to treat all cases of dropsy with digitalis in order to help the percentage that had cardiac dropsy. The constellation of symptoms known as the hyperkinetic syndrome or minimal brain dysfunction would seem also to be a final common pathway for a variety of disorders (genetic, biochemical, neurological, psychophysiological, psychogenic, etc.), some of which respond favorably to one medication, others to another, others to none.

2. *Where we want to get:* In such a situation, one naturally would like to have more confidence about the choice and dosage of medication, about diagnostic criteria, and about being able to find for *every* child an effective treatment without side effects.

3. *How we might get there:* The analogy with the better-understood clinical entity of edema leads to a clear delineation of promising lines of investigation. Such questions as these naturally emerge from the preceding clinical assessment: (a) What is the nature of the mechanism(s) by which stimulants help hyperkinetic children (when they help)? (b) What is the basic difference between the children who are helped by stimulants and those who are not? (c) What is the difference between children who are helped by stimulant A but not by stimulant B and the children who are helped by stimulant B? (d) What

clinical cues could be used to separate these children into diagnostic groups? (e) What laboratory tests can be used to distinguish such diagnostic groups? (f) How can we get the benefits of stimulants without the side effects? (g) Is there a stimulant not now commonly used that could benefit some of the children who are not helped by the currently used ones, thus reducing the residue of unbenefited children? (h) Is there a stimulant that could benefit without side effects those now benefited at the expense of side effects?

Other interesting questions, of lower immediate priority to a clinician, might be: (a) What are the causes of the hyperkinetic syndrome? (b) What are the mechanisms of symptom production? (c) Is the disorder inherited or acquired (or both)? (d) How? (e) What are the mechanisms of drug benefit? (f) Which aspects of the syndrome are primary and which are secondary results? Of course, the answers to these questions would be helpful in finding the answers to the high-priority questions. Therefore these questions are no less important but are merely of less immediate import to the clinician. Elucidation of the answers to such questions would be appropriately facilitated by collaboration with animal researchers and basic scientists, about which more will be said later.

Execution: "The Affair"

Pilot Studies: "The Courtship"

When a review of the literature fails to turn up reports of pertinent previous experience with the drug, a pilot study becomes advisable or even necessary in terms of feasibility, efficiency, and possibly ethics. The ethical considerations will be discussed in more detail later. Essentially, a pilot study may sometimes be necessary to establish an expectation of benefit that would justify subjecting a random sample of diagnosed subjects to the risks of a controlled study. Even where ethics do not require it, however, a pilot study may be useful in the decision whether the time and expense of a controlled study is worthwhile.

Often the subjects chosen for the pilot study are those for whom the usual treatments have been unsatisfactory for one reason or another. This choice is not only ethically desirable but also scientifically parsimonious. After all, there is not much point in finding another treatment that is effective only for those who have satisfactory results from the already-available treatment. If the new treatment can't help some cases in which the established treatment is unsatisfactory, it would be no practical loss to miss its efficacy in the cases that have a satisfactory response to the established treatment. (There still might be theoretical importance, but this would be more appropriately explored in experiments on animals, at least initially.) It was not hard to find some children with an obvious hyperkinetic syndrome who either had not responded satisfactorily to the usual stimulants or else had such annoying side effects that either the child or the parents regularly complained. We first tried levoamphetamine in these cases.

As we found rather promising results with these children, we began relaxing our criteria for how unsatisfactory the usual stimulants had to be in order to qualify the child for a trial of levoamphetamine. Toward the end of the pilot period, we felt justified in trying levoamphetamine on a couple of children whose response to dextroamphetamine was acceptable, merely to see if we could get even better results with levoamphetamine. The precedent for this was Laufer's (1967) clinical advice to try both dextroamphetamine and racemic amphetamine in each child to see which worked better. Thus within the pilot study there was a progression from a more cautious, stringent selection of subjects toward a more liberal use of therapeutic trials as confidence increased in the generalizability of the evidence of efficacy. The whole pilot study, in turn, was one stage in a progression toward a more generalizable confidence in the efficacy, a progression in which widespread clinical experience would hopefully be the final stage and in which controlled studies would be the penultimate stages.

Controlled Studies

The results of an uncontrolled/pilot study are subject to distortion by the selection of the patients, statistical regression, history, the Hawthorne or placebo effect, the enthusiasm of the investigator, and other influences. Therefore enough uncertainty usually remains to require controlled studies before routine clinical use is recommended. The word *control* implies comparison subjects without the treatment as a standard against which the effect in the treated subjects can be measured. For such a comparison to be valid the controls must be comparable to the treated subjects (except for treatment).

The comparability of controls to treated subjects is usually attained in one of three basic ways. (1) Individual subjects within the sample are randomly assigned to either the treatment or the control group on the assumption that random chance (with a large enough sample) will largely even out the net result of variations due to individual differences. (2) A more refined approach is the use of "matched controls," in which the subjects within the sample are paired according to the variables believed to be important and then one member of each pair is randomly assigned to the control group, the other to the treatment group. This approach seems to ensure more comparability of the two groups, but at the expense of considerable work in matching the pairs and at the risk of matching for the wrong variables, since the number of variables precludes matching for all. (3) In the crossover design each subject is used as his own control, thus supplying nearly identical groups with high comparability. History may still impair the comparability of the same-person controls, as for instance when a child's parents separate during one of the drug conditions, but we might hope that the effects of such events even themselves out as well as they do in a randomly assigned noncrossover design. Furthermore, the crossover design effectively multiplies the number of subjects in the sample because each subject can be counted under each drug condition, thus facilitating more conclusive results with a small sample. Therefore this design is often preferred where it is feasible, and we chose it for the levoamphetamine study.

As attractive as the crossover design sounds, however, it includes several pitfalls, including these. The first concerns the possible effects of the sequence of drug conditions. These are somewhat minimized by a Latin square design, which evens out the number of times each drug follows each other drug in the sequence and the number of times each drug is first, second, third, etc. Thus in the levoamphetamine studies one-sixth of the patients were randomly assigned to each of these six sequences of placebo (P), dextroamphetamine (D), and levoamphetamine (L): P-D-L, P-L-D, D-P-L, D-L-P, L-P-D, L-D-P. Another problem with the crossover design is more restricting. It is the possibility of the drug effect's being carried over from one condition through the following condition. For this reason the crossover is not a good design for testing a curative drug (e.g., an antibiotic), a drug whose test of efficacy is some definitive end point (e.g., the return of a child to school in imipramine treatment of school phobia,—Gittelman-Klein and Klein, 1971), or a drug whose discontinuance results only in delayed deterioration (e.g., phenothiazines in schizophrenia). Of course, in the latter case a study could be carried out if the drug conditions were continued long enough, but this solution introduces problems with study length and sample retention. Therefore, the crossover design is feasible mainly for drugs that suppress chronic symptoms in an immediately effective and immediately reversible manner (e.g., stimulant treatment of the hyperkinetic syndrome).

Even for stimulant treatment of hyperkinetic children there is some question about the appropriateness of the crossover design. I cannot dismiss lightly the report of some parents and teachers that during placebo condition following an efficacious active drug condition the child seems worse than before the drug was used. This effect might be explained by postulating that he just seems worse because during the active drug condition they have forgotten how bad he was before. However, it could also be a withdrawal-precipitated exacerbation of symptoms analogous to the precipitation of seizures in a seizure-prone but previously seizure-free patient by the sudden withdrawal of anticonvulsants. In such a case, the "control" (placebo) condition would really be a "drug withdrawal" condition and would not fairly reflect how well an untreated group could do. In addition to validity problems, this crossover design also raises ethical objections, which I believe are adequately answered, but which we do not have the space to explore here. This possible negative placebo bias may be partly counterbalanced by a phenomenon I have suspected in a few cases: an occasional "curative" effect of stimulants, rather than merely a reversible symptom-suppressing effect. Though space does not permit elucidating various hypothetical explanations of this suspicion, I should state that I am not referring here to the more common placebo breakup of vicious cycles (Arnold, 1973). If such a curative phenomenon does exist, it would introduce a bias in favor of the placebo when the placebo follows an active stimulant.

Placebo

Merely having a comparable control group helps correct for most variables that would bias the results. However, merely to leave the controls untreated (or to include a period of nontreatment in a crossover design) would fail to correct for one of the most interesting problems with which a drug investigator must deal. The placebo effect can sometimes work miracles of improvement on the mere basis of expectation of improvement, a positive self-fulfilling prophecy probably operating via psychosocial and psychobiological deviation-amplifying feedback (Arnold, 1973; Wender, 1968). Most drugs have both pharmacological efficacy and placebo efficacy. The latter is recognized as a valuable therapeutic tool by skilled medicine men of all persuasions, cultures, societies, civilizations, and ages and should be routinely employed to give the patient the full benefit of the drug. The placebo effect is a tribute to the importance of someone's caring enough to do something. However, it also complicates scientific assessment of new treatments. Fortunately, in drug research it can often be largely corrected for if a placebo, a matched dosage form containing no active ingredients, is given to the patient in the control condition. Under blindfold conditions this placebo will usually elicit the same placebo efficacy as the active drug, especially if the physician as well as the patient is ignorant of which is the active drug ("double blind"). Of course, the placebo itself is in a sense a treatment (a psychosocial treatment concretized into a pill), since it undoubtedly has an efficacy. However, the administration of a placebo does not compromise the value of the control group, because most studies are interested only in defining what specific pharmacological efficacy an active drug has beyond the placebo efficacy common to all drugs.

Unfortunately, placebo controls may spring leaks in the "double blindness." Any drug that has obvious and consistent side effects, such as anorexia in the case of stimulants, cannot help but tip off the experienced clinician as to which is an active drug. Therefore, Weiss *et al.* (1971) have questioned the value of the placebo in stimulant studies. From my own experience I sympathize with their skepticism. Nevertheless, I believe that such a questionable placebo control is better than a baldly untreated control, as long as we consider these reservations in interpreting the results.

Furthermore, blindness may not be as essential for eliciting the placebo effect as is generally believed. Park and his associates (1965) reported a significant placebo benefit even when patients were apprised that they were taking merely a sugar pill. At least it seems generally accepted that the physician's blindness is not necessary for some placebo effect to occur. Undoubtedly the effect with only the patient (and parent) blindfolded is not the same as with the physician also blindfolded. However, I suggest that the difference will be minimal if the physician firmly believes in placebo efficacy, as I do. Therefore, I am considering for future comparison studies the possibility of an initial short placebo "washout" as suggested by Jones and Ainslie (1966), rather than inclusion of the placebo in the double-blind crossover comparison. Only the child, the parents, and the teacher would be blindfolded during the placebo condition. Those children who maintain a good response to the placebo could be spared the necessity of the trial of an active drug. Though history in this design makes the placebo condition poorly comparable to the active drug condition, it could be justified where the drugs' comparable efficacy, rather than their pharmacological efficacy, is in question. In such circumstances the placebo condition is not needed to establish the drugs' efficacy by comparison. Its main value is to wash out some (hopefully most) of the confusing placebo effect so that the active drug conditions more accurately reflect comparative pharmacological efficacies. Thus the placebo washout with the frank knowledge of the physician, in addition to its ethical appeal, would seem more scientifically valid and straightforward than a leaky attempt at double blindness.

Selection of Samples and Validity of Generalizations

We have already noted that controlled studies are the penultimate stages in a progression of confidence in generalizations about the efficacies of drugs, beginning with the first patient treated in a pilot study. Ideally, to make the results generalizable the controlled study sample should be randomly drawn from the whole population of the designated diagnostic group. Obviously, no one clinic or practitioner could accomplish this, if for no other reason than geography. A partial answer has been multiclinic studies, pooling data from many clinics and practitioners in different geographical areas treating different socioeconomic groups. Even with this effort no study obtains a perfectly representative sample. Another approach is to select classical subjects who epitomize the clinical picture in question, thus getting a "pure culture" that more likely represents the most universal aspects of the diagnostic grouping. The pitfall of this approach is that unless the investigator screens the pure culture by the right criteria, he may actually end up skewing his sample. Therefore, this approach confidently enhances generalizability only when the diagnostic category has clearly defined, generally agreed-upon criteria. It is my feeling that minimal brain dysfunction does not qualify in this way.

Though no study enjoys a perfectly representative sample, most controlled studies strive for this goal in order to enhance generalizability. Such studies are intended as definitive. However, there is another type of controlled study that does not pretend to be definitive but rather carves a niche for itself between the pilot study and the definitive controlled study. The choice of the sample for this type of study disregards any attempt at randomness or representativeness but rather tries to prove that *some* swans are black, not necessarily trying to determine what percentage are black. This was the goal of the first levoamphetamine study. It was set up to determine if *any* hyperkinetic children had a good clinical result from levoamphetamine. No attempt was made to obtain a random sample. Some children from the original pilot study were included, as well as some children freshly referred because dextroamphetamine and methylphenidate had been unsatisfactory for them. Interestingly, though, the child from the pilot study who had the best result from levoamphetamine could not be included because he and his mother were so happy with the levoamphetamine that they would not agree to any further tinkering with the medication.

After this intermediate controlled study demonstrated levoamphetamine's efficacy on this selected sample, it became advisable to design a more definitive study with a larger, randomly collected sample. This "replication" is just now being completed. We built in the randomness by taking 30 consecutive children who were diagnosed as hyperkinetic and for whom a trial of stimulants was anticipated. My desire was to have a sample representative of the run-of-the-mill cases apt to be diagnosed and treated in the usual course of clinical practice. Even with these efforts, of course, the sample was skewed by the variables that influence whether a given hyperkinetic child is referred to a child psychiatry clinic or to a pediatric clinic or private practitioner.

Retaining the Sample

Eliciting and maintaining the cooperation of the subjects undoubtedly account for a significant proportion of the blood, sweat, and tears invested by any clinical investigator. The problem is particularly compounded in neurochemical research with children, for which the cooperation of several parties must be maintained. The parents' cooperation is at least as important as the child's, and parents must sometimes be supported in withstanding the criticism of a grandparent or a neighbor for having their child "drugged." The teacher's cooperation, at least to the extent of filling out rating forms conscientiously, is indispensable. Family therapy is sometimes necessary not only for the good of the patient, but also to make the drug study possible. Nursing the case through the difficult placebo days may tax all of the clinician's psychiatric skills. Sometimes the placebo condition (or another drug condition) has to be prematurely terminated, and clinical, ethical judgment must be exercised in determining how long an apparently unsatisfactory drug condition should be allowed to continue. I usually ask myself in such circumstances, "If this were my child, how much longer would I want to continue, knowing that this might be a placebo?"

The retention of samples is well worth the effort invested, for every patient lost introduces bias. It is better to expend the same energy in retaining one subject than to add two new subjects. Therefore one should not bite off more than he can chew in deciding on the size of the sample.

Stipends for the teacher for filling out the rating form and reimbursement for transportation for parents on a tight budget can offer these people some assurance that the investigator does not wish to impose on them. However, the best way to retain the sample is to be a good clinician, developing rapport from the beginning with the patient, his parents, and his teacher in an honest, concerned way. The investigator must believe that what he is doing is good for the individual child as well as for science. Stringer (1959) has reported on the therapeutic value of research. I personally feel that my research patients get more exact care than my others as a result of the research itself. In fact, I have occasionally set up a poor man's placebo comparison for nonresearch patients by giving them some leftover matched dosage forms and explaining how we want to determine in a blind fashion whether the medicine is really doing the child any good so that we will not need to continue it unless it is really doing something for him. Though such a single, intrasubject comparison is inconclusive for a variety of reasons (Chasson, 1967; Mainland, 1964), it can be clinically helpful for (1) cases in which it is not clear whether the child is really benefiting pharmacologically from the drug or whether it is all placebo effect; (2) cases in which the child resists taking the medicine; or (3) cases in which the parents have some scruples about "drugging" the child.

Measuring Instruments

Measurements of drug effect must be relevant to the problem being treated and not too tedious to do periodically. Since the main problem for most hyperkinetic children is in school, ratings by teachers are essential. Additional ratings seem advisable from the parents. Ideally, the ratings should include side effects.

Although "objective" behavior-rating forms, such as the ones reported by Conners (1969) and Davids (1971), boast the advantages of more complete coverage and the measurement of comparable parameters from subject to subject, they risk diluting a few important symptoms with other items irrelevant for a given child. Therefore, in addition to objective rating scales, we developed a system for rating target symptoms (Arnold, Wender et al., 1972) named by the parents in response to the question "What are the things about your child you are most worried about?" The parent quantified these symptoms at each visit, e.g., "temper tantrum three times a day," or "can sit still for only five minutes at a time." Thus changes in target symptoms from one drug condition to another could later be rated by independent, "blind" raters. Since the type and design of rating instruments will determine the later possibilities for various ways of handling data, the instruments should be chosen with this consideration in mind. In fact, it is not too early for statistical consultation at the point of choosing the rating method.

Prediction Studies

The discussion thus far has assumed that the research objective is the evaluation of a drug's efficacy, toxicity, and side effects. However, an equally important question for the Promethean clinician is the predictability of such effects, especially efficacy. Prediction studies differ somewhat in design from studies of drugs' effects. In both cases, of course, the effect of the drug must be measured or rated. However, in a study of drug effect, the measured drug effect is a dependent variable, whereas in a prediction study the measured drug effect is accepted as an independent variable with which the dependent variable of predicted drug effect is compared (to find the validity of a prediction technique). This difference has implications for what kind of controls are built into the study.

One example was our attempt (Knopp et al., 1973, "Predicting . . .") to develop electropupillography (EPG) as a physiological predictor of stimulant benefit in hyperkinetic children. Walter Knopp studied EPG tracings of light reactivity before and a half hour after a test dose of D-amphetamine in children who had been diagnosed and scheduled for a therapeutic trial of amphetamine. With no clinical knowledge of the patients, he "blindly" predicted on the basis of a previously determined hypothesis what the behavioral response would be on chronic administration of the drug. Conversely, with no knowledge of the EPG data, I (the clinician) rated behavioral effect and collected parents' ratings of effect. Thus the blindfold part of this study was not in regard to the drug condition but in regard to the EPG predictive condition for the clinician and the patients and in regard to chronic drug effect for the predictor. There was no need for anyone to be "blind" of the drug used. We were not studying whether or to what extent the drug was efficacious but how its efficacy correlated with prediction. By the same token, a placebo did not seem necessary. Of course, for some prediction studies a placebo control might be necessary, especially if the placebo response is what's being predicted. Even in this study, it might be argued that the placebo effect could produce changes both in the measured physiological predictor and in subsequent behavior. This interesting theoretical possibility is being checked in subsequent "piggyback" prediction studies attached to placebo-controlled studies of drug effects. Nevertheless, for this first study a placebo control did not seem warranted.

Thus the particular needs of a given study should determine what controls are included. Attempting to include every conceivable control regardless of need would produce an unnecessarily unwieldy design. Selection is necessary, and such selection evolves from a clear understanding of the focus of study, the variables involved, and their effect on each other.

Analysis of Results: "The Gossip"

A controlled study is only half completed when the patients have been successfully nursed through the study. Appropriate analysis and interpretation of the data is indispensable if the study is to contribute anything worthwhile, either humanistically or scientifically. There are four main aspects to the appropriate handling of data: (1) common-sense organization of the data; (2) sound statistical analysis; (3) meaningful interpretation of the statistical results; and (4) nonstatistical heurism.

For the statistical testing it is helpful to have consultation from a mathematician or statistician. However, the investigator himself should be acquainted with such things as what can be done with statistical tests, what types of tests are suitable for what types of data, and what is the minimum meaningful size of a sample for various tests. This knowledge is necessary not only for intelligent collaboration with the statistical consultant but also for planning the study for most efficient handling of data and the clearest results. Two useful books for novices are Chasson (1967) and Mainland (1964).

In the nonstatistical heuristic scrutiny of the data, patterns can sometimes be found that will give clues to more basic explanations and hypotheses for further investigation. For example, in the first levoamphetamine study it was not clear from the pooled data whether each child showed a comparable response to the two isomers, with each child doing a shade better with dextroamphetamine, or whether some children may actually have done better with levoamphetamine but were outnumbered and diluted by a larger number of children who did well only with dextroamphetamine. Eyeballing of the data revealed that in fact two of the children appeared to show a better response to levoamphetamine, while the majority of children appeared to show a better response to dextroamphetamine, and a few seemed to show comparable responses. These data suggested that the two drugs worked differently in different children by different mechanisms, thus warranting further study, with attempts to ferret out the distinguishing criteria in the children who showed a better response to levoamphetamine. We are just completing a replication study designed to focus on the distinguishing characteristics.

Interpretation of the results requires some knowledge of the limitations of the statistical tests used and the limitations of the sample in size and representativeness, a humanistic concern for clinical needs, and a pragmatic grasp of clinical possibilities. (A serendipitous intuition for the generation of hypotheses is also helpful but not necessary.) From the first controlled study of levoamphetamine we concluded only that levoamphetamine is useful for treatment of *some* hyperkinetic children (bearing in mind our mode of sample selection and our original "some swans are black" goal) and cautioned that though statistical tests did not show a difference between the efficacy of the two isomers, there might be a real difference between the two that was not detected statistically because of the small size of the sample. We stated that levoamphetamine did not seem to be the first drug of choice but that it might be useful in some children for whom dextroamphetamine was unsatisfactory.

Ethics of Neurochemical Research in Children: "The Morality"

Aside from the more irrational sentiments aroused in some laymen by the idea of "experimenting with drugs on children," there are some realistic ethical problems that must be considered. These might be roughly divided under the headings of (1) *primum non nocere* ("first, do not harm") and (2) *secundum bona non retinere* ("second, do not withhold good treatment"). The first is a well-known clinical axiom; the second is an unknown clinical axiom that I just made up to express the implicit premise of a common quandary. Both have implications for (3) informed consent and for (4) collaboration with basic scientists, including animal researchers.

Before exploring these four areas of ethical concern, we should note that prediction studies can be different from drug effect studies in ethics as well as in design and controls. For example, the electropupillographic study described under "Prediction Studies" did not require any alteration in the usual clinical management. Therefore the only ethical consideration would be if the predictive testing carried a risk, either physical (e.g., venipuncture) or emotional (e.g., leaving the child with a sense of failure). In this case it did not. If it did, the potential benefit to the individual subject would, of course, have to balance the possible pain or harm before such a study could be done on children. For the most part, however, the ethics of prediction studies seem less formidable than those of drug effect studies. Therefore the latter will be the main focus of the following discussion.

Primum Non Nocere

The axiom "first, do not harm" most obviously applies to clinical investigations of (1) new, untried drugs or of (2) old drugs for new uses, rather than of (3) old drugs for the same use.

In the case of an entirely new drug never before used on children, extensive animal experimentation (and possibly studies in adults) would, of course, be a prerequisite for an ethical clinical judgment according to the paradigm explained by Wender (1971). The clinician-investigator would multiply the probability of a benefit by its estimated importance and weigh this "product" against the probability of an untoward reaction times its importance, just as a gambler might figure the odds by multiplying a small chance times a large payoff and weighing it against a large risk of a small loss. If the estimated product for the anticipated benefit is smaller than for the anticipated risk, I do not see how the clinician-investigator could ethically proceed with such a study on children. On the other hand, if the anticipated-benefit product outweighed the anticipated-risk product, the investigator could ethically proceed, providing he made sure that consent was truly informed. Since my investigations were with amphetamine, which had been prescribed for decades for children, I did not have to be concerned with this first category.

An example of the second category, applying an old drug to a new use, might be to try penicillin for hyperactivity on the hypothesis that the behavior disorder is a toxic effect of a subclinical streptococcal infection. (To the best of my knowledge no such hypothesis has yet been proposed, but with the current trend toward novel explanations it should only be a matter of time.) In such a case, of course, preliminary animal studies would be advisable. In any event the clinician-investigator would have to weigh the possible risks (e.g., allergic reactions to the penicillin, development of drug-resistant bacterial strains) against the possibility of benefits, following the clinical probability paradigm explained above. If he decides to proceed, he must, of course, make sure consent is truly informed. A fragile case might be made that the study of amphetamine should be classed under this category of a new use for an old drug. Indeed, to the best of my knowledge at that time, it had not previously been used in pure form for the treatment of hyperkinetic children. However, as part of the racemic mixture of amphetamine's two optical isomers, it had been used for decades for the treatment of such children. Conceivably, of course, levoamphetamine in pure form might be an exceedingly dangerous drug for hyperkinetic children, being rendered harmless in the racemic mixture because dextroamphetamine acts as an antidote. However, such a possibility flies in the face of all that is known about much-studied amphetamine. For example, such a hypothesis would have to assume that levoamphetamine is more toxic than dextroamphetamine in children, even though we have evidence from studies in adult humans and in animals that levoamphetamine is not any more toxic than dextroamphetamine. It would take a more obsessive individual than I to doubt that in regard to risk, the study of levoamphetamine in hyperkinetic children falls logically into the third category.

The third category, studying the use of an old drug for a condition in which it had previously been used, logically encompassed the risk of using levoamphetamine on hyperkinetic children, even though levoamphetamine had not been specifically prescribed for that indication. There was no reason to believe that the children to be studied would be any different from the children who had in previous years been medicated with levoamphetamine as part of the racemic mixture. Therefore this isomer had already been used on the very type of patient in which it was to be studied, and if there were special dangers of its use on such patients, they should have come to attention already. Therefore, I concluded that I did not have to worry about the *primum non nocere* axiom nor give any more attention to informed consent in this regard than the ordinary clinician in the course of routinely treating such children (for what I consider routine information, see Arnold, 1973). However, in regard to the second axiom *secundum bona non retinere*, there was a problem.

Secundum Bona Non Retinere

The axiom "second, do not withhold good treatment" has long been an ethical problem for anyone who does controlled studies with people. A common objection, for instance, to a controlled study of some educational intervention, such as a new textbook or teaching method, is that if there is a good chance of the intervention's helping the children, it is not right to deprive the control group of that intervention. The same sort of criticism has been leveled at double-blind placebo-controlled studies of drugs, especially of the non-crossover variety. One mother of a neurologically handicapped child wrote this about controlled studies:

> As they relate to our children I believe that their use may actually be sometimes immoral. Every time you do one using our children, where laboratory animals might be used just as well, you have the potential of denying the children receiving the placebo and the children in the control group something which might be of great benefit to them. Remember, you are using the days, months, and sometimes even years of our children's lives that can be ill afforded when they have so many strikes against them to begin with. They will not have those days and weeks and months to live over again when you finally satisfy yourselves with your little graphs and charts.

It might be tempting to dismiss such complaints as naïve, unscientific, or even antiscientific. Certainly they are antiscien*tistic* in the sense of criticizing a religious devotion to scientific techniques, but I do not believe they are antiscientific. On the contrary, they expose a problem that a Promethean humanist must consider in scientific work with children. However, a more thorough knowledge of the complexities involved makes the elimination of control groups humanistically as well as scientifically questionable in certain circumstances.

The objections to withholding the treatment from control groups implicitly ignore the possibility that the intervention or treatment may carry some risk of harm as well as chance of benefit. Even in the area of educational interventions, there is some risk of harm if "harm" can encompass the substitution of a lesser benefit for a previously available one. The new textbook or teaching technique may be less effective than the previously established one, so that the experimental group, though benefiting to some extent by the new book or technique, does not benefit as much as it would have by the old book or technique. In drug research, we do not even have to stretch the definition of harm in this way, especially when investigating drugs whose use on children is already publicly decried by some people. In such circumstances the axiom *primum non nocere* demands a controlled study for public health reasons, and, of course, it takes precedence over *secundum bona non retinere*. Furthermore, the placebo effect can make an otherwise useless treatment appear efficacious. Without adequate controls for the placebo effect, the erroneous conclusions may be drawn that the treatment should be continued for the child in question and should be initiated for other children, possibly at some risk of harm, certainly at unnecessary expense. It should not be hard to obtain a consensus that if a drug is useless for a given disorder, it should not be taken for that disorder. In this regard the double-blind placebo study can help protect the population at large and even to some extent the individual child, especially if a crossover design is feasible. In such cases, controlled studies are in the best tradition of Promethean humanism if they meet the following conditions.

1. There should be indications from pilot studies, animal work, or previous clinical research, that the drug being studied may offer some advantage over already-established treatment, at least in some individuals.

2. Implied in the first condition is this corollary: the subjects should not be deprived of far more certain, established therapies to undergo a controlled study of a treatment that is not believed to have comparable efficacy, assuming that the risks of the old and new treatments are comparable. This at first seemed an obstacle to studying levoamphetamine. It might be argued that since dextroamphetamine (and other stimulants) significantly benefited two-thirds of hyperkinetic children, no child should be deprived of this effective treatment by being put in a study of a drug with unknown efficacy. This would have been

an insurmountable obstacle if dextroamphetamine and the other stimulants had been 100 percent satisfactory (but then there would have been no need to investigate other drugs anyway). As it was, the children who had already tried dextroamphetamine (or another stimulant) either without sufficient benefit or with intolerable side effects provided an opportunity for ethical pilot trials of levoamphetamine. The results from the pilot study then provided enough expectation of efficacy to justify a controlled study.

3. The benefit of the treatment has to be in some doubt, or at least the harmfulness of delaying a control patient's treatment long enough for the study has to be in doubt. In the presence of undoubted significant efficacy dependent on immediate treatment, the principle of *secundum bona non retinere* would preclude a controlled study, which would not be needed anyway. An example would be a treatment that results in survival for some patients who have a disease that previously had been universally fatal. To the best of my knowledge there has been no controlled study of the efficacy of appendectomy in acute unperforated appendicitis. From our present perspective such a study would appear unethical as well as unnecessary. In one sense the "control" was provided by history; before appendectomies, appendicitis was routinely fatal; with appendectomy, appendicitis is routinely survived. Of course it might be argued that something about the disease just happened to change at the same time that the operation was developed and that appendicitis would have become a nonfatal disease even without appendectomies. However, the answer for this argument is provided by accidental controls: cases that do not get medical help are still routinely fatal. The efficacy of no stimulant could approach this kind of certainty or dependence on immediate institution of treatment. Therefore any study of stimulants in hyperkinetic children would meet condition 3.

4. The principle of *primum non nocere* must be complied with as explained above, including the balancing of the risk-of-harm product against the chance-of-benefit product.

Informed Consent

Informed consent in neurochemical research with children presents several problems. First, informed consent of whom? Legally the parent (or guardian) is the one who must be informed and whose consent must be obtained for research on a minor. This legal stance is based on the assumption that the parent (1) is dedicated to the welfare of the child and (2) because of his maturity is better able to judge what is best for the child than the child himself is. Both of these assumptions are open to question in certain cases. The latter seems of questionable validity when the minor is mentally and emotionally mature and seems quite able to judge for himself what is best.

Therefore I routinely, "just to be safe," direct my explanations to the child in the presence of eavesdropping parents and obtain a verbal consent from the child before obtaining written consent from the parents.

The first assumption, that the parent is dedicated to the welfare of the child, is fortunately valid most of the time. However, troubled, troubling children can sometimes exasperate parents to a point of desperation where they may become more concerned about finding relief for themselves than about the welfare of the child. They may even take the attitude "Do whatever you want with him; it'll serve him right to be a guinea pig. If there's a slipup, sacrificing his life for medical science will have been the only decent thing he ever did with it." In these rare circumstances I question whether the parent is capable of giving a valid consent for the child. The few times I have been faced with this situation I felt obligated to assume mentally the role *in loco parentis* and ask myself, "If this were my child, would I want him in the study?" Incidentally, this is not a bad question for the investigator to ask himself about every child.

Another problem with informed consent in placebo-controlled studies is whether or not to tell the patient and his parents that one of the drug conditions will be a placebo. Of course, in a design that will require the patient to take only a placebo for a year even though it seems ineffective, disclosure seems obligatory. However, in crossover studies, in which the placebo period constitutes only a nuisance of short duration and in which every patient is also exposed to the active drugs, the issue does not seem as clear, and other considerations might take precedence over "full" disclosure. Having tried both disclosure and nondisclosure of the inclusion of placebos, I am not sure whether in such circumstances it makes much difference, either ethically or scientifically.

In the replication study we are just completing, I did not voluntarily disclose the placebo possibility ahead of time. I justified the nondisclosure by this rationale:

> Some hyperkinetic children have a good response to placebos, so that a placebo is not really "nontreatment" for hyperkinetic children. If they are to have the best chance of benefiting from this safest of all "drugs," thereby avoiding unnecessary medication with an active drug, they and their parents should not be apprised of the placebo possibility beforehand, because the placebo effect depends on strong expectations of benefit (Arnold, 1973). From my previous experience with placebo disclosure, I had no reason to suspect that knowledge of the placebo inclusion would alter anyone's decision about consent for a crossover comparison of this short duration.

I am not convinced there has been any advantage, scientific or otherwise, to proceeding this way. Many people guessed or assumed anyway that a placebo was going to be used. On the other hand, some patients and their parents in the first study forgot about the placebo idea even after being told. When a placebo was administered, a few explained their deterioration by saying that the medicine was making them worse; they perceived the placebo as a toxic drug rather than the "sugar pill" they had been told about beforehand. The net result in my impression is that roughly the same proportion of people seem to end up being aware of the placebo possibility during the actual drug trial, whether they have been told beforehand or not. Furthermore, there is some evidence that preliminary disclosure of even placebo-only treatment does not impair the placebo benefit (Park and Covi, 1965). Therefore, in any future studies I would probably disclose the placebo possibility before consent, presenting it in the terms described under "Retaining the Sample."

The Place of Animal Research

Mention of animal research may seem inappropriate in a discussion of neurochemical research in children, but actually it is very pertinent, as implied by comments throughout the ethical discussion. The current push for practical, "clinical" research as contrasted with "basic" research has tended to downgrade the importance of studies of animals. Of course, research on animals can never completely substitute for research on humans; there are limitations on the extrapolation to humans of findings on animals. However, I agree with the critical mother who said of drug studies, "Every time you do one using our children, where laboratory animals might be used just as well, [you do our children a disservice]." Obviously, certain stages of work on drugs can be done only with human subjects, just as other stages can ethically be done only with animals. However, some areas of investigation can be approached by experimentation on either humans or animals. In such circumstances it would seem ethically desirable to do as much of the work on animals as possible. As Samuel Corson has said, "You shouldn't be experimenting on children; we should first experiment on dogs (or other animal models)." This is one reason I support the expansion of work on animal models of childhood psychopathology. The other reason is that such work is scientifically and temporally parsimonious, thus hastening the time for more definitive, clinically applicable answers to the types of questions I posed in "Delineating the Questions." Animal experiments can be designed and controlled in ways either not feasible or not ethical with children.

Ideally, the work on animals should be under the direction of a full-time scientist who is receptive to clinical input and collaborates freely with clinicians but has a devotion to laboratory detail that the clinical investigator does not have time for. It is also helpful for the director and technicians in the work on animals to feel a fondness for the animals comparable to that which parents naturally feel for their children. This helps keep the animal model relevant to children.

The results of studies of animals, though, must be interpreted in light of their limitations. For example, if an animal is made hyperkinetic experimentally, the mechanism by which it was experimentally rendered hyperkinetic is not necessarily the same as that by which children are naturally rendered hyperkinetic. Even with animals that naturally show the symptoms in question, such as Corson's hyperkinetic dogs (Corson *et al.*, 1972a,b), there remains some question about extrapolation to children. The same limitations apply to responses to treatment. In my opinion, the most productive use of animal experimentation is in close collaboration with clinical investigations, so that (1) ideas derived from clinical work can be checked out efficiently in the animal model to see if they hold up under closer scrutiny and if they are worth further clinical investigation, and (2) findings from the work on animals can enjoy immediate trial applications to human subjects, with feedback for the design and direction of new animal experiments.

Summary–Epilogue

In this essay I have tried to share some of the joy and intellectual fun of my love affair with neurochemical research in children. I admit to such gratification without shame, because I think good research is spawned as much by passionate interest as by scientific precision and objectivity. I also admit unashamedly to backing into research through clinical interests, which help me define what are areas of ignorance, what type of knowledge is desired, and how it might be obtained. Such a clinical entrée suits a humanistic approach to research.

Clinical humanism alone, of course, is not adequate to the task. It must use scientific methods in execution, both for validity and efficiency. There are many areas of common interest between humanistic clinical art and valid scientific method. For instance, the retention of samples, a *sine qua non* for validity, is facilitated by humanistic clinical skills. Pilot studies that test out new ideas are both scientifically parsimonious and humanistically ethical. They constitute the logical first clinical step in a progression of drug use from laboratory and animal studies through pilot studies and increasingly sophisticated gradations of controlled studies to widespread clinical use. At each step of the way scientific, humanistic, ethical (*primum non nocere, secundum bona non retinere*) decisions must be made about the degree of risk versus the potential benefit, informed consent, the type and degree of experimental control (including the placebo), the selection of samples, the measures used, and the interpretation of results.

The analysis of results is one of the most satisfying parts of research, like opening a long-awaited surprise package. I believe that a combination of common sense, sound statistical method, and heuristic curiosity leads to the most valid, enjoyable, and productive handling of data.

ACKNOWLEDGMENT

I wish to acknowledge my debt of gratitude to many teachers and colleagues, both for encouragement and support and for many of the ideas incorporated into this chapter.

References

ARNOLD, L. E. The art of medicating hyperkinetic children. *Clinical Pediatrics,* 1973, **12,** 35–41.

ARNOLD, L. E., KIRILCUK, V., CORSON, S., & CORSON, E. Levoamphetamine and dextroamphetamine: Differential effect on aggression and hyperkinesis in children and dogs. *American Journal of Psychiatry,* 1973, **130,** 165–170.

ARNOLD, L. E., STROBL, D., & WEISENBERG, A. Hyperkinetic adult: Study of the paradoxical amphetamine response. *Journal of the American Medical Association,* 1972, **222,** 693–694.

ARNOLD, L. E., WENDER, P. MCCLOSKEY, K., & SNYDER, S. H. Levo-amphetamine and dextroamphetamine: Comparative efficacy in the hyperkinetic syndrome: assessment by target symptoms. *Archives of General Psychiatry,* 1972, **27,** 816–822.

BARCIA, A. Predicting the response of children with learning disabilities and behavior problems to dextro-amphetamine sulfate. *Pediatrics,* 1971, **47,** 73–79.

BRADLEY, C. Benzedrine and Dexedrine in the treatment of children's behavior disorder. *Pediatrics,* 1950, **5,** 24.

CHASSON, J. B. *Research design in clinical psychology and psychiatry.* New York: Appleton-Century-Crofts Division of Meredith Publishing Co., 1967.

CONNERS, C. K. A teacher rating scale for use in drug studies with children. *American Journal of Psychiatry,* 1969, **126,** 152–156.

CORSON, S. A., CORSON, E., KIRILCUK, V., ARNOLD, L., KNOPP, W., & KIRILCUK, I. *Experimental control of hyperkinetic and violent behavior in dogs.* 16mm black-and-white narrated film, Ohio State University, 1972a.

CORSON, S. A., CORSON, E., KIRILCUK, V., KIRILCUK, J., KNOPP, W., & ARNOLD, L. E. Interaction of amphetamines and psychosocial therapy in the control of violence and hyperkinesis in dogs. CINP 8th Congress Abstracts, August, 1972. *Psychopharmacologia, Supplement,* 1972b, **26,** 55.

DAVIDS, A. An objective instrument for assessing hyperkinesis in children. *Journal of Learning Disabilities,* 1971, **4,** 499–501.

GITTELMAN-KLEIN, R., & KLEIN, D. F. Controlled imipramine treatment of school phobia. *Archives of General Psychiatry,* 1971, **25,** 204–207.

JONES, M. B., & AINSLIE, J. D. Value of a placebo washout. *Diseases of the Nervous System,* 1966, **27,** 393–396.

KNOPP, W., ARNOLD, L. E., ANDRAS, R., & SMELTZER, D. Predicting amphetamine response in hyperkinetic children by electronic pupillography. *Pharmakopsychiatry,* 1973, **6,** 158–166.

KNOPP, W., ARNOLD, L. E., & MESSIHA, F. Gilles de la Tourette's Disease: Implications for research in Huntington's chorea. *Advances in Neurology,* 1973, **1,** 135–145.

LAUFER, M., & DENHOFF, E. Hyperkinetic behavior syndrome in children. *Journal of Pediatrics,* 1967, **50,** 463–464.

MAINLAND, D. *Elementary medical statistics.* Philadelphia: Sanders, 1964.

PARK, L. C., & COVI, L. Nonblind placebo trial. *Archives of General Psychiatry,* 1965, **12,** 336–345.

POPPER, R. Science: Problems, aims, responsibilities. *Federation Proceedings,* 1963, **22,** 961–972.

SATTERFIELD, J., CANTWELL, D. P. LESSER, L. I., & PODOSIN, R. L. Physiological study of the hyperkinetic child. *American Journal of Psychiatry,* 1972, **128,** 1418–1424.

SNYDER, S. H., TAYLOR, K., COYLE, J., & MEYERHOFF, L. The role of brain dopamine in behavioral regulation and the actions of psychotropic drugs. *American Journal of Psychiatry,* 1970, **127,** 117.

STRINGER, L. A. Research interviews with mothers as entry into primary prevention. *American Journal of Public Health*, 1959, **59**, 485–489.

WEISS, G., MINDE, K., DOUGLAS, V., WERRY, J., & SYKES, D. Comparison of the effects of chlorpromazine, dextroamphetamine, and methylphenidate on the behavior and intellectual functioning of hyperactive children. *Canadian Medical Journal*, 1971, **104**, 20–25.

WENDER, P. *Minimal brain dysfunction in children*. New York: Wiley, 1971.

WENDER, P. Vicious and virtuous circles: The role of deviation amplifying feedback in the origin and perpetuation of behavior. *Psychiatry*, 1968, **31**, 309–324.

IN OSLER'S DAY
IT WAS SYPHILIS

As is so often the case, the research with which I have been identified had an odd and tortuous beginning. Chance has played an overwhelming role. The medical school to which I went, then known as the Long Island College for Medicine, was a perfect illustration of a trade school rather than a component of a university. Since I had early conceived the thought of becoming a pediatrician, it was my good fortune, in the course of a variety of contrived roles, to meet up with two residents in pediatrics who were university-minded and a cut above their peers. One was Dr. Harold Eisenberg and the other was Dr. Martin Glynn. They kept an eye on my progress and I consulted with them toward the end of what was then the standard two-year internship. Dr. Glynn both guided and paved my way toward a pediatric residency in the prestigious New York Hospital. The time this was to begin was a year past the completion of my internship, and of this year, six months were already planned to be devoted to a term in communicable diseases and tuberculosis at the then-flourishing Kingston Avenue Hospital for Communicable Diseases. This left six unsettled months before the much-desired residency at the New York Hospital was to begin. At this juncture, Dr. Eisenberg offered a suggestion. In his day pediatric residents of the Long Island College Hospital got their communicable disease experience in a hospital with a famous name (the Charles V. Chapin Hospital) in a place that was little known to most of us (Providence, Rhode Island). In the course of his experience, he had come across a unique and curious setting known as the Bradley Home, which devoted itself to the emotional problems of children, and he suggested that with six months to spare, this could be a very interesting placement. One thing led to another, and newly married and in the dead of winter (and also in the throes of a new world war), a most hazardous journey found us in Providence, Rhode Island.

What was then the Bradley Home had a most interesting background and history. Its donors, Mr. and Mrs. George L. Bradley, had established it as a memorial to the child whose name it bore. Apparently she, the only child of

M. W. LAUFER, Bradley Hospital, Riverside, Rhode Island.

these well-to-do and concerned parents, had suffered some kind of encephalopathy that, in her early childhood, had left her mentally retarded, cerebral-palsied, and epileptic. Her parents, with all their wealth, found no resource available for her. In their wills they express the hope that their home and their estate might be used so that from the suffering of this one child might come comfort and hope for many. The first board of trustees seeking to carry out their will enlisted as their prime consultant Dr. Arthur H. Ruggles, who was then both the superintendent of Butler Hospital and a professor of psychiatry at Yale. Impressed by the numbers of European children who had suffered epidemic encephalitis in World War I and who survived to display sequelae of most intractible behavior combined with physical impairments, he proposed that this institution should be designed to care for children in this country who had been afflicted in the same way. They would thus have the same sequelae, close enough to the problems presented by Emma Pendleton Bradley herself to fulfill most appropriately the wishes of the donors.

With this in mind, the Bradley Home was built like an orthopedic hospital of the day with the expectation that its program would be diversified and strengthened by the addition of pediatricians, psychiatrists, and psychologists. From the very outset the psychologist provided a link with Brown University, and the chief psychologist of Bradley was also of professorial rank at Brown. As Brown's was an experimental, physiological, nonclinical department, psychologists at Bradley were of the same nature. These psychologists were of the highest order, beginning with Herbert Jasper, Docteur des Sciences of the Sorbonne, who became one of the two founders of encephalography in this country and was followed by Donald Lindsley, Ph.D., whose career in neurophysiology, in neurological psychology, and in electroencephalography is most illustrious.

With this background, children were admitted to Bradley Hospital from the outset on the basis of neurological and orthopedic disability but also because they had difficult or intractable behavior.

With such a scope in mind, the staff at its inception consisted of pediatricians, headed by Dr. Charles Bradley, and psychiatrists whom Dr. Ruggles imported from the adult private mental hospital that he headed, Butler Hospital.

Regrettably, this represented an uneasy mixture with explosive potentialities roughly equivalent to that of the atomic bomb. The ensuing explosions steadily escalated and eventually resulted in the fiery departure of the psychiatric component, leaving the pediatricians under Dr. Bradley to assume total responsibility. Parenthetically, one of the psychiatrists who spun off in the contemporary white heat was Dr. Leolia Dalrymple. She became a training analyst with the Boston Psychoanalytic Society and Institute and in that capacity analyzed the author of these notes, who sometimes wondered whether she thought she had Dr. Bradley or Dr. Laufer on the couch.

With the background that has been described it is understandable there would be frequent reference to the "organic driveness" of Eugen Kahn or to reminiscences of post mortem studies on victims of encephalitis lethargica and comments as to lesions in the "periventricular gray."

By the time the author of this chapter arrived to assume the role of resident, World War II was in full operation. Personnel were already being drained off in various directions and were hard to replace, and the previously flourishing cerebral palsy component or service was beginning to wind down. While there was a definite concern for the psychological life of the children and inner-personal and inter-personal components that might have led to their admission, the concern for organic components continued to be marked. All children had a most exhaustive physical examination, which included as careful a neurological examination as was feasible. All children had an electroencephalogram.

Work with EEG had begun in 1933 under Herbert Jasper, who came to Bradley to head its psychology department and to be a professor in the department of psychology at Brown University. He was developing an actual operating department of electroencephalography at the same time that similar work was going on at the Massachusetts General Hospital under Dr. F. Gibbs and his wife-collaborator, Erna Gibbs, along with Dr. W. Lennox. Dr. Jasper was succeeded in both roles, at Bradley and at Brown, by the equally illustrious Donald B. Lindsley, who was responsible for this area at the time described by these notes. At this time also, amphetamines were being used on a routine basis—though no clear clinical indications for their use were in vogue at the time. There was no doubt that in some children the results were quite startling. When Dr. Bradley was questioned concerning these results and why this agent should have such an effect, he communicated the concept that the children came to Bradley because of difficult behavior, which was their way of showing that they were desperately unhappy or unsatisfied in their lives; that amphetamines are euphoriants and that as the children were enabled to feel happier as the result of the medication, there was less need for them to display their deviant behavior, whether withdrawing or aggressing. This rationale allowed the consideration of the use of amphetamines in almost any situation, and so it could be tried in a liberal manner.

Having seen that amphetamines could indeed be useful, trainees at Bradley tended to make use of this medication wherever they went. Unfortunately, they often found that results did not warrant continuation of it and heard from others, "This stuff has been tried and it doesn't work at all. I don't think Bradley's ideas are worth very much." After the usual cycle of disillusionment, I could not but reflect that there had indeed been cases in which the results had been most worthwhile. This unsatisfactory situation led to a nagging desire to elucidate guidelines for the use of this medication and also to understand, if at all possible, why it should be useful in the first place.

While such concerns were germinating, my military service intervened. Among other things, this involved a period of service as neuropsychiatrist and electroencephalographer at a rather unique army hospital in the Zone of the Interior, which was really equivalent to a university or a teaching hospital. This was the Mayo General Hospital at Galesburg, Illinois, which was within relatively easy reach of Chicago. Some of my studies carried out on electroencephalograms and head injury provided occasions for visits to Chicago, which also allowed an awareness of the pioneering work of Ward Halsted at the University of Chicago. He was there developing a battery of tests to provide a psychoneurological basis for evaluating and localizing brain pathology. The results of his work were so interesting as to stimulate a young ex-enlisted man, who was one half of the psychological component of the Mayo General Hospital, to visit and look into the work of Halsted. This young man was Ralph M. Reitan and this marked his launching into a sphere of activity that has been very productive, first in conjunction with Halsted (the Halsted-Reitan battery) and since in many developments for which he himself has been responsible.

· By 1946, with the help of Dr. Bradley and Dr. Ruggles, it was possible for the author to leave military service and to return to what was then the Bradley Home, as clinical director under Dr. Bradley. At that time and for a few years yet to come, there were still individuals who had been at Bradley from its very inception in 1931 and readily told tales of the past to eagerly listening ears. The account that follows is derived from that time and from encounters in various parts of the country over the next 10 years. Some of these reports may be apocryphal, but, in essence, they are as follows.

In the early days of Bradley, it was hoped that abnormalities of the structure of the central nervous system might be found to be responsible for the children's difficult behavior and that therefore, neurosurgical approaches might be useful. Partly with this concept in mind, it was said, a routine procedure after the admission of children was to perform a pneumoencephalogram upon them. This often resulted in unhappy sequelae and, in particular, in complaints of severe headache. In a desire to diminish this effect, it was conceived that agents that would increase the blood pressure could conceivably increase the rate of restoration of cerebral spinal fluid and thereby diminish the headaches. A newly recognized vasopressor was Benzedrine. In good scientific fashion this medication was tried, not only for children who were suffering from postpneumo headache but also in control children who had not recently undergone this procedure. The story goes that these children themselves noted that sudden and unexpected increments in the ability to handle arithmetic began to appear, and the youngsters began to refer to this medication as the "arithmetic pills." Responding to the children's observations, the staff then began to explore more carefully the behavioral resultants of the use of this medication, and, it is said, this exploration led to its eventual use as a treatment modality.

Given the total context of concepts such as "organic driveness," of the openness to the possibility of an organic basis for disturbed behavior, and of the repeated demonstration that these medications did indeed do something useful for certain children, the background was laid for bringing together a number of disparate observations.

Dr. Bradley himself contributed by his work in a paper with Dr. Rosenfeld (Rosenfeld and Bradley, 1948), in which he delineated a syndrome of: (1) unpredictable variability in mood; (2) hypermotility; (3) impulsiveness; (4) short attention span; (5) fluctuant ability to recall material previously learned; and (6) marked difficulty with arithmetic. All these were related to early asphyxia and anoxia. No mention was made in this paper of the relationship to treatment modalities, but this paper was a final stimulus to the developing thought that the amphetamines had their useful role in dealing with what was then tentatively called the "organic syndrome."

Dr. Bradley left for Oregon in the same year as the appearance of this paper. In his absence, the struggle to reach some kind of acceptable conceptualization of what these medications were doing and why they were doing it led to a review of his writings to that time. The first, the very first article ever written on the use of amphetamines in children's behavioral problems, appeared in November 1937. It is hard to believe, but it is now 36 years that these medications have been in use. In that report, Dr. Bradley discussed 30 children whose behavior ranged from schizoid to aggressive and assaultive. He recounted a variety of useful results and tried to offer some rationale for these. It is of surpassing interest that in this very first article he suggested that the medication might stimulate higher inhibitory levels in the central nervous system and thus reduce involuntary activity through increased voluntary control. A concept such as this has recently been advanced with increasing emphasis! He also cautioned that evaluation of the child and of the medication were needed so that one would not cover up underlying psychologically based conditions.

There was a lapse of four years until his next article, written with Margaret Bowen, his faithful collaborator (1941). At that time he reported upon a larger series, now 100 children. Trying to determine how it was possible that schizoid and withdrawn children on the one hand and aggressive, attacking children on the other were both brought closer to a desirable median, he felt that he now had to drop the previous suggestion of stimulation of higher inhibitory, cortical mechanisms and turn to the one that had become current at Bradley—that is, that amphetamine, in essence, made children feel better, so that they could act better. Once more, however, he cautioned that the use of this medication did not replace either psychotherapeutic or environmental manipulation and that it should be used only with the utmost care by physicians with adequate background and training.

Pursuit of the problem of what amphetamines did and for whom now came under two conflicting influences. Previous comments have indicated that the Bradley Home of old maintained a respectful concern for organic contributions to behavior and even provided a haven for children whose problem was primarily organic, such as epileptics and children with cerebral palsy. At the instance of Dr. Bradley, the cerebral palsy component at Bradley, which had been quite prominent, was spun off into what eventually became the world-famous Meeting Street School. The neurological components of what had been Bradley were placed in the hands of and fostered by Dr. Eric Denhoff, who had been a trainee at Bradley during the regime of Dr. Bradley himself. His association with the Bradley Home continued and helped to keep the neurological components prominent.

In the meantime, the author of this chapter, while maintaining his respect for the organic aspects, felt that the psychodynamic ones needed even more prominence than had been the case and sought the opportunity for psychoanalytic training at the Boston Psychoanalytic Society and Institute. In the context of those times, consideration of the organic aspects was viewed as essentially antipsychoanalytic, so this training represented an influence in contradiction to the organic concerns previously noted. If I may reminisce, this was a very uncomfortable situation in which to be. Even to hint to fellow candidates that there might be an organic component of significance in some of the children under discussion was an invitation to be dealt with in a manner remarkably close to ostracism.

My resultant feelings of isolation were significantly relieved when one of the faculty of the institute, who had a significant background of experience in training on the British psychoanalytic scene, directed the attention of the candidates to the work of Melanie Klein and the furor polarizing around her and her ideas. This work, in turn, brought about a greater awareness of what seemed to be the greater overall receptivity in British psychoanalytic thought to the role of varieties of influences, including organic ones. Incident to this greater exposure to British psychoanalytic thought, was an awareness of the careful and broad-guaged experimental work of E. James Anthony. This made an initial impression, which became more compelling as the years passed, that it was possible to adhere to psychoanalysis while still considering the role and virtue of other concepts.

At any rate, in the midst of my uncertainty and confusion resulting from the clash between "dynamic" thinking and the constant reminders stemming from clinical experience with what seemed clearly to be organically impaired youngsters, and while I was still struggling with unformed ideas that suggested that there must be a significant role for the diencephalon in the problems with which we were confronted, the electroencephalographic journals brought into focus the work of Gastaut (1950). He had brought into clinical usefulness a functional test known as the photo-Metrazol threshold. In his succinct words, "Photo-Metrazol activation is a clinical neurophysiological test which provides a method of the exploration of certain sub-cortical structures, among which the most important are those of the diencephalon and most especially of that of the thalamus [p. 249]." His procedure consisted of recording an electroencephalogram while simultaneously injecting Metrazol intravenously and flashing a stroboscopic light into the eyes of the patient. Any individual treated in this way eventually displays an end point that consists of a simultaneous myoclonic jerk of both arms and a spike-wave burst in the electroencephalogram. Calculation of the number of milligrams of Metrazol that brings about this response, as against the weight in kilograms of the patient, gives the photo-Metrazol threshold, measured in milligrams per kilogram. In adults a normal range of the amount of Metrazol required to bring this response about was readily established. In humans and in animals with thalamic dysfunction it could be shown that there was a lower photo-Metrazol threshold, or that it took less Metrazol per kilogram of body weight to evoke the response. Moreover, in situations in which there was a unilateral dysfunction of the diencephalon, there was shown to be a lower threshold on the involved side and a normal threshold on the uninvolved side.

The explanations offered or perhaps the hypothesis offered in this paper and a companion one by Gastaut and Hunter (1950) about the significance of this test and the abnormalities noted with it could not help but resonate with previous poorly formed speculations as to the rationale for the development of the hyperkinetic picture and tentative speculations as to the role of the amphetamines in altering it. These speculations in turn stemmed from the old and oft-restated comments on "organic driveness" and "involvement of the periventricular gray."

Gastaut (1950) pointed out that stimulation of the optic pathways by means of a stroboscope ordinarily results in trains of responses ending in the occipital cortex. However, when the patient was treated by intravenous administration of Metrazol, something different developed. Electrical paroxysms appeared in the frontal lobe, far from the occipital region, to which they could come only by divergence from the optic pathways through synaptic connections whose resistance had to become significantly lowered under the influence of Metrazol on diencephalic pathways. Apparently intravenous Metrazol acted to facilitate synaptic transmission in the thalamus, opening connections that in normal conditions are functionally impermeable. While cautioning against any strict interpretation of this conjecture and indicating that it really was not factually correct, Gastaut and Hunter (1950) did say, "It is as if there had been a short-circuit [p. 284]."

These comments evoked many reverberations (even though Gastaut's concepts might not be accepted today). For instance, if there was indeed an involvement of the diencephalon in the hyperkinetic syndrome and this newly reported measure reflected integrity of function of the diencephalon, then conceivably hyperkinetic children might show some alteration of the photo-Metrazol threshold. Moreover the picture evoked by Gastaut's words, of an effect of Metrazol in allowing irradiation of impulses over larger areas of the cortex, could not help but bring to mind the striking mode of behavior of children who seem hyperkinetic shortly after birth and who seem to respond in a mass way and an excessive way to almost any stimulus—almost as if stimuli, for them, do irradiate over their cortex.

To a mind mulling over these suggestions other bits of evidence came pouring in, all seeming to fit together coherently though not completely. This was the time of my beginning awareness of the significance of the work of Magoun (1952), which stressed the role of the ascending reticular activating system in the brain stem, preserving central alertness through its ascending functions, and facilitory influences on lower motor outflows to its descending functions, in interaction with the cerebral cortex. Such roles would seem to have a pertinent connection with children who are overalert and overactive.

My increasing preoccupation with the diencephalon received an added impetus from the observations of Arey and Dent (1953). Their post mortem studies in 35 fetal and 102 neonatal deaths revealed 11 premature live borns, but no stillborns, with intraventricular hemorrhage. Arey and Dent indicated that these were all a result of subendymal hemorrhages, usually located about the terminal vein between the caudate nucleus and the thalamus. While they thought it probably innocuous, they also noted that subependymal hemorrhages were occasionally encountered about the terminal vein of the thalamus in the absence of intraventricular hemorrhage. In speculating on the causes of these, they cited the concept attributed to Schwartz (1927) that the head of the newborn is subjected only to atmospheric pressure, while the rest of the body sustained intrauterine pressures, resulting in negative pressure or a suction effect, with venous engorgement in the brain and the rupture of vessels. In this contribution, therefore, Arey and Dent were pointing to a significant area and also offering a concept about causation. Present concepts (Shetty, 1973) suggest that periventricular hemorrhage is probably from the thin capillary network (cerebral capillaries have a single layer of endothelial lining in the human newborn) rather than any particular vein.

Moving from such anatomical and pathological considerations, the next item began to suggest neurohumoral components. Marrazzi (1953) pointed out that in central brain synapses, acetylcholine facilitates synaptic output, while adrenalin/noradrenalin reduces it. Amphetamines, he suggested, produce similar effects by enhancing in some way the concentration or activity of adrenaline.

Next came some significant clinical contributions by psychoanalysts. Frosch, along with Wortis (1954), commented on the similarity of the symptom picture among hyperkinetic youngsters and children seen after postencephalitic behavior disorders, resulting from an exanthamatous disease or after head injury. Forsch and Wortis noted that they could not help but relate these children to adults and explosive-impulsive components, who often display abnormal EEG findings. This relation led them to feel that some impulsive character disorders in later years have an organic component, while some have not. The breaking through of an impulse, then, depends on a sufficiency of control apparatus. Insufficiency might result from a direct impairment of control apparatus or an increase in the strength of an impulse (whether this be physically or psychologically mediated). Frosch and Wortis commented that one might see neurological evidence of lower-level damage, hypothalamic involvement, etc. These might influence the flow of impulses to the cortex, perhaps permitting an overwhelming of cortical control apparatus, leading to an insufficiency.

In a possibly analogous mode of thinking Bellak (1955), drawing on his own observations and those of Loretta Bender and of Margaret Schonberger-Mahler, pointed to a holistic concept, which he applied to schizophrenia. He considered the role of organic factors with a physical causation and organic factors secondary to distortion of the mother–child relationship as well as to purely psychogenic problems—all conceivably playing a role in chronic schizophrenia. Such a holistic type of thinking seemed increasingly applicable to childhood hyperkinetics as well.

Still, I had a nagging concern over the fact that so many children who presented the picture that we were coming to recognize so readily and that we later characterized as "hyperkinetic impulse disorder" presented no clear diagnostic evidence of involvement of the central nervous system and had nothing in their history that would provide an acceptable etiological statement. One consistent point was that they tended to be first-born males. Some helpful suggestion came from an exhibit and discussion with the same Schwartz (1957) who had earlier been quoted by Arey and Dent. His exhibit stated tersely: "Birth is brutal." Again, he discussed direct injury and direct and indirect effects of the "lower pressure" on the head or the "release principle." His statement that almost every baby born normally suffers some disturbance of cranial and cerebral circulation as a result of the "release effect," especially involving the vein of Galen, and that late effects may involve cavitation, contraction from cicatricial shrinking, etc., seemed to offer an explanation both of causation and of the frequently noted delay in the onset of symptoms.

By this time, a great deal of both internal and external tension was developing. We were confronted with numbers of children, referred for a variety of problem manifestations, many of whom seemed to resemble those we were beginning to describe as hyperkinetic. The problems of many of these children seemed to be related to hyperkinetic factors but often were not limited to such factors. We felt impelled to do what we could to help these children by means of the medications that had proved useful for others, and for these, too, they often seemed of value. Yet we were using medications whose mechanism we did not understand in children for whom there was no clear or acceptable diagnostic maneuver. Since so many of the bits and pieces that we had accumulated pointed to some role of the diencephalon, we were almost literally impelled to make use of the photo-Metrazol technique described and explained by Gastaut (1950). This seemed to be almost ideal for our purposes. Unfortunately, his work had been done on adults and there was very little in the literature having to do with children.

We had to make some fundamental exploration of Gastaut's technique. We had to make sure that we could adapt it to children and that the results were consistent and reproducible. We could not feel justified in attempting this technique with children who had no problems for which the outcome might be of any significance. To us this meant that we were limited to the emotionally disturbed children who were patients at Bradley and in whom we could keep the factor of emotional disturbance constant while differentiating among the total group as between those who seemed to have some organic component and those who did not.

This led to our first published report (Laufer et al., 1954). This delineated the specifics of the procedure, described a sample, and established the reliability by retest. An "organic" versus a "nonorganic" grouping was established, a mean threshold was determined for each, and a cutoff threshold was delineated that could discriminate between organic and nonorganic with a minimum degree of error. It was noted that the children with "organic syndromes," when off the amphetamines, had a threshold of 4.8 milligrams per kilogram. The same children, when receiving amphetamines, had a level of 6.7 milligrams per kilogram, which was identical with the level determined for emotionally disturbed children with no discernible organic component. These findings seemed clearly to indicate that the children with organic syndromes had some measurable and discernible abnormality of diencephalic function and that amphetamines had a measurable effect upon this threshold. This report would seem to provide some solid factual basis for the hitherto much-debated and scoffed-at role of the amphetamines.

These findings were incorporated in our first attempt at an overall, definitive statement (Laufer et al., 1957). This depicted the clinical syndrome of hyperactivity; short attention span and poor powers of concentration; variability; impulsivity; irritability; and explosiveness. The frequent concomitant presence of poor schoolwork was explained as partly reflecting the hampering effects of the behaviors described and a partly a result of visual-motor difficulties. The complex of symptoms was thought to be related to diencephalic dysfunction, especially that of the hypothalamus, even while it was recognized that each and every item depicted could have other causes. We again pointed out that in the hyperkinetics, the mean for the Metrazol threshold was 4.54 milligrams per kilogram, a highly significant difference from the mean photo-Metrazol threshold of 6.35 milligrams per kilogram in nonhyperkinetic, emotionally disturbed children. Further, treatment with the amphetamines caused a shift among hyperkinetics from a mean of 4.8 milligrams per kilogram to a mean of 6.7 milligrams per kilogram, a distinctly significant result. In as much as the clinical picture, and also the low photo-Metrazol threshold and its alteration by amphetamines, could be found in individuals without historical evidence of classical traumatic or infectious factors, not only a variety of prenatal components were postulated, but also a variant of Schwarz's thesis under the heading of the "squeezed-lemon hypothesis."

A number of possible themes were also adduced in an attempt to conceptualize the mechanisms by which any of these factors might result in the clinical picture that was so striking. Once more, the theme was that of diencephalic-cortical relationships. At that time it seemed more reasonable to place the major site of difficulty in the diencephalon, while assuming that some normal process of development would take place in the cortex that would eventually render this region less subject to being overwhelmed by the dysfunctioning diencephalon.

This concept viewed the diencephalon as normally serving to route, sort, and pattern impulses that came in from peripheral and central receptors, not only diverting them to appropriate cortical areas but also giving them significance, weight, and valence (such as when a sleeping mother could sleep through the quantitively loud noise of the sanitation department rattling garbage cans under her window, while waking at the quantitatively minute noise of her baby). The hypothesis further assumed that when the diencephalon was injured or dysfunctional, there was lesser resistance to transmission at its synapses, so that the infant or child could be overwhelmed by and at the mercy of stimuli flooding in from peripheral or central receptors.

Such a mechanism had been hinted at by Watson and Denny-Brown (1955), indicating that subcortical structures, especially thalamic, when diseased, allowed a breakdown of synaptic coordination channels and were thus associated with instability of synaptic resistance. Our viewing of the difficult and sometimes catastrophic behavioral phenomena resulting from this condition led to our appreciation of the impact it must have upon adults, siblings, playmates, and others exposed to such behavior and the consequent emotional turmoil and poor self-image of the hyperkinetic child, further worsening his behavior. Incidentally, we came to this view at a time when the *tabula rasa* theory of child rearing and behavior still held sway—when any behavioral difficulty in a child was seen as a result of malignant impulses originating from his parents' unconscious hostilities and distortions. For our hyperkinetic children, at least, we were suggesting that the child had something to contribute to the equation. We in no way eliminated a consideration of feelings, however!

Because of the frequently associated scholastic difficulty, this original paper included the concept, subsequently dropped, that a specific learning disability was always a concomitant. The paper also attempted to conceptualize the role of action of the amphetamines. As Marrazzi (1953) had indicated that these agents could "inhibit or lower the level of synaptic transmission" in the diencephalon and P. B. Bradley (1957) had located the "site of action as possibly related to the brain stem reticular activitating a system of Magoun," we suggested that these effects might counteract the previously postulated increased ease of transmission at the synapses of the diencephalon.

With all these neurophysiological concepts, the paper also cautioned that emotional factors must still be considered and called for an end to the then all-too-current "all-or-none" kinds of thinking.

This paper was quickly followed by a more clinical paper (Laufer and Denhoff, 1957), which was the first to use the term *hyperkinetic impulse disorder* and also made the first attempts to depict it as one of a number of syndromes that could result from a variety of causes—such as maldevelopment, malformation, and malfunction, occurring *in utero*, during the process of delivery, or in the first few years of life. We called these syndromes the *syndromes of cerebral malfunction*.

In this paper we had come to recognize that scholastic difficulties might be behavioral in origin but that they might also represent a concomitant specific learning disability. This was also the first attempt at some specificity in age relationships, stressing that the condition under discussion might be outgrown anywhere from ages 8 to 18 and indicating that it always was outgrown. We gave hints that this was a process of maturation (neither intellectual nor sexual) but no clear indication as to what this process might be.

We also studied the emotional aspects, resultants, and concomitants more closely. Work from various sources had suggested that infants who do not have abundant and flexible mothering would have unrelieved tensions and grow up to be tense adults who expected unhappiness. It was suggested that since these infants could overreact and be unduly sensitive to normal stresses and stimuli, it would be very hard for even an experienced mother to meet their needs. Greenacre (1952), by the way, had postulated that accidents of and at birth might have much to do with the form and pattern of anxiety, the ability to sustain anxiety, and the molding of personality attributes.

In the context of those times, the mother had been schooled to regard the infant's reaction to her as of one special and overwhelming significance, with the baby being the "litmus paper," so to speak, that would by some unerring process determine her worth as a mother and as a female. Against such a background, a new and untried mother of a firstborn would be particularly apt to react catastrophically to the unsatisfiable and unsatisfying characteristics of the hyperkinetic newborn—feeling and expressing the devastating thought, "My baby rejected me from birth." This was but one of the many sources of painful and negative interaction between parent and child that contributed so much to the eventual clinical picture. As a result, we observed that proper work with such children and such cases might call upon the total armamentarium of the child psychiatrist and the allies with whom we needed to work, including special educational help for the child, psychotherapy for the child, and casework for the parents.

As more and more attention (and contention) was drawn by the concepts heretofore stated, there seemed to be both undue emphasis upon and adverse reaction to the rubric *brain damage* and confusion about what might be attributed to this devastating term. This state of affairs led to the first published article (Denhoff *et al.*, 1959) on what was henceforth to be designated as the "syndromes of cerebral dysfunction." This article listed the host of possible consequences not only of injury but also of maldevelopment (to which heredity was later added as a possible contributor), of altered structure, of delayed maturation, and of malfunction (even deriving from emotional stresses!). We hoped that this list would replace the objectionable terms *brain-damage* and *brain-injured*, and we also emphasized that not just one but several concomitant deviations in the same child could stem from the same cause.

Although the concept of the hyperkinetic impulse disorder became increasingly familiar, somehow there was a widespread impression that by some magic this condition disappeared at puberty and could not therefore afflict adolescents. In the hope of counteracting this misconception, I presented a study in 1962 that focused on the forms of this condition and consequences by which it might be manifested in adolescence.

Through all these articles, it must be confessed, there ran the theme that this condition was *inevitably* outgrown, though its end point gradually crept up from 18 to 20. This inevitability, however, was soon called into question, first in a very thoughtful article by Hartocollis (1968). He pointed out that psychiatrists usually seek evidence of organic causes in psychiatric patients, primarily to rule out such items as tumors and also as an alternative to psychological factors and causation. Any suggestion of an organic *component* would be readily discarded by those physicians who choose to concern themselves primarily with a patient's feelings, thinking, and behavior. He reported on a group of 54 patients, ages 15 to 25, who were admitted to the Menninger Clinic as inpatients for behavioral reasons and who were then referred for neuropsychological testing because of a suspicion of organic causes, a possibility considered only after their admission. From among this group, 15 were selected whose scores on a neuropsychological test battery were in the mid range—neither the highest nor the lowest.

All showed impulsive behavior, restlessness, hyperactivity, concrete thinking, difficulty with mathematics or reading, lability of mood, irritability, excitability, and sometime violent outbursts or suicidal attempts. In most of these cases the history showed these characteristics to have been present since childhood. Problems tended to develop as these people progressed in school, with an inexorable progression of behavioral and academic difficulties and personality changes. Hartocollis characterized them as having a low threshold to stimulation and concluded that those who functioned in this way might need special attention and protection.

Hartocollis stressed that it was hard for parents and clinicians to accept that some forms of cerebral dysfunction could exist alongside intellectual adequacy. Lastly, he said, where there is intellectual adequacy, the patient may be more unhappily aware of limitations in his performance than if he were significantly retarded.

Hartocollis commented on the resistance of physicians to the possibility that a disturbance might be organic rather than psychogenic and that it might have many roots. It might also have many unfortunate consequences, including unrealistic expectations or total reliance upon the patient's efforts to alter his own situation, analogous to the past expectations of his parents. Resistance to such possibilities cannot help but lead to unhappy reflections on what it is that leads physicians to forsake their heritage, to omit and ignore the role of the central nervous system in the area they place foremost in their consideration, and simultaneously to depreciate and denigrate organic components, in an unhappy perpetuation of an unscientific either–or kind of thinking. This approach seems particularly odd when coupled, as it so often has been, with an assertion of an essential primacy over other, allied disciplines, such as psychology, social work, and nursing.

Another, somewhat-related article was the one by Quitkin and Klein (1969) dealing with behavioral syndromes in young adults that are related to possible minimal brain dysfunction. Quitkin and Klein prefer to refer to "behavioral soft signs," such as cognitive and executive malfunctions, with delay in developmental milestones, hyperkinesis, learning disorder, social disorganization, inattentiveness, concreteness, and memory defect. They commented that these are all perfectly recognizable but do not point to any specific neurological lesion. They quote others as suggesting that organic components lessen resistance to environmental factors in an augmentation model. They describe a behavioral picture ("impulsive-destructive") that correlates with a childhood history suggestive of hyperkinetic behavior disorder. In noting our suggestion that the hyperkinetic picture wanes with adolescence, they suggested that their findings indicate that this is not necessarily so.

Indeed, despite our previous assertions, it is not necessarily so! Not only others, but we ourselves have seen a very few cases continuing into early adult life. This phenomenon again raises the question of what it is that finally puts an end to the clinical evidence of this condition, and experience certainly makes it clear that it is neither puberty nor any arbitrary time. We continue to suspect that the operative mechanism is the final completion of myelinization of the cerebral cortex, especially as there are reports that indicate that this may not finally occur until age 30. One way of testing this hypothesis is to check on the parameters of cortical-evoked responses in hyperkinetic versus age-equivalent, nonhyperkinetic children. Satterfield and his associates (1973) reported that "minimal brain dysfunction children" have longer latencies and lower amplitude-evoked responses than do normal age-matched controls, suggesting that these differences may represent a delayed maturation of the central nervous system in such children. This is a hint in the right direction, but no one has yet done a long-term developmental study on the pattern of development of cortical-evoked responses in hyperkinetic children.

Meanwhile, emerging studies have begun to offer some hope of better understanding of the actual neurophysiological mechanisms involved in the favorable results from the use of amphetamines and methylphenidate in the treatment of the hyperkinetic. These studies have emanated from the laboratories of Snyder, Taylor, and their colleagues and of Axelrod and Wender, who presented such theories as part of an entire, fascinating book on the topic of minimal brain dysfunction (de la Cruz et al., 1973). These studies suggested that amphetamines both release catecholamines at synaptic junctions and block their reuptake. There seemed to be a differential implication of both noradrenergic and dopaminergic pathways. It was suggested that if dextrorotatory and levorotatory amphetamines are equal in their effect, then dopaminergic mechanisms are involved. If, however, it takes three to four times the amount of levorotatory amphetamine to effect results equivalent to those of dextrorotatory amphetamine, this was felt to suggest that noradrenergic mechanisms are being tapped. Once again, attention was returning to synaptic functioning in these children.

At this juncture, there was a good deal of excitement in the press and many pontifications in psychiatric and other literature suggesting that the use of medications for hyperkinetic children was a criminal assault upon them, their families, and their rights, and that actually, the medications were being used to dampen the normal high spirits and alertness of childhood, which were being put to the test by inadequate and coercive school systems and teaching methods.

It was therefore particularly electrifying to learn from Corson et al. (1971) that he had become aware of naturally occurring hyperkinetic, untrainable dogs in which amphetamines inhibited overactivity and aggressiveness, while sedatives and tranquilizers did not. This finding was followed by a black-and-white 16mm sound film produced by Corson *et al.* (1972) and dramatically narrated by L. E. Arnold. It depicted seven naturally occurring hyperkinetic dogs that also had problems in learning. Some were, in addition, aggressive—one in a spectacular manner. This one failed (as did the others) to respond to any approach, including any other pharmacological agent, till dextroamphetamine was administered, to which his positive response was equally spectacular. The violent behavior disappeared before the hyperkinetic behavior. Also, there were differential responses to different doses. An equally striking observation was that normal dogs were *made hyperkinetic* by the medication. A later paper published by the same group (Corson *et al.*, 1973) reported that *one* dog required three to four times as much levorotatory amphetamine as dextrorotatory amphetamine for hyperkinesis, while both forms of medication were equally effective for aggression. These results (in *one* animal) could conceivably mean that the dopaminergic systems were involved in aggression and the noradrenergic systems in hyperkinesis. These authors speculated that hyperkinetic dogs might suffer from hypoarousal, with overactivity serving as a reparative means of providing afferent input. In other words, they ask, "Do amphetamines provide essential neurotransmitters which hyperactive dogs attempt to obtain via afferents from muscular activity?" Suggesting that the medication also facilitates information retrieval, they comment that the effects may not be paradoxical at all but actually normalizing.

In regard to the first point, that overactivity provides a substitution mechanism, we must recall that in humans our description of the syndrome of hyperkinetic impulse disorder listed a variety of components in addition to hyperactivity. One of them is distractibility. It may be significant that distractibility can be seen by itself without the presence of hyperactivity and that when it is present, it, too, generally responds favorably to the use of amphetamines. To us this suggests that some different mechanism is involved.

The interesting point about information retrieval brings to mind our concept of the nature of the learning problem in young schoolchildren who are only hyperkinetic and do not also have a concomitant specific learning disability. Actually, in the first three grades learning is equivalent to memorizing and not to thinking. It is as if the data bank of a computer were being charged so that it could later be programmed. *Learning* means not only remembering but remembering on a long-term rather than a short-term basis. There does seem to be a short-term and a long-term memory. In the untreated state a hyperkinetic child is often unable to focus his mind on something long enough for it to be transferred from the short-term to the long-term memory system. In essence, he hasn't "learned," so he can't retrieve.

In this and a later article (Arnold *et al.*, 1973) the same group returned to the theme of differential affects on aggression and hyperkinesis in children and in dogs, commenting as before that levo- and dextrorotatory amphetamines are equally potent in dealing with aggression but that dextroamphetamine is three to four times as potent as levoamphetamine in calming "nervousness." These are very interesting speculations, but there are some aspects that may as yet be unelucidated. Most of the studies of this nature compare dextro- and levorotatory amphetamine. In our own work, we have observed and commented that there seems often to be a remarkable specificity of response among hyperkinetic children who present pictures that on the surface look indistinguishable. In them all (not some) components seem to respond favorably in one case to dextroamphetamine and in other cases to racemic amphetamine. Having been aware of and puzzled over this for a long time, we thought it reasonable to assume that in those who respond well to racemic amphetamine, but not to dextroamphetamine, the potent agent must be levorotatory amphetamine.

In 1949 it was possible to obtain the levorotatory form on an experimental basis as Laevedrine. This was tried in what must be admitted to be a small number (recalled as being 10) who responded to racemic amphetamine. However, they showed equally unfavorable results with Laevedrine as they had with dextrorotatory amphetamine! We ceased the experimentation at that time, but we could not help but wonder whether racemic amphetamine may have in some children specific effects that are not exhibited by either of the optical isomers.

Another article from the same group (Arnold et al., 1972) made a useful attempt to localize some of the tracts and pathways involved. For dopaminergic tracts they suggested one running from the substantia nigra to the corpus striatums and others running from the brain stem (near the interpeduncular nucleus) to the nucleus accumbens in the septal region of the limbic forebrain and in the olfactory tubercle (implicated in the mediation of emotional behavior) or to the caudate nucleus and connecting tracts, in particular, for its role in mediating activity.

In the meantime the devoted work of a dynamic young Irish child psychiatrist, Paul McCarthy, allowed the accumulation of information concerning the later history of a number of individuals, now adolescent or older, who had received amphetamine treatment in earlier years. His findings as of 1973 (Laufer, 1973) as to success in life and failure to bring about lifelong "dependence upon drugs" were relatively reassuring.

After a period in which it seemed that only C. Bradley and those he influenced were concerned with this picture, there has been increasing interest in it. There have been some highly interesting psychiatric studies of the nature of the child's inner psychic responses to this condition and the need for careful differentiation of this state from other, more usual psychopathological states. These are summarized to some extent in relatively recent articles. Wender (1971) has published an entire book devoted to this topic. Book reviews have called attention to the recent appearance of *MBD: The Family Book About Minimal Brain Dysfunction* (Gardner, 1973). An entire volume of the *Annals of the New York Academy of Sciences* has been devoted to the topic of minimal brain dysfunction (de la Cruz *et al.*, 1973). There have been an issue of *Seminars in Psychiatry* on the topic of minimal cerebral dysfunction in children (Walzer and Wolff, 1973) and an issue of *Pediatric Annals* on "The Hyperkinetic Syndrome and Minimal Brain Dysfunction" (Laufer, 1973).

The use of the term *minimal brain dysfunction* has seemed to contribute to some confusion. It has seemed to us that this confusion could be minimized by more general acceptance of the overall concept of *syndromes of cerebral dysfunction*, which can include the hyperkinetic impulse disorder and specific learning disability. Potential confusion can come about from varying uses of the term *minimal brain dysfunction*. For some it seems to be equivalent to the hyperkinetic picture. For others it seems equivalent to the learning disability. And for still others, it may refer to both. The concept of the syndromes of cerebral dysfunction, on the other hand, carries the clear implication that either of these syndromes may occur in isolation as well as together. As we previously stated, "to view these two syndromes as always occurring together can be confusing and lead to improper treatment considerations. For instance such a view could result in all children with learning disability being given medications, which would be most improper and, on the other hand, in treating all hyperkinetics with educational measures, which might be inadequate [Laufer, 1973, p. 12]."

In retrospect, this has been a most interesting path to follow. My clinical observations led to armchair speculation, fortified by an omnivorous appetite for the literature and large doses of serendipity. Tension over the armchair speculation, unfortified by experimental or laboratory evidence, led to a delving into neurophysiology and some actual clinical and laboratory work that seemed at least to begin to place the hyperkinetic impulse disorder syndrome on a firmer pathophysiological footing.

My high index of suspicion about the occurrence of this syndrome in turn required careful differential diagnosis to determine the presence of other components of psychogenetic origin not associated with this picture. The all-encompassing nature of the sad sequelae and complications of this syndrome required increasingly intimate work with and knowledge of the speciality and methods of special educators, psychologists, social workers and speech and language personnel, neurophysiologists, neurologists, etc.

Much has been learned in later years, but we *still* do not know all the steps in the mechanism whereby the hyperkinetic impulse disorder creates its effects, how medication modifies it, and what brings about the eventual outgrowing of the condition.

Still it can be said, as Osler did years ago, that "to know syphilis is to know medicine." To know the hyperkinetic impulse disorder and the other syndromes of cerebral dysfunction is to know every aspect of our field of child psychiatry, from the psychodynamic to the most exquisitely organic. Would that we could know more!

References

AREY, J. B., & DENT, J. Causes of fetal and neonatal death with special reference to pulmonary and inflammatory lesions. *Journal of Pediatrics.* 1953, **42**, 1–25.

ARNOLD, L. E., KIRILCUK, V., CORSON, S. A., & CORSON, E. O'L. Levoamphetamine and dextroamphetamine: Differential effect on aggression and hyperkinesis in children and dogs. *American Journal of Psychiatry,* 1973, **130**, 165–170.

ARNOLD, L. E., WENDER, P. H., McCLOSKEY, K., & SNYDER, S. H. Levoamphetamine and dextroamphetamine: Comparative efficacy in the hyperkinetic syndrome. *Archives of General Psychiatry,* 1972, **27**, 816–822.

BELLAK, L. Toward a unified concept of schizophrenia. *Journal of Nervous and Mental Diseases,* 1955, **121**, 60–66.

BRADLEY, C. The behavior of children receiving benzedrine. *American Journal of Psychiatry,* 1937, **94**, 577–585.

BRADLEY, C., & BOWEN, M. Amphetamine (Benzedrine) therapy of children's behavior disorders. American Journal of Orthopsychiatry, 1941, **11**, 92–103.

BRADLEY, P. B., & HANCE, A. J. The effect of chlorpromazine and methopromazine on the electrical activity of the brain in the cat. *Electroencephalography and Clinical Neurophysiology,* 1957, **9**, 191–215.

CORSON, S. A., CORSON, E. O'L., KIRILCUK, V., KIRILCUP, J., KNOPP, W., & ARNOLD, L. F. Differential effects of amphetamines on clinically relevant dog models of hyperkinesis and stereotypy: Relevance to Huntington's chorea in advances in neurology. 1. In A. Barbeau, T. N. Chase, and G. W. Paulson, (Eds.), New York: Raven Press, 1973.

CORSON, S. A., et al. Effects of d-amphetamine on hyperkinetic untrainable dogs. *Federation Proceedings,* **30**, 1971.

CORSON, S. A., et al. Black-and-white sound film, 16mm. Experimental control of hyperkinetic and violent behavior in dogs. Narrated by L. E. Arnold. 1972.

DE LA CRUZ, F. F., FOX, B. H., & ROBERTS, R. H. (Eds.). Minimal brain dysfunction. 205: Annual New York Academy of Sciences, 1973. (396 pages)

DENHOFF, E., LAUFER, M. W., & HOLDEN, R. H. The syndromes of cerebral dysfunction. *Journal of the Oklahoma State Medical Association,* 1959, **52**, 360–366.

FROSCH, J., & WORTIS, S. B. A contribution to the nosology of the impulse disorders. *American Journal of Psychiatry,* 1954, **111**, 132–138.

GARDNER, R. A. *The family book about minimal brain dysfunction.* New York: Jason Aronson, 1973.

GASTAUT, H., & HUNTER, J. An experimental study of the mechanism of photic activation in idiopathic epilepsy. *Electroencephalography and Clinical Neurophysiology,* 1950, **2**, 263–387.

GASTAUT, H. Combined photic and Metrazol activation of the brain. *Electroencephalography and Clinical Neurophysiology,* 1950, **2**, 249–261.

GREENACRE, P. *Trauma, growth and personality.* New York: W. W. Norton, 1952.

HARTOCOLLIS, P. The syndrome of minimal brain dysfunction in young adult patients. *Bulletin of the Menninger Clinic,* 1968, **32**, 102–114.

LAUFER, M. W. Cerebral dysfunction and behavior disorders in adolescents. *American Journal of Orthopsychiatry,* 1962, **32**, 501–506.

LAUFER, M. W. Long term management and some follow up findings on the use of drugs with minimal cerebral syndromes. *Journal of Learning Disability*, 1971, **4**, 519–522.

LAUFER, M. W. The dynamic syndrome and minimal brain dysfunction. *Pediatric Annals*, 1973, **2**, 6–86.

LAUFER, M. W., & DENHOFF, E. Hyperkinetic behavior syndrome in children. *Journal of Pediatrics*, 1957, **50**, 463–474.

LAUFER, M. W., DENHOFF, E., & RUBIN, E. A. Photo-Metrazol activation in children. *Electroencephalography and Clinical Neurophysiology*, 1954, **6**, 1–8.

LAUFER, M. W., DENHOFF, E., & SOLOMONS, G. Hyperkinetic impulse disorder in children's behavior problems. *Psychomatic Medicine*, 1957, **19**, 39–49.

MAGOUN, H. W. An ascending reticular activating system in the brain stem. *American Medical Association Archives of Neurology and Psychiatry*, 1952, **67**, 145–154.

MARRAZZI, A. S. Some indications of cerebral humoral mechanisms. *Science*, 1953, **118**, 367–370.

QUITKIN, F., & KLEIN, D. F. Two behavioral syndromes in young adults related to possible minimal brain dysfunction. *Journal of Psychiatric Research*, 1969, **7**, 131–142.

ROSENFELD, G. B., & BRADLEY, C. Childhood behavior sequelae of asphyxia in infancy. *Pediatrics*, 1948, **2**, 74–84.

SATTERFIELD, J. H., LESSER, L. I., SAUL, R. E., & CANTWELL, D. P. Electroencephalographic aspects in the diagnosis and treatment of minimal brain dysfunction. *Annals of the New York Academy of Sciences*, 1973, **205**, 274–282.

SCHWARTZ, P. Birthtrauma as a cause of mental deficiency, Exhibition at APA Annual Meeting, Chicago, 1957.

SCHWARTZ, P. Die traumatischen Schädigungen des Zentralnervensystems durch die Geburt: Anatomische Untersuchungen, Ergebn. d. inn. Med. u. Kinderh, 1927, **31**, 165.

SHETTY, T. Personal communication. Assistant Professor of Medical Science, Brown University Medical Program, 1973.

WALZER, S., & WOLFF, P. H., (Eds.). Seminar on minimal cerebral dysfunction in children. *Seminars in Psychiatry*, 1973, **5**.

WATSON, C. W., & DENNY-BROWN, D. Studies of the mechanism of stimulus-sensitive myoclonus in man. *Electroencephalography and Clinical Neurophysiology*, 1955, **7**, 341–356.

WENDER, P. Minimal brain dysfunction in children. New York: Wesley-Interscience, 1971.

DEVELOPMENTAL
RESEARCH

INTRODUCTION

It would seem to be the most natural thing in the world for the child psychiatrist, with his often-proclaimed emphasis on development, to undertake developmental research, but quite surprisingly this is not the most populated area in the general field of research in our discipline.

Sander has carried out basic work in laying a solid foundation for the relatively new subspeciality of "infant psychiatry," and he has set about it in a way that makes it a model for further studies. The main reason is that he appears to have many of the attributes that are associated with the good researcher. He is quiet unless he has something pertinent to say; cautious in assessing novel developments; precise in describing his own work; careful in his interpretation of data; attentive to new suggestions from others; and altogether remarkably competent. Although psychoanalytically trained, he is essentially an empirical investigator whose dynamic understanding has increased his sensitivity to what he is observing in the laboratory, but he sensibly leaves the theory outside when he enters the research situation. It may be that someday he will be able to bring his work into line with psychoanalytic theories of development, but currently he is not quite ready for that. With so many investigators concentrating their efforts on the primary unit of mother and infant, one begins to question whether anything new can still be said about it. However, the nicest thing about empirical research is that it constantly generates new data, and there is an equally good chance for new data to generate new theory. In this sense empirical research has a clear advantage over "metapsychologizing" from the armchair. In his studies Sander has focused on the infant's state, the mother's state, the synchrony between the two, and the regulatory mechanisms of the system that optimally should function not too perfectly nor too imperfectly for good infant development. He has tried to describe a psychophysiological matching between two unlike organisms that need to reach a mutual equilibrium and understanding. The complexity of the model is such that the investigator is hard put to devise methods for disentangling the various regulatory operations, but the data appear to provide good evidence of "the embeddedness of the human infant in a microscopic interactive regulative system as well as a macroscopic one." This certainly sounds like a good base for making further progress.

Call is also concerned with the adaptive processes at work in the mother and infant relationship and with the infant's activity and assertiveness in finding satisfactions for himself in the new extrauterine world. The "nuclear" ego involved has fascinated Call for many years, especially the congenital variations in its capacities. There is no doubt, given the right amount of support in terms of time and money, that he will follow his "snout hypothesis" far beyond the end of its nose. He differs from Sander in one striking respect: he is much more inclined to look at his data, even in their rudimentary form, within the context of psychoanalytic theory, and he constantly reaches out into the future of the infant to wonder how his current findings will help to shape later clinical developments. He is thus a more psychoanalytic investigator than Sander and more ready to make the "mysterious leap" from basic observation to sophisticated theory. For example, it would be difficult for Sander even to bring himself to consider the significance of his findings for future transference and countertransference reactions in the psychoanalytic situation. Science, however, has always been ready to harbor both kinds of scientists, the cautious and the intrepid, and has profited handsomely.

The work of Chess is so well known as hardly to need any introduction. Her developmental studies have become a byword in the field, and it is difficult these days to present a paper dealing with etiology without making at least some reference to her "constitutional" theory. Like so many others, she is a clinician who has "backed into research" because of the many unanswered questions that confronted her in her daily clinical work, but she has remained primarily a clinician. For this reason she appears singularly free from the snide, deprecatory attitudes toward clinicians (and their well-known susceptibility to hunches) that mar the work of "purer" researchers. She seems right in suggesting that amateurism has no place in serious investigation and that the transformation of clinician into researcher comes with "the realization that data analysis is of primary importance, definitely not to be done in the evening after a full day's work plus everything else that happened up to the moment of putting the children to bed!" This comment also provides us with an intriguing insight into the pressures that play upon the woman-mother investigator. The family of the researcher is seldom considered as part of the research environment, and yet Chess has provided us with evidence of how important it can be. She and her husband have been close co-workers, and it was observing their four children and the "differences" they showed from birth that led to their fruitful developmental hypotheses. The incident of the "squeaking door" suggests that it takes more to be a researcher than to be a mother; one needs to be a mother with a very special type of mind, endlessly curious about phenomena and ready to put ideas to the test. These kinds of mothers are probably not very common in the general population! Her research work has been clearly governed by the Pavlovian dicta of gradualness, modesty, and passion, since it is these very qualities that make her contribution one of the most fascinating and revealing in the book.

INFANT AND CARETAKING ENVIRONMENT

INVESTIGATION AND CONCEPTUALIZATION OF ADAPTIVE BEHAVIOR IN A SYSTEM OF INCREASING COMPLEXITY

Louis W. Sander

Introduction

The assignment of bringing together one's "research perspective, research philosophy, methods, and findings" in one autobiographical account presents some rather obvious and many more subtle difficulties. It is obvious that such a contribution cannot be in the usual format of a scientific paper. And it is difficult to generate a personal synthesis and at the same time to offer it as a research contribution. It has seemed feasible for me only to try to organize and communicate in some reasonably concrete way the course that my work and thought have taken over the last score of years. During that score of years my career in clinical child psychiatry has become largely a commitment to certain problems of early developmental research, in particular, a concern with the question of organization itself in personality development.

A Red Thread

The opportunity that research in child psychiatry presented to me was of gaining at least some perspective of a dismayingly complex universe, one that is rapidly becoming more complex as the knowledge of every aspect of the bio-

LOUIS W. SANDER, Professor of Psychiatry, Boston University School of Medicine, Boston. Dr. Sander is supported by NIMH Research Development Program # K5-MH-20, 505. The data reported were obtained during project support NIMH # 898C1, NIMH # 3325 and NICHD # 01766. Work carried out during current support by The Grant Foundation, New York, has contributed in a major way to the viewpoint presented herein.

logical process widens. From my original dismay has emerged the conviction that what it is essential to understand is the way coherence, integration, or "unity of the organism" can be achieved and maintained in an individual engaged in interactions with surroundings of great and apparently increasing complexity.

I assume that the synthesis Dr. Anthony has asked for concerns those gaps between the more formal and objective communications of my scientific publications. These gaps contain the personal information, influences, and rationalizations referred to by Polanyi (1959) as the "personal coefficient of knowledge." In his discussion of Polanyi's position Wallerstein (1973) described this aspect of the world of natural science as related to "realities created by acts of perspective and interpretation." He went even further to propose that "even the world of natural science is a man-created reality, a particular way of looking at and giving meaning to the facts of nature [p. 18]."

In fact, the recent address given by Robert Wallerstein as outgoing president of the American Psychoanalytic Association provides a most fortuitous frame of reference for an essay intended, as I have assumed, largely for an audience of psychiatric professionals. In this paper Wallerstein pursued the relatively neglected problem of the construction of the world of outer reality as itself a "psychic instance," pointing to the necessity of going beyond the notion of an outer reality as an "average expectable environment" in conceptualizing psychic organization. He argued that it is insufficient now to make such a generalizing assumption in formulating the role of the ego as mediating among an id, a superego, and an *outer reality*. Wallerstein concluded that

> until recently, cultures, no matter how different, each contained a conservative tradition: that children reared within the reality of each, could expect to complete their days within that system of demands—the basis for the conception of the stable and the average expectable. It is in our generation that our life task has become fundamentally different: to survive successfully within a reality matrix in which the *adaptive requirements* are being radically and varyingly transformed within the lifetime of each of us as individuals, rather than slowly over the many generational history of a people. In maintaining our *psychic integration* under such circumstances, we need all the understanding that psychoanalytic study of all the interacting pressures upon us can give [pp. 31–32].

For such an understanding are needed new, more detailed, and more explicit conceptualizations of the adaptive process in relation to personality development, especially conceptualizations that can account for psychic integration in the face of an increasing complexity, both within the individual and in his encounter with his environment. Just as information—processing models, introducing cybernetic control in regulation, have replaced hydrostatic models of behavior organization, so also relatively simpler biological models of adaptation such as those based on the use of an "average expectable environment" may have to be replaced by more inclusive formulations.

Biologists long have been thinking about the problem of organization of behavior, extending the framework provided by a concept of adaptation. A wealth of leads has been offered from this source for students of interpersonal adaptation, such as those given by Mason[1] (1968) or Ashby (1952). Psychopathology can be viewed as a failure of integrative mechanisms just as easily as it can be viewed as a consequence of conflict. However, as Mason has pointed out, just as in biological research relatively less attention has been paid to problems of synthesis than to those of analysis, so in psychiatric research less attention is given to understanding the genesis of ego strength than is given to the genesis of conflict.

When one views the empirical data of human interpersonal behavior, he finds disturbingly paradoxical functions that must be accounted for in the same individual. Both integration and differentiation must be accounted for by the same model. Can factors introducing complexity also provide mechanisms for synthesis and simplification? Can more sophisticated models of adaptive behavior representing processes of basic regulation also suggest more adequate models for the so-called "higher functions" of the human, functions such as cognition, self-awareness, or "inner perception."[2] In fact, polarity in the arrangement of the forces with which the adapting organism must cope are so ubiquitous in the natural world (e.g., night and day, heat and cold, activity and rest, input and output) that it would not be surprising if a key to the comprehension of adaptive mechanics in development could be found in the organism's confrontation with and resolution of oscillating or opposing tendencies.

For me, the traditional training and concerns of clinical psychiatry initiated the guiding questions and provided research direction. The primary concern of the psychiatric clinician is with "the person"—an essential coherence synthesizing components interacting in the greatest complexity. In the therapeutic encounter, if the sensing of and the attention to the facilitation of essential coherence is neglected in favor of any one element over others, the therapeutic process soon becomes compromised or obstructed. The central question arises almost at once: How are the events in an interpersonal interaction to be related to the generation of changes in the organization of a

---

[1] In his discussion of research in relation to the biological problems of synthesis and organization, W. A. Mason has provided a comprehensive perspective, an inspiration, and an example of the way sufficient empirical data can be accumulated to bear directly on problems of biological organization and to suggest relevant models.

[2] Von Holst (1950), an investigator of insect behavior, has raised some of the same questions that the psychiatrist has. Given the same exact configuration of movement of a limb or muscle, which is at one time passively moved and at another time actively moved by the organism, how are these movements centrally distinguished? In other words, how does the organism distinguish what happens to him from what he makes happen? In Von Holst's conceptualization are included many clues relating intention, perception, consciousness, etc.

personality, especially to improvement of the integration of its component parts—its coherence? In the early 1950s the way the organization of a child's character became established was attributed largely to the effect of the maternal character on the actual caretaking interactions of a mother with her child. The above question, stimulated by speculations about the therapeutic process, could be as easily asked about the developmental process: How do the events in the rearing interaction influence the organization or coherence of the child's personality in the first place? Might there be basic processes by which interpersonal interaction influences organizing functions in the human that are common to both levels of inquiry? Much theory revolves around the role of "object relationships" in this process, and synthesizing conceptualizations[3] have outlined the major steps in the development of object relationships, not at all a simple concept in itself. However, in the early 1950s few had looked in any systematic way at any appreciable sample of individuals for the actual course of events taking place between mother and infant over the first few years.

A Longitudinal Naturalistic Perspective of Interaction Between Infant and Mother

It seems now purely a stroke of good fortune that shortly after I had completing training in child psychiatry at the Judge Baker Guidance Center and the J. J. Putnam Children's Center, Dr. Eleanor Pavenstedt invited me to join her group as a research psychiatrist. The opportunity to participate in a detailed naturalistic study of the early mother–child relationship was a most fortunate beginning for my experience in developmental research and is only part of the larger debt that I owe to Dr. Pavenstedt. It was in 1954, some time after she had founded the Boston University Child Guidance Clinic, that the longitudinal study entitled, "The Effect of Maternal Maturity and Immaturity on Child Development" (Pavenstedt et al., 1954) was launched under her direction. The aim of the project was primarily to contribute to clinical child psychiatry. Its hypotheses reflected an awareness of and a commitment to holistic issues in a conceptualization of organization in developing personality. For example, one of the hypotheses of the project proposed "that the degree to which a mother perceives and interacts with her child as an 'individual in its own right' will correlate directly with the level of maturity of her personality and with the level of maturity reached by her child at six," (each of these clusters being defined in terms of variables described on the observational level).

The effort to document such a proposal one way or the other gives evidence of the clinician's confidence that he can make inferences from a synthesis of clinical material, as well as evidence of a certain aplomb in confronting the

---

[3] See Erikson (1950) et al., Hartman et al. (1946), Mahler, (1968), and Spitz (1959).

many levels of inference involved. This effort also illustrates again the essential place of synthesis in the attitude of the clinical-therapeutic approach to the psychiatric enterprise. Synthesis, after all, may not be a pitfall to be skirted in the name of science but the very essence of that which we seek to understand in early developmental research.

A brief description of this initial naturalistic longitudinal project is given here as a background for discussion of the work that led from it:

Beyond the documentation of a natural history, the groundwork of a body of data was laid, which made it possible to ask specific questions of the role of developing object relationship in the ensuing organization of the child's personality. The design of subject groups, the systematic schedule of observations, tests, and interviews, and the guiding hypotheses made this possible. The subjects consisted of 30 primiparous mothers, meeting basic criteria for normality. There were selected during their second and third trimesters of pregnancy from a general hospital prenatal clinic over a three-year period. The selection was on the basis of closeness of agreement of a detailed characterologic assessment of each with one of three maternal character profiles which had been drawn up to represent the most mature, the most immature, and a middle group. It was expected that the contrasting behaviors exhibited in child-rearing by these three different groups of mothers would provide an empirical basis for studying the relationships between events experienced by a child and features of his or her character at an outcome point, namely, the first year at school or the sixth year of life. It was considered that *outcome* in the development of a personality organization in the child could not be judged from empirical data before such organization had sufficiently consolidated. Therefore, the guiding hypotheses of the study, which related maternal character variables, interactional variables, and variables defined for the child's characterological development at six, were proposed *only* in terms of an outcome to be assessed during the child's first year at school. The application of hypotheses to the data depended on detailed definition of both maternal and child character variables in terms of empirical criteria derived from behavioral observation and clinical experience.

As has been pointed out, the investigation of relationships by this method is a type of clinical research, depending on the synthesis of evidence and depending on a level of inference by which psychoanalytic concepts can be applied in categorizing and assembling empirical data. A feature of a longitudinal study such as this, which is one of its greatest strengths, is that its repeated observations at different times and under a variety of circumstances can provide the data from which such inference reasonably can be drawn. The redundant and consistent becomes apparent, as does any deviation, once a trend has become established in the data.

A most intensive schedule of data collection was carried out, with remarkably little missing data, by a multidisciplinary team, which numbered as many as 15 at one point. The contacts were spaced at regular intervals every two to four weeks for the three to four years during which the most intensive sequential data collection was carried out. Beside the variety of contacts, and their regular repetition, upon which we relied to provide a fair picture of the child and his or her relationships in different situations and environments, objectivity was enhanced by: 1) Tape recordings of interviews, which followed an associative anamnesis in the first half-hour and a standard sequence of items in the second; 2) Three standardized observational situations consisting of well-baby examinations, developmental tests, and play interviews; 3) The use of multiple observers (one for mother's behavior, one for child's behavior and one for the running sequence); 4) Pre-defined observational categories.

Although it had been designed and initiated as a 10-year investigation with hypotheses relevant only to an outcome at age six, the entire project was terminated approximately at its midpoint, when necessary further funding could not be obtained. Completed data had been collected on some 22 subjects over the first 36 to 40 months of life with consistent data on the remaining 8 only through the first 1½ to 2½ years of life. Needless to say, the transcription of all tape-recorded interviews, dictated observations, home visits, and testings, examinations, play interviews, etc., resulted in voluminous data on each pair, which although remarkably encompassing became equally difficult to organize, reduce, analyze, and communicate. The problem remaining in 1959, then, was to analyze these data without the hypotheses, part of the design, or any of the outcome data. Nevertheless the struggle with this problem provided most of the incentive for the research that has followed. Although we could not know at the time, by dint of the rather enormous personal effort of Dr. Pavenstedt and her colleagues, later on a detailed outcome observation[4] was carried out anyway over the first year at school for the 22 subjects having the most complete early data.

In salvaging the extraordinarily rich documentation of interaction and development over the first three years of life, we felt we should at least communicate something of the striking range of behaviors we had encountered in the rearing observed in our three subject groups. In making comparisons we wanted to stay at the level of observed behavior in mother–infant interaction. But short of 30 case histories, how could these essential differences be defined and compared systematically from one mother–infant pair to the other over a three-year span? What were the salient variables and how were they to be related over time?

As a solution at least for communicating the essential clinical differences between the courses followed by the different infant–mother pairs—we formulated an epigenetic sequence of the adaptive issues negotiated over the first three years in the interactions between each mother and infant. The sequence was common to all pairs, but the actual behaviors, through which the adaptive adjustments were carried out, were idiosyncratic (Sander, 1962, 1964).

The sequence and its rationale represented the interweaving of ideas about the adaptive process from a wide variety of sources—from the work of others and from our own experience of interviewing mothers and observing their interactions with their babies. The basic perspective was the biological viewpoint of the living organism: from the cell upward, living organisms are actively self-regulating and, at the same time, of necessity exist in a continuous intimate exchange with essential support factors provided by the surround. There is an obvious polarity inherent in this view: attention to either cannot

---

[4] This research was supported by the Supreme Council of the Scottish Rite.

be given at the expense of the other. There are mechanisms of active self-regulation and there are essential factors whose source is provided by a surround.
The content of behavior must be accounted for in a specific context.

A most useful resolution of this polarity rests on cybernetic theory. The
information—processing model is applied to the adaptation between the self-
organizing components—the infant and the mother—and the adapted state
then consists of a relatively harmonious coordination between them, consistent
with the conditions for existence of each. With one component, the infant,
rapidly growing and consequently rapidly changing, new qualities and quantities of infant behavior are constantly being introduced into the content of
interaction. The regulation of infant functions, based on behaviors that have
become harmoniously coordinated between mother and infant, will become
perturbed with the advent of each new, and usually more specifically focused
and intentionally initiated, activity of the growing infant. Thus adaptation or
mutual modification on a new level is required. Since the behavioral innova-
tions by the infant are often aimed at a progressive assumption of control of
situations as a part of the widening of his scope of self-regulation *vis-à-vis* the
environment (i.e., he becomes more vigorously alloplastic), these changes im-
pinge critically on the mother's long-established strategies of self-regulation
(i.e., especially strategies for the control of extrinsic variables as a means of
regulating her own intrinsic variables). The interactional picture is best organized in terms of the epigenetic sequence in which this progression of
relative coordinations is achieved.

The levels that represent this sequence on the basis of empirical data were
selected from the experience of interviewing the mothers regularly and
systematically over the first three years of their participation in the longitudinal study. It became apparent that each mother was experiencing times of
relatively greater worry and stress, which were then followed by times of relatively greater harmony in her role as a mother. After we had followed 10 or 15
of the mothers, we could even begin to predict, for a given age, the area of
stress or the area of success the mother might report. A perspective emerged,
and a relatively simple sequence of the usual course of interactional events[5]

[5] It should be kept in mind that this is an account of interaction and is not intended as a summary
of developmental steps. Furthermore, any *interactional* sequence will be seen to parallel the
developmental sequences proposed by others, e.g., Mahler (1968). These will be touched upon
briefly below and referred to in part; it should be evident, however, that within the scope of this
paper a comprehensive cross-referencing cannot be undertaken. The interaction is between a
growing infant who has arrived with a particular endowment in regard to the regulation of its
functions and a maternal character whose various facets will reveal themselves at different points
as the infant differentiates new capabilities for determining his actions. The sequence illustrates a
progressive differentiation, on the part of both the mother and the infant, of behaviors constituting their exchanges—a progressive differentiation of increasing complexity. The fact that a sequence of adaptive issues between mother and infant was proposed primarily as a way of organizing observational material for analysis, does not mean an unawareness of or disinterest in
the contribution of other figures (e.g., fathers) or other influences in the child's interpersonal environment.

TABLE 1
Adaptive Issues Negotiated in Interaction between Infant and Caretaker

Issue	Title	Span of months	Prominent infant behavior that became coordinated with maternal activities
I	Initial regulation	Months 1–3	Basic infant activities concerned with biological processes related to feeding, sleeping, elimination, postural maintenance, etc., including stimulus needs for quieting and arousal.
II	Reciprocal exchange	Months 4–6	Smiling behavior that extends to full motor and vocal involvement in sequences of affectively spontaneous back-and-forth exchanges. Activities of spoon feeding, dressing, etc., become reciprocally coordinated.
III	Initiative	Months 7–9	Activities initiated by infant to secure a reciprocal social exchange with mother or to manipulate environment on his own selection.
IV	Focalization	Months 10–13	Activities by which infant determines the availability of mother on his specific initiative. Tends to focalize need-meeting demands on the mother.
V	Self-assertion	Months 14–20	Activities in which infant widens the determination of his own behavior, often in the face of maternal opposition.
VI	Recognition	Months 18–36	Activities (including language) that express perceptions of own state, intentions, and thought content.
VII	Continuity (conservation of self as active organizer)	Months 18–36	Activities rupturing and restoring coordination on an intentional level. (Intended and directed aggressive behavior in equilibrium with directed initiations aimed at facilitating restoration of interactional concordance.)

could be consolidated. The sequence is listed in Table 1 with the time span in the longitudinal course over which it was most usual for the adaptation to occur.

For evaluation of the data collected, each of the adaptive levels listed was worded as an open-ended question, an "issue"[6] to be negotiated between infant and caretaker, which represented the degree to which harmonious coordination was reached by the pair in relation to the interactional behaviors designated for that level and over the time span indicated.

Issue I: Basic Regulation

In the first three months of life the mother's worries usually concern the problem of establishing, by her caretaking procedures, a regulation of the basic functions of her infant, such as feeding, sleeping, and elimination, so that they become both relatively predictable and relatively comfortable for her as well as harmonious with the household. Effects during this time appear to be bidirectional or reciprocal—infant on mother and mother on infant—with changes or modifications of behavior mutually conforming. An initial, reciprocally chained contingency consists of change of infant-state–caretaker intervention and *vice versa*. The "state" of the infant represents a first level of synthesis of coherence within the multiple physiological subsystems of the infant and is characterized by periodicity or rhythmicity. This suggests that influences modifying state regulation in the neonate obey rubrics that determine phase control of biologic rhythms. Phase synchrony between mother and infant in regard to the periodicities of relative activity and quiescence of each represent a second level of synthesis, now within the regulatory system instead of the individual. One of the features most idiosyncratic during the first three months is the extent to which the infant is helped or compromised in beginning to determine aspects of his own regulation. On the part of the mother trial-and-error learning gives way to ideas of what "works" and to the feeling of confidence that she now *knows* her baby's needs and can specifically meet them, while not jeopardizing her own needs and the remaining obligations of her day.

Issue II: Reciprocal Activation

The second three months—fourth, fifth, and sixth—are usually a period of relative delight, in which reciprocal behavior and reciprocal conformity be-

[6] For each issue several categories of items were individually rated as evidence for or against the adaptation and the degree of harmonious adjustment that had been reached. All evidence that could be discovered in the record both for and against was extracted and drawn on in the evaluation of the items. Agreement between independent analysts on the evaluation of such major trends, when taken in these large time blocks and based on extensive and repeated documentation, is not impossibly difficult (Sander, 1969).

come more differentiated and actively directed by each. The mother develops active social reciprocations with her infant around the spontaneous development of smiling play. Both come to participate in this with delight and mounting expressions of exuberance as the period wears on. It is proposed that the affect of joy and delight, as a concomitant of reciprocal social chaining, is established here as the criterion indexing the occurrence of an interpersonal "fitting together." The total and vigorous involvement of the infant's voluntary motor system as part of heightened social play represents a new and additional mechanism of behavioral integration for the infant in relation to affect. At the same time the principal activities of caretaking, such as diapering, dressing, or the beginning of spoon feeding, are being accomplished more and more through active reciprocal coordination of the actions of each. Anyone who has tried to feed a five-month-old his cereal knows the coordination it involves—and the effort needed by each to achieve it. The emergent active, and for the most part now voluntarily controlled, contributions of the infant to the organization of behavioral configurations are here carried out in relation to direct and immediate coordinations with the actual motor configurations of the mother, rather than, as somewhat later on, accomplished as a consummation of intrinsically held, goal-directed schemes.

Issue III: Infant Initiative

The third three months—the seventh, eighth, and ninth—find the infant expressing increasingly clear, independent, directed initiative of his own to explore the world as his motor apparatus develops and creeping is possible. It is assumed that what is appearing here, at the time of emergence of object constancy (in Piaget's sensorimotor theory), is the beginning guidance of behavior by inner imagery. The strength of intentionality or goal-directedness in guiding action here first becomes recognizable at times when exploratory aims are blocked. The mother experiences a first *active* bifurcation in the direction of the child's initiative: toward her, or away from her.[7] This early level of active independent organization of his world often meets a very basic ambivalence in the mother. The baby's activity can be interpreted as aggressive, rejecting, or naughty on the one hand, or precocious, gratifying, and stimulating on the other, with consequent patterns of reinforcement or interference becoming characteristic for the pair.

[7] The emergence of an initial level of autonomy from a previously more "symbiotic" relationship has been described by Mahler (1968) as the "hatching" process. The relationship of these interactional levels to the phases of autism, symbiosis, and separation-individuation proposed by Mahler involves a somewhat different perspective from which the progress of change in behavioral organization over these time spans also can be viewed. The relevance of one of these perspectives to the other would require extensive additional discussion, which is not possible in this paper.

The presence of a basic 24-hour state regulation in the infant, maintained by already stabilized and adapted exchanges with the caretaking environment at this age level, should permit a relative "disjoin"[8] of the active exploratory initiative of the infant. The already-adapted exchanges need no longer come into the arena of interactional modifications. On the other hand, in the presence of instability in infant states or in the caretaking environment, there would be a tendency of regulatory needs to preempt the infant's action in the service of restoring the stability of basic functions.

Issue IV: Focalization

Over months 10, 11, 12, and 13 the advent of locomotion and the extension of the capacity to direct one's own activity and express specific intentions by it sets up the opportunity for the child to settle the extent to which his mother is available to him. This is an availability as a specific response to the child's bid—not just care in general. It begins the intended manipulation of a person now, instead of an object, and is associated with a potential widening of the bifurcation of directions of reinforcement or interference begun in the previous issue.

One mother will be gratified by this special knowledge of her baby's needs for her and her capacity to act specifically on them. Another mother experiences the child's directed and more specific, intended demands at this time as exceedingly threatening—something to be escaped from or defended against. The ambivalent availability of the mother, which may have been subtly evidenced earlier, may now be dramatized openly as her limits begin to be set. If her limits are consistent and constructive, we find the mother has a certain confidence that even if she yields to her child, the child will eventually turn away from her to wider horizons of his own. The pressure the child exerts at this time varies with the ambivalence of the mother in responding to him. If her availability is certain, he can turn to greater novelties; if she tries to run away, he is demanding; if she reacts to threat by aggression, his demand may provoke her attack or her surrender. Thus is illustrated the im-

[8] In Ashby's model (1952) "disjoin" represents the temporary and semi-independence (i.e., partial or relative independence) of a subsystem, which is made possible by a rich network of constancies in the system. Inasmuch as over these months there appears to be a rather exquisite sensitivity of the infant to inhibition by the mother, there should be an advantage to the infant if his active exploratory function of building sensori motor schemata is not too "richly joined" to basic physiological regulation, insuring that the effect of a mismatch does not become catastrophic. It may be that the basic physiological implications of experiencing a "mismatch" may be determined by the level of "disjoin" or exploratory functions over this chronological period. Failure of a rich network of constancies through this period to permit such a disjoin perhaps accounts for the significance of the "depressive position" in the dynamics proposed for this period (Winnicott, 1954). The relevance of Ashby's model is made clearer in Glassman (1973), "Persistence and Loose Coupling in Living Systems."

portance of a concept of balance or equilibrium for negotiating the levels of adaptation.

This extension of scheme building to an active manipulation of the mother as a total person occurs at the close of the first year. In the first year of life maternal responsivity has traditionally been viewed as experienced by the infant in terms of whatever particular need was in ascendancy at the moment—the "part object." This state of affairs may eventuate in a "fragmentation" of object relations, if this unifying issue of "focalization" is not adequately negotiated. Thus we encounter another of the multiplicity of mechanisms by which synthesis or integration is effected when developmental change is viewed from the perspective of adaptive behavior in an infant–caretaker system.

The successful negotiation of a reasonable set of conditions for, and of limits to, a predictable availability of the mother has appeared from the study of our material to be closely associated with a *preservation* of the same basic affect of delight that has marked interpersonal "fitting together" since issue II. Depending on adequate negotiation of the issue of focalization, the same affect becomes available for the next in sequence, namely the turning of investment and attention to widening mastery of the world beyond the mother.

Issue V: Self-Assertion

In the 14–20-month period there emerges a new capacity of the child to organize his world actively, to assert himself, and to widen his initiative to determine and select his own direction of activity. The child's aim at this time often seems to be to possess the initiative for its own sake. When his directions tend to run counter to the mother's wishes or the household rules, the issue is raised of the degree to which or the areas in which this assertion will be successful. There appears to be a shift in the content of the toddler's awareness during this time, and he becomes more sensitive to various visual and auditory stimuli and to events within his own body. Spitz (1957) has proposed that during this period the toddler has a heightened awareness of his own intentions; at the same time his wishes are being restricted as part of the imposition of rules and the constraints of socializations. Spitz associates this process with the emergence of the "I" experience.

The child's initiative, obviously, is not *all* in a direction away from or contrary to the mother but is balanced by bids for reciprocation with *her*. The probability of success for the latter he has been determining in the previous issue, a probability that now provides the context in which he can pursue his own inner intentions and the independent plan of action stemming from them. This pursuit extends the bifurcation of direction of investment toward and away from the mother begun in issue III. The heretofore relatively coherent progression of adaptations based on the differentiation of new levels of coordination with the mother through the reinforcement of matching reciprocations with her is now complicated by gratification and reinforcement arising from the successful realization of the toddler's own inner idiosyncratic intention, goals, and plans of action. It will be seen at once that if the previous reinforcement and gratification have been connected with the achievement of a reciprocal exchange with the mother, we are now encountering a new phenomenon. The appearance of success and gratification begins to become evident as the infant maintains his own inner aims even if they are in opposition to rather than in reciprocation with the mother. In other words, guidance of behavior on the basis of the pleasure of realizing inner aims can take precedence at times over the more familiar (pleasurable) reinforcement of finding a coordination with the parental caretaker. Whereas before this period the child has reacted to separation as an upsetting event, now he himself initiates separation, both physical and psychological. The importance of a stable basic regulation has to do with a context in which the child can begin dimly to recognize his own role in determining action, i.e., that he is pursuing his *own* intention rather than reacting to a lead. The emergence of autonomy as here proposed is based on the further differentiation of awareness—especially that of inner perception, which sets the stage for the "disjoin" of the self-regulatory core. The next two issues are particularly concerned with this process.

Issue VI: Recognition

At the beginning of the second year of life and over approximately the same time span as the previous step, the other side of the bifurcation becomes evident as the rapid development of secondary-process functions heralds a new level of increasingly differentiated communication between infant and mother. Speech and the child's capability of predictably communicating inner experience and intentions so they can be read by the empathetic mother make possible a confirmation for the child of his inner perceptions in an actual exchange. This is communication based on a new level of inner awareness rather than the sensorimotor level of physical objects or of direct encounter. The development of speech is a necessary condition for interactions that can now idiosyncratically and specifically convey the child's experience of his own feelings, his fantasies, his play objectives, etc.[9]

The issue here is how much the mother and child will develop and broaden their reciprocal coordinations on this level, especially in the face of the

[9] The relevance of issues VI and VII to Mahler's (1968) rapprochement subphase and the establishment of "libidinal object constancy" is that the two issues are constructed here as a concurrent polarity necessary for a "decentering formulation" in the structuring of constancy of self as a framework for subsequent self-regulation. These points will be taken up to some extent below.

disharmony consequent to this issue of self-assertion and the subsequent related behaviors of directed aggression, which will be described in the following step. The stimulus to develop a new level of communication may arise in part from its success in maintaining reinforcement through reciprocity with the mother on a new level of symbolic representation and language, while the older, sensorimotor avenues of interaction now become involved in the disruptive encounters.

The label we have given to this aspect of the sequence of adaptive coordinations in the progression of mother–infant interactions is *recognition*. It gives ascendancy to a new level of awareness in negotiating adaptation for both mother and toddler. The experience of coordination (here matching of a particular communication between partners) must constitute a first level in the experience of self-recognition, namely, realization that another can be aware of what one is aware of within oneself, i.e., a shared awareness. It is assumed that this level marks the beginning potential for awareness of a self-organizing core within—actually a core that from the outset has been operative in the service of regulation at the more biological level but is now in a position to be accorded a new priority in the guidance of behavior. Thus, while the progression of interactions can be looked on as belonging to an ontogeny of regulation, it involves and even may in part rest upon an ontogeny of awareness. Negotiation of this issue sets the stage for the establishment through the next step in the epigenetic sequence of continuity or constancy in the content of self-recognition (self-constancy being analogous to the object constancy of Piaget's sensorimotor theory).

The importance of this phase for later adaptive flexibility in the personality is that self schemata cannot be modified without, at least for a time, an access to perception or awareness. Further, the achievement of a basic capacity for eventual self-recognition provides a basis for a sense of *continuity* in the human organism. This permits relatively greater independence from variation in outer or environmental regularities, upon which organisms at a more primitive level depends for stability.

Issue VII: Continuity or "Self" Constancy

In the latter half of the second year the bifurcation in the progression of interactions with the mother widens with the appearance of a new quality in aggressive and destructive behavior.[10] This is a quality of directedness and

[10] Again it must be recalled that this framework has been derived from data collected from a particular white urban population at a particular point in social change affecting this particular population. It was our impression that every step in the impact of the multiple potentials inherent in the maternal character eventually is acted out in clear and decisive behavior in interaction with her toddler. Thus the transmission of maternal "dynamics" in actual behavior is not a mystery if one has access to a sufficiently detailed longitudinal picture, suggesting an approach to the adaptive specificity that Wallerstein (1973) has called for in understanding developmental organization of ego.

intentionality in these behaviors, which up to this time have been seen usually as more immediately reactive to frustration or externally imposed conditions. Now they appear elective and initiated by the child in directed and provocative moves, often at some time removed from the defining of a rule or "don't"— most often first toward objects of the material environment and then toward the mother in the testing of an intended interpersonal encounter.

The restoration of a previously adapted equilibrium between toddler and caretaker environment, which has been perturbed by the child's new capacity to carry out intentionally destructive and directed acts of aggression, provides the condition necessary for a key experience of "reversal" in regard to self-constancy. The intentional disruption of previously reinforcing and facilitating exchanges with the caretaker disrupts the toddler's newly consolidating self and body representational framework. Reexperience of his own coherence, again at his own initiative or by outreach from the caretaker, provides a situation from which "self" constancy as an inner structure can be established. An interactional equilibrium in the infant–caretaker system is critical in terms both of providing the experience of the taking of a contrary position and of still providing the experience of specific recognition by the familiar caretaker when the intention resumes to restore facilitating reciprocation again. The necessity for reversibility in establishing self-constancy on the basis of "self-schemata" as "operations," in Piaget's sense, gives a rationale for some of the child's employment of directed destructive or aggressive behavior in the second 18 months of life. Should the caretaker be unable to differentiate or fail to aid in restoring the facilitating self as the toddler had previously experienced it, the toddler's own familiar "good self" as a constant frame of reference would be impaired. In conceptualizing this issue as related to and immediately following issue VI, we envisioned the process as paralleling the notion of reversal in Piaget's sensorimotor theory, whereby operations become abstracted from action and thus freed for new combinations in thought.[11] The self-representation as a scheme has been discussed by Sandler and Rosenblatt (1962) and in this issue can be considered as gaining abstraction and thus mobility as an operation. Self as active initiator or as active organizer is thus "conserved."

The difference between mother–infant pairs in the way such directed intentional aggression was handled was striking in the range of tolerance to intolerance of any such testing. The ambivalent mother, who is in considerable doubt about setting her limits, permits more than another, but eventually she too comes to the point of standing her ground, usually by an angry display long overdue. After this, if the prior step has been negotiated, there follows an

---

[11] This has been suggested by Spitz (1957); "The achievement of the faculty of judgment on the level of the capacity to signify 'no,' either by gesturing or by word will be found to correspond to the achievement of reversibility in terms of Piaget's Theory (1936) [p. 144]."

abating of the intensity and frequency of elective and provocative clashes with her.

An issue depending on experiences of "reversal" in establishing self-constancy, and introduced by the new capacity for directed aggression, may or may not be negotiated. The longitudinal data lead us to believe that optimally there may be an age-appropriate span to which this consolidation is limited. After 30–36 months the child becomes increasingly able to anticipate and consequently to *conceal* inner content that has been so ingenuously revealed in the expression of his intentions and wants between 15 and 30 months, associated at that time with an awareness shared between infant and caretaker via expectations held in common by both. After this age level, concealment (and "defense") renders inaccessible, even to the child himself, the awareness providing a relatedness between the elements necessary for this essential step.

This sequence of levels constructs an *ontogeny of interactive regulation* in the infant caretaker system, at each level involving new elements that represent integrations of old accomplishments epigenetically. The sequence suggests as well as ontogeny of awareness, the characteristics of which are becoming organized through the sequence of adaptations. As increasing numbers of elements enter the repertoire of coordinated behaviors and expectancies and constitute new contexts for action, even finer discriminations become targets of exploration and scheme formation and are drawn into the interactive regulatory process. Research contributions to an ontogeny of awareness have already begun in investigations based on the use of the novelty or surprise reaction in early infancy (Bower, 1972; Charlesworth, 1964) or the focusing of attention (a major means of regulating motility even in the neonate), especially the patterns of attentive focus developing in the exchanges between infant and caretaker (Stern, 1971). Piaget (1973) has commented on the role of both conscious and unconscious aspects of early cognitive development, basing this theoretical position of the relationship of consciousness in scheme formation to the assumption, which he attributes to Claparede, that it is mismatch that provokes arousal and conscious experience. This is essentially the same notion as that proposed by others also (e.g., Hunt, 1961; Von Holst, 1950).

In tracing the extension of sensorimotor scheme-building of the infant in interaction with his caretaking environment, we have followed the emergence of his increasingly clear intentionality. Spitz (1957) suggests that this sets the stage for the emergence of the self at around 15 months of age in terms of the toddler's perception (awareness) of his own intention during the restriction of his volitional execution of his intended aims, an experience frequent at 15 months. Certainly the perception of, or inference of, direction of intentionality continues to play a major role in the regulations of interpersonal behavior. In the concept of the emergence of the self framework[12] as an essential self-regulatory mechanism in the second 18 months of life, much remains to be clarified regarding access to awareness, particularly the relationships between "inner" perception and feedback to expectations or goal-directed activity, i.e., the child's synthesizing of readouts of his own state as *context* and goal-directed activities as *content*.

Recapitulation and Summary of Issues

The *first* issue, in which coordination between activities of infant and caretaker takes place (months 1, 2, and 3), is the level of the basic regulation of infant states. Idiosyncrasies in the organization of the self-regulatory characteristics of each partner demand a certain specificity in the modifications necessary for achieving harmonious reciprocal coordination, with wide variation to be found in different infant–caretaker pairs in the role accorded infant cues in determining the adaptation.

The *second* issue (months 4, 5, and 6) concerns the timed "fitting together" of the more active, voluntarily directed reciprocal behaviors characteristic of social (smiling) play and of the caretaking interactions of this period (e.g., diapering, bathing, and feeding of solids). The affect of joy or delight becomes established as a criterion for precision in the matching of interpersonal reciprocations.

The *third* issue of coordinations (months 7, 8, and 9) concerns the adjustments between infant and caretaker necessary to accommodate the more active initiation by the infant of the now more evidently intentional, goal-directed activities and the rapid acquisition of a widening repertoire of motor skills. Patterns of facilitation and interference (i.e., regulation) of infant initiative and intentionality become defined.

The *fourth* issue in which interaction must be coordinated between infant and caretaker (months 10–13) concerns the extension of the manipulatory activities of the infant from the area concerned with material objects to one concerned with active, intentionally directed manipulation of the responses of persons, especially the caretaker. The extent of availability of the caretaker's response to an intentional bid of the infant is being determined and is thus, in the usual mothering situation, determining the extent to which and the conditions under which the chief regulatory element of the infant's environment, namely, the caretaker, can come within his repertoire of active self-regulatory schemata.

The *fifth* issue (months 14–20), at the time of new gains in locomotor freedom, requires adjustment between infant and caretaker in terms of those

---

[12] See Spiegel (1959); also for his review of the self in relation to psychoanalytic metapsychological considerations.

new self-assertive behaviors of the infant deliberately (intentionally) initiated against the wishes and limitations of the caretaker. The restriction to volition at this time appears to be associated with an especially keen awareness of the intention, or inner motivational state, that is being frustrated.

The *sixth* issue (extending over the second 18 months of life) concerns coordinations achieved on the level of newly appearing "secondary-process" functions in the toddler, of representation and expression, stemming from his "inner" perception of his own intentions and his own state, his own fantasies or wishes, etc., and depending heavily on the development of language for communicability. In the "fitting together" at this level, the toddler can experience that another is aware of what he is aware of within himself, providing an experience of personal recognition in a shared awareness and possibly facilitating a consequent capacity for self-recognition. Relatively stable infant–mother coordination at this level provides a context in which basic strategies can become established, allowing the child to use this awareness of "inner" events to guide his own behavior.

The *seventh* issue, paralleling the previous issue in time (the second 18 months of life), concerns the adjustment being made in regard to directly provocative, aggressive, and destructive behavior. The dimensions of the affect of anger in the caretaker environment come in for active exploration, exposing the toddler's self framework, which is being consolidated in issue VI, to disruption. Restoration can be initiated by either the toddler or the caretaker, but it is proposed that (reciprocal) coordination at this level provides essential experiences of continuity of the self framework, especially when the toddler's interaction is in the context of his being in, or taking, a contrary position *vis-à-vis* the caretaker.

Conceptualizations of Adaptive Behavior

The rationale for proposing an epigenetic sequence of interactional adaptations as an approach to the understanding of emerging character organization is suggested by a number of widely different sources. These sources can be but briefly touched upon here. They are intended as a stimulus for the reader's reflection on the sequence of interactional issues and on the relevance of an adaptive model. Behavioral details of interpersonal interaction can be ordered by such a model and hypotheses suggested that relate idiosyncrasies of adaptation with idiosyncrasies of character organization. This is not intended as a comprehensive review of relevant literature but includes only a most limited selection from those sources that have contributed to this viewpoint.

From the psychoanalytic point of view, Erikson's (1950, 1959) proposal of an epigenetic sequence of adaptations through mutual and reciprocal adjustments between infant and caretaking environment was the basis of his concept of a sequence of stages in personality development. This contribution opened a whole new vista for the conceptualization of mechanisms responsible for "ego" development. Basically the sequence of adaptations proposed in our work can be seen as merely filling in the smaller details of Erikson's first two issues of basic trust and autonomy, and as implementing his basic plan[13] of adaptive behavior in a biologic system, in which we discern four basic assumptions.

1. A lawful relationship connects the actual characteristics of behavior of the interactors in the infant–caretaking situation and the organizing of certain features of the child's personality during that time.

2. There is a balance between the polarities constraining the interaction, with a crucial alternative or "issue" for each stage determining the direction of the outcome and settled by decisive encounter.

3. In the history-dependence of the organic system a generalization of early, more specific adaptive strategies later on broadly underlies the biases of ensuing adaptations (e.g., organ mode to social modality).

4. With increasing complexity consequent to growth and differentiation, there are necessary corresponding capabilities maintaining a coherence or unity of the individual—i.e., "ego identity" and, later on, "integrity." Just what mechanisms underlie these capabilities has been of central interest.

The interactional, adaptive framework is only a leaf taken from the biologist's notebook. The biological literature is the major source of data and the conceptualizations of adaptive mechanisms in systems consisting of components in exchange. Adaptation most basically can be envisioned as being determined by mechanisms related to maintenance of the regulation of functions of each partner. The *bonding* between the interacting components, which keeps them exchanging as an enduring system, stems from the requirement that regulation of the intrinsic processes of each be provided by the properties and activities of the other. In other words, on the simplest level exchange (interaction) is determined by a requirement for regulation. One of the perspectives that the biological approach provides is that the concept of the "unity of the organism" relates to an organism functioning in its proper environment, i.e., its situation of evolutionary adaptation. A major difficulty in conceptualizing at the psychological level arises from a tendency to view the organization of behavior as the property of the individual rather than as the property of the more inclusive system of which the individual is a part.

The notion of an epigenesis in adaptive behaviors within a biological system has been elaborated from the viewpoint of embryologists, for example, in the work of Bertalanffy (1952), and Weiss (1949). The former, a principle architect of "systems" theory, has pointed out that from the most primitive

---

[13] Also see Spitz (1959).

level upward, two features characterize all matter that can be said to be living, namely, "primary activity" and "organization." Adaptation cannot be conceived of adequately as a simple matter of cause and effect, stimulus and response, or the passive enduring of proximity. The living machine must be considered as already running, the complexly governed interactions with its support system already being specified as the conditions for the living state.

At the cellular level Weiss (1949) explored the neuroembryological mechanisms of adaptation governing the relations between the central and peripheral components of the nervous system and formulated the viewpoint of adaptation that has been the most useful. His definition (1969) of a *system* in the sense in which it is being used here clarifies a number of points:

> Pragmatically defined, a system is a rather circumscribed complex of relatively bounded phenomena, which within these bounds, retains a *relatively* stationary pattern of structure in space or of sequential configurations in time in spite of a high degree of variability in details of distribution and interrelations among its constituent units of lower order. Not only does the system maintain its configuration and integral operation in an essentially constant environment, but it responds to alterations of the environment by an adaptive redirection of its componental processes in such a manner as to counter the external change in the direction of optimum preservation of its systemic integrity. . . . The complex is a system if the variance of the features of the whole collective is significantly less than the sum of variances of its constituents. . . . In short, the basic characteristic of a system is its essential invariance beyond the much more variant flux and fluctuations of its elements of constituents. By implication this signifies that the elements, although by no means single-tracked as in a mechanical device, are subject to restraints of their degrees of freedom so as to yield a resultant in the direction of maintaining the optimum stability of the collective. The terms "coordination," "control" and the like, are merely synonymous labels for this principle [pp. 11–12].

And in relation to the central thread of this essay, one might add the term *integration.*

From the vast contribution of investigations in the areas of ethology and animal behavior have come a number of widely inclusive perspectives of interactive regulatory mechanisms constituting adaptive behavior in the organism–environment system and relevant to both phylogeny and ontogeny (e.g., Hinde, 1966, Uexküll, 1934). The most relevant work of T. C. Schneirla (1959) and his colleagues has seemed to be their study of the mechanisms by which "ontogeny progressively frees processes of individual motivation from the basic formula of prepotent stimulative intensity relationships." (See also Rosenblatt et al., 1961.)

Cybernetics and its offshoot, information-processing theory, have provided a body of more formalized conceptualization by which the adaptive and self-organizing behavior of biological systems can be represented. This formalized conceptualization has been of enormous influence in bringing a wide range of phenomena under simplifying propositions that model much of the apparent complexity of the living process:

One of the basic notions is that the system possesses inner criteria to which new inputs are matched. A certain "error signal" results if there is a mismatch. This activates effector apparatus which can then carry out activities to reduce the error signal. If these activities repeatedly require certain modifications necessary to achieve a match (e.g., on encountering consistent features of the environment) the modifications become part of the inner criteria. The criterion (or schema) then comes to represent the organism–environment relationship more precisely. Miller, et al. (1960), have expressed these points in their concept of the TOTE unit as the basic unit of behavior. The cogency of the information processing model for the developmental process has been suggested by D. MacKay (1956). He proposes that an inner criterion on which an error signal is based must itself have an ontogeny, differentiating more specifically from earlier more global routines. The information-processing model provides a means of visualizing the organization of self-modifying system, which can take a changing relation to environment into account in terms of changes within itself as it maintains goal direction. In his application of the model to an understanding of neurophysiology and especially the regulatory function of the brain stem, Pribram (1963) emphasizes the optimal response of the system when such changes take place relatively slowly and by small increments. This provides an optimal "error signal" to which the system is best suited to respond. The concept of an error signal optimal for acquisition of new behavioral schemata sheds further light on the picture we have drawn of regulation and its relation to the sequence of interactional issues.

The governing in biologic systems is in large part carried out through cybernetic or feedback control in which part of the output is fed back as input to the system, and, in terms of its match or mismatch with a criterion governs ensuing output. Such systems tend to oscillate and are usually in a continuing cycle of variation requiring constant input to maintain the limits congenial to any enduring existence of the system. This input can be provided by a second cybernetic system so a given state in one system provides the criterion for the control of the other, each system then setting a bias on the other, locked, so to speak, in a reciprocating or phase-synchronized relationship (Sander, 1969).

Contributions of cybernetic theory and the information-processing model to the problem of adaptive and integrative mechanisms have been suggested by a wide variety of investigators (e.g., Bowlby, 1969; Von Holst and Mittelstaedt, 1950). Hunt (1961) has provided a most comprehensive perspective of the relevance of the information-processing model in organizing data that relate early experience to cognitive development and especially to the conceptualizations of Piaget. In 1965 Hunt broadened this perspective in stating his theory of intrinsic motivation and proposing its role in psychological development. In this theory he suggests a three-stage epigenetic development of intrinsic motivation in the infant.

Piaget (1936) anticipated far in advance, and yet in detail, the essentials that have been described above for the information-processing model. His sensorimotor theory first combined the essential elements of the model in implementing his preoccupation with the mechanisms of adaptation.

Piaget's "schema" obviously proposes a basic mechanism of integration. For the schema all prior experiences of a particular kind are drawn upon in determining the necessary modifications to achieve a consistent match in a new accommodation. In other words, by means of schemata the history of the system is integrated with the present context in organizing the final common path of action.

Polarity and the processes of the equilibration of polarities (e.g., decentering) form a central theme by which integration is carried further. Piaget (1969) summarized the three lessons that he drew from biology and that have never ceased to illuminate his thinking:

> The *first* is that all adaptations of the organism . . . imply the closest interaction between organism and environment: . . . No subject without action on objects and no objects without a structuration contributed by the subject. . . . [The *second* is that] any biological adaptation implies two *poles* by virtue of these interactions, on the one hand, it is an accommodation, i.e., a temporary or lasting modification of the organism's structures under the influence of external factors; [and on the other] . . . A complementary pole, the assimilation pole, which has the task of integrating external factors into the organism's structures. . . . A third analogy is obviously necessary: if biological or cognitive adaptation requires two poles, they both tend toward total harmony by means of successive equilibrations. From the embryological regulations, whose fundamental stage Paul Weiss called "re-integration," or from the numerous cybernetic circuits described by Waddington at the heart of his "epigenetic landscape," up to the self regulations which the study of mental development is continually bringing to light, we find a quite remarkable continuity. . . . We are struck by the generality of these vital fundamental processes, whose knowledge is just as indispensable to the psychologist as to the biologist.

There is currently much interest in applying sensorimotor theory to the process by which the child gains lawful relationship with aspects of his interpersonal environment (see Escalona, 1963; Gouin-Decarie, 1965; Hunt, 1961). The polarity referred to by Piaget (Piaget & Inhelder, 1969) in the development of "object relations" is the polarity of *self* and *other*. The decentering of affectivity onto the other as an alternative to the self is part of a single integrated process correlated with cognitive decentering.[14]

The chronology of interactions described above and the correlated epigenetic sequence of adaptive issues can also be viewed as an effort to apply Piagetian concepts. The concept of *equilibrium*, for example, can be here represented empirically in the achievement of stable interactional coordinations. These levels of adaptation provide a sequence of contexts permitting widening options (increasing selectivity) from which a next level of dif-

---

[14] In an application of Piagetian concepts to the developmental analysis of interpersonal behavior Feffer (1970) discusses decentering in terms of reciprocating *role* schemata (e.g., giving–taking and punishing–being punished). The polarity of concern in our viewpoint, on the other hand, is that between self-as-coherent (confirmed or reinforced) and self-as-dispersed (negated or extinguished), the polarity being then resolved in recognition of self-as-having-option-to-initiate. This formulation is particularly relevant in conceptualizing the genesis of narcissistic personality disorder.

ferentiated volition can take off in building interpersonal coordinations and schemata of interpersonal relations.

An application of Piagetian concepts to the empirical material of our longitudinal study, as assembled under issues VI and VII, can be suggested. These contrasting interactions represent a polarity, i.e., interactional coordination versus divergence. (In psychoanalytic terms this could be expressed as the polarity of libidinal and aggressive drives or, in Mahler's formulation for this age period, as the polarity existing in the rapprochement subphase of the separation–individuation process.) In terms of our emphasis on an ontogeny of awareness in focusing the infant's initiation and intentionality, the harmony achieved in the negotiation of the sixth and seventh issues should be considered also in its relation to emerging self-awareness (see Spitz, 1957) and the establishment of an initial conservation or constancy in the structuring of self. Here there is opportunity for an inner decentering between polarities of self-awareness: the self as facilitated and coordinated (issue VI) and the self as negated and not coordinated (issue VII). If the interactive regulation existing between the toddler and his caretaking environment allows an *option* for *exercise* of *choice*, or behavior initiated by the toddler, a conservation of self-as-initiator or of self-as-active-organizer should harmonize the polarity. The failure of a self-constancy here would leave the child vulnerable to polar oscillations in terms of the interaction that happened to be current, a vulnerability in regulation that would powerfully determine that child's subsequent adaptive strategies.

Finally, Ross Ashby's (1952) conceptualization and mathematical derivation of the "origins of adaptive behavior" provides a remarkable model for adaptive behavior in an increasingly complex system. Drawing on the same Bourbaki school of mathematics as did Piaget, Ashby provided a mathematical derivation for usable definitions of many of the usually imprecise terms thrown about when we speak of adaptation, systems, regulation, etc. In addition he derived principles of adaptive mechanics that account for some of the usually more difficult areas to be explained in adaptive behavior—for example, system, regulation, essential variables, the law of requisite variety, channel independence, adaptation time, use of the recurrent situation, temporary and partial independence, and the mechanism of disjoin of a subsystem made possible by constancy or stability (richness of equilibria) within a complex system. This mechanism of disjoin makes possible differentiated adaptations with the environment at the level of subsystems, so that perturbation of or in the "disjoined" subsystem does *not* spread to the rest of the organism.

If we approach the early organization of infant behavior in terms of principles of adaptive behavior in an infant–caretaker system, the problem of coherence or integration takes on a somewhat different color than when it is considered as one of the many functions of the individual to be attributed to his "ego." A whole array of mechanisms becomes evident that contributes to the "coherence" of the organism functioning within the caretaking system to which it is adapted. In fact, different contributions can be identified for each of the seven issues.

The adaptations appropriate to each level may contribute basic interpersonal strategies or interactional parameters in the sense that they become characteristic constituents of the interactive regulations involved in later, more differentiated interpersonal adaptations. The adaptations related to each issue do not represent something established once and for all, but they are successive contributions to the maintenance of a continuous regulative process in interpersonal interactions.

Mechanisms of synthesis and integration must advance *pari passu* with increasing differentiation if "adaptation time" (Ashby, 1952) is not to become unduly prolonged. Ashby suggests that under conditions providing a richness of "regions of stability" or equilibrium in interactive regulation, the self-organizing core could itself gain relative "disjoin" as a subsystem and thereby possibly a "temporary and partial independence." Under these conditions such a subsystem would be capable, within limits, of participating in ensuing perturbations of adaptive encounters with the surround without the perturbation's spreading over the whole complement of subsystems that constitute the more basic biological functions of the individual. Ashby's argument thus provides the rationale that a "self" or a self-organizing subsystem is essential to the regulation of adaptive behavior in a system at the critical level of complexity.[15]

---

[15] Complexity in behavioral adaptation should increase with the richness of the behavioral repertoire available (the law of requisite variety; see Ashby, 1958), thereby increasing the number of possible selections of appropriately differentiated behaviors when conditions permit options (i.e., in Ashby's terms conditions that do not displace "essential variables" from their regions of stability; such displacements would limit selectivity by preempting behavior to restore basic regulation). Such necessary complexity appears to accompany complexity in social interaction and communication. For example, a provoking question, motivating the detailed investigations by Dr. D. Ploog (in a personal communication to the author) and his colleagues regarding communication in the squirrel monkey, is why such a relatively small creature with such a relatively simple habitat has evolved such highly complex communicational behavior. If Ashby's model is right, the advantage gained in predator avoidance or food gathering for the squirrel monkey may be less important than the gain in complexity of repertoire, regions of stability, and, consequently, selectivity made available for the self-organizing function. The critical step in human evolution may have been at the point of both complexity and stability at which the organism's own "state" itself became conscious, i.e., both coherent enough and recurrent enough to become a criterion for match.

The information-processing model, in the general sense being used here that it is mismatch that leads to perception and consciousness, indicates that an ontogeny of interpersonal regulation must indeed be also an ontogeny of awareness. For both, the conceptualization of the infant and the caretaking environment as a system is central, with an ontogeny of awareness depending heavily on characteristics of "state" as context and on goal-oriented activities as content.

Investigation of Interactive Regulation in Three Infant–Caretaking Systems

The longitudinal study, therefore, led to a viewpoint about how to apply conceptualizations of the adaptive process to early human development. It is a particular viewpoint of adaptive behavior by which data from the first 18 months of life can be related to the second 18 months of life and the biological level can be related to the psychological level. Therefore in 1963, when the opportunity arose through the National Institute of Mental Health research development program to begin a new program of investigation, we decided to study the infant and caretaker as a system with a more detailed examination of the mechanisms of regulation, their relation to interactions and to events within the system, and their changes over time. One of our findings when we rated and assessed the sequence of infant–mother interactional issues was that the characteristics of negotiation of the first issue tended to predict the negotiation of subsequent issues, at least through issue VI. In other words, if we assessed the characteristics of adaptation between the partners right at the outset, when the system was first getting underway, we might gain basic insight into the idiosyncracies of adaptation that that particular system might show at subsequent levels of coordination, and something like an adaptive potential or adaptive capacity for any given infant–mother pair might be indicated.

To investigate differences in adaptive progress in different systems, one should have access to some striking but uniform contrast in infant–caretaker "fitting together," which should not be confounded with differences in endowment of the infants. The contrast in harmony of "fitting together"ideally

TABLE 2

Design for Investigation of Interactive Regulation in Three Infant–Caretaking Systems

Group	N	Caretaking period 1 (0–10 days)		Caretaking period 2 (11–28 days)	Caretaking period 3 (29–56 days)
A	9	Nursery		Single caretaker (X or Y) rooming in	Foster home
B	9	Single caretaker (X or Y) rooming in		Single caretaker (Y or X) rooming in	Foster home
C	9	0–5 days	6–10 days		
		Natural mother rooming in	Natural mother at home	Natural mother at home	Natural mother at home

should be studied only over a limited time span, so that the extent of recovery from perturbation to the system can be examined. For such an investigation we wanted measurement that would be reasonably precise without upsetting naturalistic observation. The subject samples to be observed also had to provide a contrasting analysis without experimental manipulation. Three samples of normal infant–caretaker pairs were chosen for study, nine pairs to be in each sample. The first two samples had specific contrast in caretaking condition; the third sample consisted of neonates reared by their own experienced, multiparous mothers. We used five principal methods of data collection over the first two months of postnatal life to get parallel observation of several infant variables and several caretaker variables that would be quantitative and would occur frequently enough and over a long enough time span to permit the identification of significant changes in values or the appearance of a regular recurrence or a relative stability of values.

Design

The study[16] sample consisted of three groups of nine normal[17] infants each (Table 2). Two groups were composed of infants given up by their mothers for adoptive placement and cared for by surrogate mothers. Of these the infants in group A spent the first 10 days in the newborn nursery being cared for by the usual nursery staff (multiple caretaking) on a fixed 4-hour nursery feeding schedule. These infants were then shifted to an individual rooming-in arrangement in a regular hospital room, where each infant was cared for by a single caretaker on a demand schedule 24 hours a day for the next 18 days. At the end of the first four weeks the infant was placed in a regular agency foster home and was there followed for a second four-week period.

The infants in group B (also going to adoptive placement) went directly into rooming in (usually 24 hours after delivery), where they had a first single surrogate-mother caretaker from day 2 through day 10 and were shifted to a second such caretaker from day 11 through day 28. These infants were always on a demand schedule while cared for in the hospital. After the first four weeks they also went to foster homes, where we continued to observe them for a second four weeks.

Group C was composed of infants of experienced, multiparous mothers. These infants were cared for by their own mothers, in rooming in for five days,

---

[16] "Adaptation and Perception in Early Infancy," USPHS HD01766, carried out in collaboration with G. Stechler, Ph.D., H. Julia, Ph.D, and P. Burns, M.D.

[17] Normality was precisely defined and controlled by prenatal history, observation of delivery, and postnatal examination.

and then were followed at home for the remainder of the eight-week study period.

Groups A and B were designed to elicit differences in infants cared for *over the first 10 days* by multiple caretakers on a rigid feeding schedule, i.e., one not allowing modification of timing of caretaker intervention, in contrast to caretaking by single caretakers on infant-demand feeding schedule. The subsequent caretaking conditions (from day 11 onward) were the same for groups A and B, i.e., single surrogate mother rooming-in 24 hours per day and infant-demand feeding. The assignment of infants to the two groups and to the two nurses who did most of the rooming-in surrogate mothering was unbiased. Group C provided a basis for comparison rather than a strict control group. Obviously home rearing by a mother differs in many ways from hospital and foster rearing. Group C was designed to provide normative data for the parameters measured, with which to compare the more closely monitored group A and B infant–caretaker pairs.

Methods of Data Collection

The four methods employed are briefly described.

1. *Around-the-clock observation.* Experience with the infants and the mothers in the longitudinal study impressed us with the obvious fact that adaptation between a mother and her infant is not carried out only in the time units customarily sampled in mother and infant observations but in all 24 hours of the day. "Relationship" must first involve *living together.*

Observation around the clock can be carried out if one considers that the continuous observation of even one variable of a complex system provides an observational window on the state of that system over time. For example, if one could measure automatically, around the clock and day after day, only the infant's presence in or absence from the bassinet, one could derive a great deal of information about the pattern and the change in pattern of caretaking events. Couple this variable with one monitored from the infant while in the bassinet—for example, time of the occurrence of crying—and one has a means of observing interactions between infant and caretaker.

Essentially, the monitor was a recording bassinet, operating without instrumentation of the baby; it utilized an Esterline-Angus event recorder moving at 12 inches per hour to record continuously, by separate pens in parallel, several channels of digital inputs. These represented (a) small summations of infant activity obtained via an air mattress, a strain gauge, an amplifier, and an integrator system; (b) infant crying (occurring while the infant was in the bassinet); (c) the caretaker's removal of the infant from the bassinet, the duration of the removal, and the return of the infant to the bassinet; and (d) the proximity of the caretaker to the bassinet.

2. *Observation of time of onset of awake state and sleep state for group A and B infants during the first month of life.* These observations of clock time of major change of state were made by the registered nurses acting as surrogate mothers with high reliability in terms of a simple dichotomous definition based on eyes' remaining open or closed over a span of at least five minutes. These observations by nurses fully accustomed to 24-hour duty and to accurate charting permitted an around-the-clock correlation of the monitor with the observed state and gave information about the periodicity of state changes in the infant—their day–night distribution and the striking individual differences between infants who had been reared by the same surrogate mother.

3. *Observation of feeding interaction.* Daily during the first month of life and twice weekly during the second month, a feeding was observed and recorded in real time on a Rustrak 4 key event recorder. The feeding was divided into three phases: prefeed, feed proper, and postfeed. Coded entries recorded various infant states; mutual regard between infant and feeder; infant regard of feeder's face; postural change for feeding, burping, visual regard, or "other"; insertion and removal of nipple; onset and end of sucking; signs of infant distress; intensity of stimulation, etc. These measures were mostly durations and frequencies. The amount of formula taken was recorded for each period of "nipple-in time" by having the feeder put the bottle down on a scale instead of the table.

4. *Systematic observations of infant behavior on experiencing visual stimuli.* Approximately twice weekly in the first month and weekly in the second month of life the infant was presented a series of stimuli, each for a one-minute duration, at a 10–12-inch distance, with a 15-second interstimulus interval. The stimuli consisted of the following sequences: (a) a line drawing of a face; (b) the experimenter's face still, (c) nodding, (d) in full social approach using smile, voice, and movement to elicit infant attention, (e) a line drawing again, (f) the mother's face still, (g) nodding, (h) social, (i) a line drawing again, (j) the experimenter's face still, (k) nodding, (l) social, (m) a line drawing again. Using the same Rustrak 4 key event recorder, occurrence and durations of the following behavioral categories were made in real time: look, look–excite, look–excite–vocalize, look–excite–smile, look away, eyes closed, fuss. "Looking" included any orientation of infant gaze to the whole stimulus or any part of it, including its periphery and including gaze with one eye only. The testing of the infant was carried out only in optimal states of quiet alertness.

The analysis of data generated by these many variables, which were measured repeatedly on the three groups of neonates over their first two months of life, cannot be covered within the scope of this chapter. A number of findings have been reported (Burns *et al.*, 1972; Sander, 1969; Sander and Julia, 1966; Sander *et al.*, 1969, 1970, 1972), and others will be reported in the near future. Many of the findings are relevant to the adaptive process in an interactive regulative system, contributing toward answers to basic questions although not fully answering them. For example, one asks: How early does an interactional bonding between infant and caretaker become established? Which infant variables appear to play a primary role in this process? What are some of the effects on the adaptive process of a limited perturbation of the system at this early point?

In regard to the first question, our evidence confirms the impression that a "bonding"—that is, a specific adaptation between the infant and the individual providing sole care—is established within the first 10 days[18] of postnatal life. In this adaptation it is assumed that the infant's idiosyncracies of regulation have become coordinated to some extent with the caretaker's idiosyncracies. This adaptation was shown by the immediate and significant rise in 24-hour crying output on day 11 for group B infants, who had experienced a change in surrogate mother on that day, an increase in crying that persisted a number of days. (The same two surrogate mother nurses cared for all but one of the group B infants. Each new infant subject admitted to the study was assigned to one or the other alternately in an unbiased way, so that on day 11 infants went as often from nurse A to nurse B as from nurse B to nurse A.)

The feeding data demonstrated the same effect of change of caretaker on day 11 for group B as did the crying variables. "Distress events" during feeding, which over the first 10 days of life had settled down for group B infants to a low level relative to the number occurring for infants in group A, also showed a sudden, significant, and persistent rise at day 11 for the group B infants. (Distress events consisted of the number of episodes during the feeding of spitting up, crying, gagging, vomiting, turning away, etc.) In current research we are pursuing the question of which variables will be the most sensitive indicators of perturbation of the initial coordination with a single caretaker.

In regard to the second question, certain infant variables do appear to play a primary role in the interactions through which regulation is carried out. The important variables are those related to the various "states" of the infant. These evidence oscillation or periodicity, both in the active and quiet cycles of REM and N-REM sleep and in the longer epochs of wakefulness and sleep. It seems evident that the sequence infant-state-change–caretaking-intervention is a first and most basic contingency and that caretaker-intervention–infant-state-change is an equally basic contingency, which bonds or links the pair in reciprocal regulation from the very outset. We have encountered marked individual differences in the length of the gross sleep and awake epochs characteristic of

[18] Regulatory exchange between infant and mother has existed from conception onward. Anderson (1973) has stressed the critical role of the initial hours post partum with possibly enduring consequences to the way the transition to postnatal regulation is accomplished.

each infant. The relative length of these two epochs is significantly intercorrelated, suggesting the existence of individual differences in an epoch "duration factor." The modification of the overall lengths of sleep and awake epochs and of their day–night distributions is one of the important sites of adaptive pressure as the caretaker seeks to bring her infant's 24-hour temporal organization into some coordination with the 24-hour pattern of events in the household. The data suggested that the shifting of epoch length toward shorter or longer periods may be related to the style of caretaking of the particular nurse who is doing the surrogate mothering.

Research on biological rhythm has made a key contribution to the conceptualization of the adaptive process and the temporal organization of interaction in the system. This contribution is an insight into the control of the phase relations of oscillating systems, which makes synchrony between them possible. Phase control involves quite a different array of mechanisms from those included in the traditional stimulus–response or learning perspective (see Aschoff, 1965). Franz Halberg (1960) has concluded that "Temporal organization of physiologic function usually involves a circadian time structure, with great although not unlimited plasticity. . . . By synchronization with environmental routines integrative circadian systems gain adaptive value. Temporal coordination in physiology has both integrative and adaptive facets. Periodicity analysis provides for resolution of adaptation as a function of integration and vice versa."

Figure 1 shows the progress of infant and caretaker variables over the first 10 days of life in the nursery (group A) and in the single-caretaker rooming-in situation (group B). Not only do crying and motility continue to increase under the nursery (group A) condition, but they remain greatest in the 12 night hours. In the rooming-in (group B) condition, not only are motility and crying at a much lower level and not only does a shift occur between days 4 and 6 to their predominance in the 12 *day* hours, but also a synchrony appears between the larger epochs of activity and crying in the infant and both the time of occurrence of and the duration of caretaking interventions.

That "temporal coordination in physiology has both integrative and adaptive facets" has been documented beautifully, for both the normal and the neurologically at-risk neonate, by the work of H. Prechtl (1968) and his colleagues. These investigators have obtained simultaneous recordings from a number of physiological subsystems during extended six- to eight-hour polygraphic studies of neonate's cycling through subphases of sleep. The group of infants designated as hyperexcitable (and those who have been found later to pose greater behavioral difficulty in rearing) is found to show poorer "coherence" or synchrony between physiological subsystems at the points of change as they pass through REM to N-REM cycles. The distinctness of

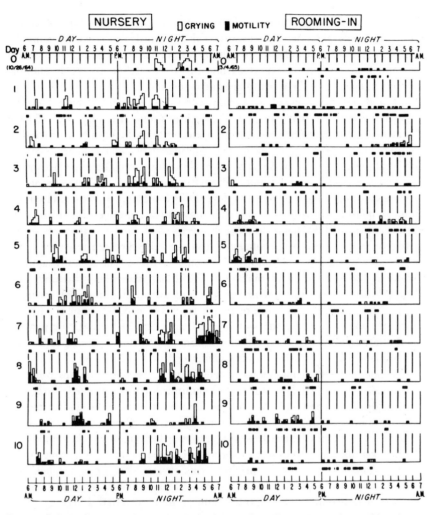

Fig. 1. Relative frequency, duration, and distribution of motility, crying, and caretaking pips as measured by the activity and interactional monitor for a nursery and a rooming-in baby for the first 10 days of life. Caretaker intervention for each baby and for each day of life are represented by the black marks directly below the solid lines indicating day of life.

states in these infants is less clear than in the normal infant, making it difficult for the caretaker to read the cues indicating which state the infant is in. These are cues that usually guide the mother in selecting which intervention is in order or, indeed, whether an intervention is in order. The "state" itself, then, represents a summation or an integration of multiple subsystems comprising the infants' physiology. Phase synchrony between the cycling infant states and episodes of caretaker activity constitutes a next order of integration in the system. Variables that indicate the state of the infant[19] may be among the most critical for assessment of both mechanisms of regulation in the infant and progress of adaptation between infant and caretaker.

The design described above has allowed us to chart the course of sleeping and waking over the first month of life, both in group A infants (who did not experience caretaking response as contingent on their changes of state) and in group B infants (whose caretaking was contingent on their changes of state). Day–night organization of sleeping and waking (i.e., sleeping more between 6 P.M. and 6 A.M. and waking more between 6 A.M. and 6 P.M.) became statistically significant within the first 10 days of life for group B infants but not for group A infants. However, within a few days after group A infants had been transferred from the nursery to the contingent caretaking environment of the surrogate mother who was rooming-in (on day 11), they abruptly showed a precocious advance in 24-hour periodicity, with a significantly greater day–night difference in the organization of sleep and wakefulness between days 11 and 25 than was shown by group B infants during this time. Interestingly enough, this reaction of advance or precocity was shown mostly by the female infant, the male infant tending to show his most rapid progress in day–night differentiation when he had had the contingent caretaking of the group B condition during the first 10 days of life (Sander et al., 1972).

Although group A infants had exposure to a noncontingent environment only during the first 10 days of life, they continued to show marked differences from the group B and C infants over the remainder of the investigation (to end of second month of life). One of the most noteworthy differences was the variability between babies when they were examined week by week. Significant stability of rank order from week to week was never obtained for group A infants in terms of a number of variables, e.g., crying, sleeping, and "looking" time on perceptual testing. In other words, stable individual differences were less evident in group A. On the other hand, stable individual differences were most striking in the group C infants, in whom the interactional idiosyncracies between infant and caretaker for a number of variables (e.g., crying before intervention) were already most strikingly evident by the end of the first 10 days. An illustration of the stability of rank ordering of subjects within groups over weeks 2–8 is given by Kendall's coefficient of concordance. Although group B and C infants showed different degrees of stability depending on the stimulus presented, group A infants never achieved a significant rank order correlation over these weeks for any of the stimuli used in the perceptual test, nor for rank

---

[19] Escalona (1962) was one of the first to call attention to the central significance of the infant's state for both investigator and mother. A current report by Anders and Hoffman (1973) assesses the neonate in terms of sleep–wake states.

ordering in terms of time spent crying during the presentation of visual stimuli. Both groups B and C had coefficients of concordance greater than the $p < .025$ level of significance for these stimuli.

The history dependence of the infant–caretaker system is illustrated also by other effects of first 10-day experience shown during the ensuing weeks. For example, group A infants evidenced significantly greater crying over the two months of the study in reaction to the presentation of visual stimuli on the perceptual test, indicating lower tolerance than the others in this situation for this particular kind of visual stimulation (i.e., the human face; see Figure 2). In relation to the notion of a connection between the consistency or stability of the system and the progress of visual discrimination or differentiation of the infant's reaction to visual stimuli, only the group C infants, reared from birth by their own mothers, showed a significant difference over the two months in the amount of time spent looking at the mother's face during the perceptual test in comparison with the amount of time spent looking at the stranger's face. In approaching interaction in the system from the viewpoint of an ontogeny of regulation, these data support the suggestion already made, that one is dealing also with an ontogeny of awareness. Furthermore, from this piece of evidence one might say that greater specificity and stability in initial adaptation may be associated with the earlier development of a more differentiated discrimination. From the adaptive viewpoint, however, an early and highly precise fitting together may create certain vulnerabilities for the infant should the system become unstable or be disrupted later. To place a value judgment on behavior from the perspective of adaptation, one must know the environment and the adaptive tasks that the infant will be encountering later.

The research approach that we have been reviewing has provided a rich

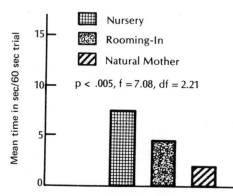

FIG. 2.   Infant fussing during perceptual test for all stimulus presentations over weeks 2–8 of life, showing caretaker group differences (Stechler, 1973).

source of hypotheses and possibilities for new research aimed at a better under-standing of the early organization of behavior and perhaps eventually per-sonality. Although work is still going on in the study of data obtained in the prior projects, survival in the research world demands new projects and new data. The same general direction has been continued, that of investigating mechanisms of the adaptive process in an infant–caretaker system, but employing advances in technology and new methods.

In a current project being supported by the Grant Foundation entitled "An Investigation of Change in Infant–Caretaker Interaction over the First Two Weeks of Life," the monitoring bassinet has been further advanced in design so that from the prone but otherwise free-lying infant in the bassinet, the occurrence and duration of five states of the infant can be recorded around the clock, along with time of occurrence and duration of caretaking inter-vention. The five states are awake and active, awake and crying, transitional sleep, REM sleep, and N-REM sleep. The continuous 24-hour record ob-tained is interfaced with computer tape storage through an optical scan system that makes possible analyses of the complex sequence and the time series as well as the usual statistical analysis of variables. The monitor discriminates a range of differences in state regulation between infants within the normal range and allows study around the clock of changes over the first week of life in sleep cycling and in longer sleep–wake epoch characteristics. The monitor now promises to be an instrument that will make possible a quantitative study of the ontogeny of regulation in at-risk infants of various types and a way of evaluating a variety of caretaking regimens that will optimize their early course of development.

As part of the same project, receiving Grant Foundation support, new methods of precise analysis of interaction between the infant and his interper-sonal world have been developed by Dr. William Condon. Dr. Condon has developed a method of independent frame-by-frame analysis of sound track and film track of neonates who have been filmed in the awake and active state while being spoken to by an adult or for whom speech is being played on a tape recorder. The frame numbers of the two tracks match, so that an analysis can be made of the points at which change in movement configuration and in speech occur, for example, at word or phoneme boundaries. As early as 12 hours after birth there is evidence of synchrony at microsecond levels between the movements of the awake and active neonate and these linguistic components of human speech (Condon and Sander, 1973). Dr. Condon's work constitutes evidence for a wholly unexpected microscopic level at which bonding in the infant–caretaker system is taking place, and it opens a whole new systems approach to the acquisition of language and to the paralinguistic aspects of communicational behavior. Stern's (1971) film analysis at the micro-second level of the regulation of head turning and facing behavior between mother and infant indicates that at 3½ months initiation of facing behavior by one or the other can be reciprocally regulated at interactional levels of less than a half second.

Recapitulation

These current findings provide evidence of the embeddedness of the human infant in a microscopic interactive regulative system as well as a macroscopic one. The first question that comes to mind might be: How does the individual ever extricate himself from the obligatory demands on behavior that this necessity for continuous regulation imposes. However, the question is misleading, since one is never extricated from the life support system or the exchanges that it provides as long as life prevails. One asks, rather, how regulatory interactions are incorporated into behavioral organization in a way that provides a measure of relatively stable continuity in the presence of both a varying environment and a changing organism, so that new modifications and adaptations can continue to differentiate within a reasonably brief adaptation time. Ashby's (1952) model of adaptive behavior in complex polystable systems, along with other, already-existing ideas, has been drawn upon in the construction of an interactive regulative perspective that encompasses the behavioral coordinations necessary for regulation both on the more biological level of the first (18) months and on the more psychological level of the developments of the second 18 months that are related to functions such as language, representation, and inner awareness.

At each level we have tried to pay attention to the mechanisms of integration and synthesis that are represented by the interactive coordinations relevant to regulation at that level. In an epigenetic sense the relative harmony of reciprocal equilibrium between partners in the system sets the stage for active differentiation of a next level, and finally for the partial and often temporary independence or "disjoin" of a self-regulatory subsystem. These subsystems are accessible in some degree to more conscious levels of function and synthesize feedback elements related both to the ongoing "state" and to active goal-direction. Intrinsic, matching criteria provided as a consequence of the disjoin constitute a new basis now for continuity and self-constancy. Perturbations of the system requiring adaptive modifications can begin to be limited to modification in the "self" framework instead of requiring modifications at all levels of linkage, including the biological level. Disjoin requires a certain complexity ("requisite variety") of stable equilibria and in this sense provides a solution for the initial, seemingly paradoxical, features of complexity and coherence mentioned at the outset.

The synthesis of a number of views of the adaptive process appears to offer a way to order empirical interactional data of considerable diversity and complexity and to provide a hypothetical framework that can be applied to the ordering. The focus becomes centralized on the problem of regulation and its connection with the exchange between component parts of a system and with the necessity to define and determine the regularity or the relative stability of variables, as well as to determine the introduction of new behaviors. Obviously, in working from the empirical approach, one tends to carry observation and analysis to ever-finer levels but hopefully remains equally sensitive to concurrent determinants of synthesis and coherence.

References

ANDERS, T., & HOFFMAN, E. The Sleep Polygram: A potentially useful tool for clinical assessment in human infants. *American Journal of Mental Deficiency*, 1973, **77**, 506–514.

ANDERSON, G. C. Paper presented at annual meeting of the International Society for the Study of Behavioral Development, Madison, Wisconsin, 1973.

ASCHOFF, J. Response curves in circadian periodicity. In J. Aschoff (Ed.), *Circadian clocks*. Proceedings of the Feldafing Summer School. Amsterdam: North Holland Publishing Co., 1965.

ASHBY, R. *Design for a brain.*, London: Chapman and Hall, Ltd., 1952. See also Ashby, R., *Design for a brain.*, 2nd Ed., Science Paperback, 1970, (Distributed in U.S.A. by Barnes and Noble, Inc.).

ASHBY, R. *An introduction to cybernetics*. London: Chapman & Hall, 1958.

BERTALANFFY, L. VON. *The problem of life*. New York and London, 1949.

BOWER, T. G. R. Object perception in infants. *Perception*. 1972. Vol. 1, pp. 15–30.

BOWLBY, J. *Attachment and loss*. New York: Basic Books, 1969, Vol. 1.

BURNS, P., SANDER, L., STECHLER, G., & JULIA, H. Distress in feeding: Short-term effects of caretaker environment of the first 10 days. *Journal of the American Academy of Child Psychiatry*, 1972, **11**, 427–439.

CHARLESWORTH, W. R. Instigation and maintenance of curiosity behavior as a function of surprise versus novel and familiar stimuli. *Child Development*, 1964, **35**, 1169–1186.

CONDON, W., & SANDER, L. Synchronization of neonate movement with adult speech: interactional participation and language acquisition. *Science*, 1974, **183**, 99–101.

ERIKSON, E. H. *Childhood and society*. New York: W. W. Norton, 1950.

ERIKSON, E. H. Identity and the life cycle. *Psychological Issues*, 1959, **1**, 50–101.

ESCALONA, S. K. The study of individual differences and the problem of state. *Journal of the American Academy of Child Psychiatry*, 1962, **1**, 11–38.

ESCALONA, S. Patterns of infantile experience and the developmental process. *The Psychoanalytic Study of the Child*, 1963, **18**, 198–201.

FEFFER, M. A developmental analysis of interpersonal behavior. *Psychological Review*, 1970, **77**, 197–215.

GLASSMAN, R. B. Persistence and loose coupling in living systems. *Behavioral Science*, 1973, **18**, 83–98.

GOUIN-DECARIET. *Intelligence and affectivity in early childhood*. New York: International University Press, 1965.

HALBERG, F. Temporal coordination of physiological functions. *Symposia on Quantitative Biology*, 1960, **25**, 289–310.

HARTMAN, H., DRIS, E., & LOEWENSTEIN, R. M. Comments on the formation of psychic structure. *Psychoanalytic Study of the Child*, 1946, **2**, 11–38.

HINDE, R. A.. *Animal behavior: A synthesis of ethology and comparative psychology*. New York and London: McGraw-Hill, 1966.

HUNT, J. McV. *Intelligence and experience*. New York: Ronald Press, 1961.

HUNT, J. McV. Intrinsic motivation and its role in psychological development. In D. Levine (Ed.), *Nebraska Symposium on Motivation*. Lincoln: University of Nebraska Press, 1965.

MACKAY, D. M. Towards an information flow model of cerebral organization. *Symposium on Cerebral Activity, Advancement of Science*, 1956, **42**, 392.

MAHLER, M. *On human symbiosis and the vicissitudes of individuation*. Vol. 1: *Infantile Psychosis*. New York: International University Press, 1968.

MAHLER, M., & McDEVIT, J. B. Observations on adaptation and defense in statu nascendi: developmental precursors in the first two years of life. *Psychoanalytic Quarterly*, 1968, **37**, 1–21.

MASON, J. W. Over-all hormonal balance as a key to endocrine organization. *Psychosomatic Medicine*, 1968, **30**, 791–808.

MILLER, G. A., GALANTER, E., & PRIBRAM, K. *Plans and the structure of behavior*. New York: Henry Holt, 1960.

PIAGET, J. *The origins of intelligence in children*, English Translation. New York: International University Press, 1936.

PIAGET, J. & INHELDER, B. The gaps in Empiricism. In Koestler, A., & Smythies, J. R. (Eds.), *Beyond reductionism—New perspectives in the life sciences*. Boston: Beacon Press, 1969, 118–160.

PIAGET, J. The affective unconscious and the cognitive unconscious. *Journal of the American Psychoanalytic Association*, 1973, **21**, 249–261.

PIAGET, J., & INHELDER, B. *The Psychology of the Child*. New York: Basic Books, 1969.

POLANY, M. *The study of man*. Chicago: University of Chicago Press, 1959. (As quoted by Wallerstein.)

PRECHTL, H. F. R. Polgraphic studies of the full term newborn. In, H. Bax & R. C. MacKeith (Eds.), *Studies in infancy clinic in developmental medicine*. London: Heinemann, 1968.

PRIBRAM, K. Reinforcement revisited: A structural view. In M. R. Jones (Ed.) *Nebraska Symposium on Motivation*. Lincoln: University of Nebraska Press, 1963.

ROSENBLATT, J. S., TURKEWITZ, G., & SCHEIRLA, T. C. Early socialization in the domestic cat as based on feeding and other relationships between female and young. In B. M. Foss (Ed.), *Determinants of infant behavior*. London: Methuen; New York: Wiley, 1961.

SANDER, L. W. Issues in early mother–child interaction. *Journal of the American Academy of Child Psychiatry*, 1962, **1**, 141–167.

SANDER, L. W. Adaptive relationships in early mother–child interaction. *Journal of the American Academy of Child Psychiatry*, 1964, **3**, 231–264.

SANDER, L. W. The longitudinal course of early mother–child interaction: cross case comparison in a sample of mother–child pairs. In B. M. Foss, (Ed.), *Determinants of infant behavior IV*. London: Methuen, 1969.

SANDER, L. W., & JULIA, H. L. Continuous interactional monitoring in the neonate. *Psychosomatic Medicine*, 1966, **28**, 822–835.

SANDER, L. W., JULIA H. L., STECHLER, G., & BURNS, P. Regulation and organization in the early infant-caretaker system. In J. R. Robinson (Ed.), *Brain and early development*. New York: Academic Press, 1969.

SANDER, L. W., JULIA, H. L., STECHLER, G., & BURNS, P. Continuous 24-hour interactional monitoring in infants reared in two caretaking environments. *Psychosomatic Medicine*, 1972, **34**, 270–282.

SANDLER, L. W., STECHLER, G., BURNS, P., & JULIA, H. Early mother infant interaction and 24-Hour patterns of activity and sleep. *Journal of the American Academy of Child Psychiatry*, 1970, **9**, 103–123.

SANDLER, J., & ROSENBLATT, B. The concept of the representational world. *Psychoanalytic Study of the Child*. New York: International University Press, 1962.

SCHNEIRLA, T. C. An evolutionary and developmental theory of biphasic processes underlying approach and withdrawl. In M. R. Jones (Ed.), *Nebraska Symposium on Maturation*. Lincoln: University of Nebraska Press, 1959.

SPIEGEL, L. A. The self—the sense of self and perception. *The Psychoanalytic Study of the Child*, 1959, **14**, 81–109.

SPITZ, R. A. *No and yes—On the genesis of human communication*. New York: International University Press, 1957.

Spitz, R. A. *A genetic field theory of ego formation.* New York: International University Press, 1959.

Stechler, G., Infant looking and fussing in response to visual stimuli over the first two months of life in different infant-caretaking systems. Presented at *The Society for Research and Child Development,* Philadelphia, 1973.

Stern, D. N. A micro-analysis of mother–infant interaction. *Journal of the American Academy of Child Psychiatry,* 1971 **10,** 501–518.

Uexküll, J. Von A stroll through the worlds of animals and men. In C. H. Schiller, (Ed.), *Instinctive Behavior- The Development of a Modern Concept.* New York: International University Press, 1934.

Von Holst, E., & Mittelstaedt, H. Das Reafferenz Prinzip. *Naturwiss,* 1950, **37,** 464–489.

Wallerstein, R. S. Psychoanalytic Perspectives on the Problem of Reality. *Journal of the American Psychoanalytic Association,* 1973, Vol. **21,** 5–34.

Weiss, P. The biological basis of adaptation. In J. Romano (Ed.), *Adaptation.* Ithaca, N.Y.: Cornell University Press, 1949.

Weiss, P. The living system: Determinism stratified. In A. Koestler & J. R. Smythies (Eds.), *The Alpbach Symposium 1968—Beyond Reductionism—New perspectives in the life sciences.* Boston: Beacon Press, 1969.

Winnicott, D. W. The depressive position in normal emotional development. *Collected Papers D.W. Winnicott.* New York: Basic Books, 1954.

THE ADAPTIVE PROCESS IN EARLY INFANCY

A RESEARCH ODYSSEY

The inclination of a clinician to become involved in systematically organized, investigative work is rare, and the path leading in that direction is never obvious. Such an inclination develops during a lifetime of personal and educational experience. It is accompanied by many false starts, incompleted projects, exploratory dabblings, and flirtations before the event or series of events that only in retrospect can be recognized as the beginnings of a project destined to occupy the bulk of an investigator's time, talent, and creative resources for years to come. In this sense research is very much like a love affair. It may be very short-lived or it may become a lifelong passion, not without its disruptions and moments of desperation. In what follows I shall tell the story of what has become my own research passion, including sidelights and attitudes that have not found expression in publications up to this time.

It was during the summer of 1959 that I began to study, in a much more systematic way than previously, the process of behavioral adaptation in the infant and in the mother–infant relationship. The literature in child development and pediatrics had until that time stressed the passivity of the newborn infant except for reflexive and random behavior. Psychoanalytic drive theory, and the hallucinatory wish-fulfillment thinking and the primary model of thought derived therefrom, placed primary emphasis on the sucking and consumatory aspect of the feeding situation, i.e., the experience of satisfaction. Only very recently had these basic assumptions about the newborn infant been successfully challenged. Peter Wolff had demonstrated in 1959 that the newborn infant was capable of complex visual following and brief periods of awake atten-

---

JUSTIN D. CALL, Professor and Chief of Child Psychiatry, Department of Psychiatry and Human Behavior, College of Medicine, University of California, Irvine; Analyzing Instructor and Senior Faculty, Adult and Child Psychoanalysis, Los Angeles Psychoanalytic Society and Institute, Los Angeles.

tiveness and responsiveness to the environment. Ethological studies had shown *how* adaptation and survival of the species involved instinctually organized behaviors "released" by specific cue stimuli at critical periods in development. This work by Konrad Lorenz, Nicholas Tinbergen, and Carl von Frisch (awarded the Nobel Prize for Medicine for 1973) had served to challenge infant observers with identifying analogous species-specific survival behaviors in the human infant.

I had not accepted the emphasis placed on the infant's passivity and the dominance of random behavior, and I believed that the newborn infant was capable of making a specific adaptation to the feeding situation. As a pediatrician I had been impressed with the smoothly articulated mouth and snout behaviors of the premature infant, which facilitated rapid adaptation to tube feeding. Many infants soon swallowed the tube, apparently capable of inhibiting the gag reflex, and sucked contentedly on the tube just as older infants might upon a pacifier. I had observed that breast- and bottle-fed newborns began to participate actively in the feeding process soon after birth, using the neurophysiologically precocious snout apparatus with its associated hand–mouth, hand to bottle, and hand to breast activities in locating, approaching, and attaching to the breast or the bottle.

A paper by Leo Rangell (1954), which explored the role of the snout in establishing and maintaining the state of poise in interpersonal contacts, provided an important bridge between these observations in the newborn and psychoanalytic theory on the development of object relations. While observing infants in the newborn nursery, we began gradually to adopt a frame of reference to which we referred as the "snout hypothesis." We were searching for changes in the infant's snout behaviors that might reflect specific responses to the process of being fed.

We soon discovered in spending long hours at the cribside that the spontaneous behavior of the infant, including the state of arousal and hand to face movement, was fully as interesting and quantifiable as were such reflex behaviors as rooting, sucking, the hand–mouth reflex (Babkin, 1958), and grasping. Clinical observations of the feeding situation in the newborn had convinced me that a detailed microanalysis of filmed mother–infant interaction during the earliest phases of the feeding process would reveal *how* these adaptively available, spontaneous movement patterns and reflexes in the infant could be used by the infant in the service of locating, approaching, and attaching to the breast or the bottle. We learned during the first half of the summer of 1959 that we could induce a state of quiet attentiveness in most fullterm, irritable infants by swaddling them. It became apparent that when the infant was in the state of quiet attentiveness there was a greater economy of hand-to-mouth movement and a greater capacity for visual following behavior.

Anticipatory Approach Behavior

Chance observation of one particular mother–infant pair during the summer of 1959 was fateful for the future of our project. On the third day of life, Mrs. D., who had successfully breast-fed her infant on day 1 and day 2, lifted her baby to the breast; as she did so, the infant opened his mouth and turned his head toward the nipple prior to any stimulation on the infant's face. It appeared that the infant could actively participate in the process of finding the nipple and attaching his mouth to the nipple independently of any stimulation of the reflexogenic zone for rooting. We called this *anticipatory approach behavior* (Call, 1964) and spent the next three summers systematically observing a sample of 17 mother–infant pairs to determine the varieties of anticipatory approach behavior and the conditions under which it occurred in breast- and bottle-fed infants. A detailed film study of each feeding from birth through the age of four days in 17 mother–infant pairs revealed that the occurrence of anticipatory approach behavior in the infant was dependent upon an adequately everted nipple-areola-breast configuration, close bodily contact with adequate but nonrestrictive head support, at least one or two satisfying feedings prior to the one in which anticipatory behavior was observed, and offering the breast or bottle while the infant was awake and attentive. It was possible to confirm that such anticipatory approach behavior did in fact occur in 11 of 17 mother–infant pairs. More important was the finding that in several infants specific modifications of rooting behavior occurred that corresponded in an adaptive way to a particular mother's method of holding and introducing the nipple into the baby's mouth. Thus not only did the infant show the capacity to adapt generally to an average expectable environment reflecting his *state of adaptiveness* at birth, but he also demonstrated his capacity to adapt to his specific mother. This latter specific "fitting in" Hartmann (1939) refers to as the *process* of adaptation.

The Nuclear Ego

These observations led me to formulate a theory about how the nucleus of early ego functions begins. I postulated internal stimuli impinging upon the inner face and external stimuli impinging upon the outer face to activate congenitally available or developmentally acquired, conflict-free, hereditary ego constituents, such as discharge thresholds, the perceptual apparatus, the neurophysiological templates for memory, and motoric activity, including reflex and congenitally available movement patterns. I reasoned that once the infant had gained the capacity to anticipate a future event, such as a feeding, the presence of an organized series of memory traces linked with adaptive motoric activity must be implied. In the case of anticipatory approach behavior, those memories would include memory of the mother's holding position, which is associated with memory of motoric action and a kinesthetic image (nonvisual) of the infant's own active approach movements. Since these approach activities involve a combination of movement patterns and reflex behavior, they may be spoken of as a quasi-reflexive motoric adaptation to the mother's feeding style and are adaptive elaborations and integrations of inborn, available movement patterns and reflexive activity. These early sensorimotor adaptations are not simple, conditioned, reflexive acts. Certain reflex components are exaggerated and others are eliminated. In order for this adaptation to occur, the object, i.e., the breast or the bottle nipple (and the experience of satisfaction associated with sucking thereon), must be identified, remembered, hallucinated, and actively sought both prior to feeding, when drive tension is increased and clues from the holding mother signal the appearance of the drive object in the outer world, and when feeding is interrupted. It will be noted that this theory relies upon Freud's assumption of "congenital variations in ego" equipment (1937) and Hartmann's further elaboration of this concept (1939). The breast or bottle nipple may be considered a cue stimulus that elicits the integration of already instinctually organized behavior (reflexes) with nonreflexive movement patterns, both of which are influenced and shaped by environmental experience, i.e., the holding position of the mother, the specific characteristics of the nipple, and the components of rooting behavior, which received optimal stimulation. It should be emphasized that this earliest series of adaptive behaviors does not depend on nor is it integrated by visual gestalts. This theory of nuclear ego formation should be distinguished from Glover's (1943) concept of multiple ego nuclei, which coalesce to form an inner ego core.

Visual Bonding and the Nonvisual Experience

The role of vision in organizing all other perceptual experience endows visual experience with a prepotent influence in the development of mental representations of the outside world. Smell, taste, touch, movement, warmth, and the experience of satisfaction itself eventually become synthesized in terms of a visually identifiable object. Mental representations of objects remain fragmentary and uncertain for a prolonged period of developmental time in congenitally blind children (Fraiberg, 1969). Such children eventually learn to identify objects using their hands and audition in place of vision. Sighted children who become blind or partially sighted children, who have a visual template available to them with which to organize ongoing experience in visual terms, have much less difficulty in identifying objects and stabilizing mental representations of them. The prepotence of vision in organizing experience should not blind the observer to the significance of nonvisual experience. The essence of an object, that is, its inherent nature and meaning, is largely determined by coanesthetic modes of perception (Spitz, 1945). Diacritical modes of perception, such as vision, audition, and fingertip discrimination, serve more to locate and identify an object than they do to determine its inherent nature, especially the pain–pleasure aspects of an object. The nucleus of early ego hypothesized here predates the prepotency of vision as an organizer of experience.

By the fourth day of life vision begins to play an important role in locating the breast or the bottle. On that day significantly more time is spent in awake states than before. The eyes open before feeding, and the amount of time spent in awake, visually attentive states rapidly increases from them on. Prior to that time anticipatory approach behavior is observed in most babies in which the conditions for its development is optimal. The rapid increase in the capacity for visual attentiveness after the fourth day has been documented (Wolff and White, 1965). When vision is used during the feeding situation, the infant soon seeks his mother's face and particularly her eyes as she seeks visual contact with him. Visual bonding of mother and child thus begins. The mechanisms of how visual bonding takes place in the context of need satisfaction during feeding is an area ripe for systematic study. The implications of these early mechanisms of ego development are significant for the evolution of the child's subsequent course in object relationships and subsequent development of ego functions.

Anticipation of the experience of satisfaction in nursing precedes visual bonding. Unsuccessful or distressful nursing experience is reflected by the infant's turning of the head, body, and eyes away from both the nipple and the mother's face and eyes, thus delaying and distorting the establishment of the visual bond between mother and infant within the context of the experience of satisfaction.It should be emphasized that the experience of satisfaction in early infancy is a dyadic one, especially for the breast-feeding mother, who experiences relief, warmth, and tranquility from being successfully nursed by her infant. The significance of nonvisual experience in the evolution of object relations is reflected in the nature of visual bonding behavior and later in reports of visual imagery that can be understood as the manifest content of underlying nonvisual experience. Visual imagery, as observed in the Isakower phenomenon and in hypnagogic experience or during free associations during the controlled regression of analysis, should be examined in terms of discontinuities and disruptions in need-satisfying experiences. One hypothesis would be that such fragmentary visual experience is a visual representation of traumatic events connected with need satisfaction. Such visual imagery, like the dream following a traumatic neurosis, is a belated attempt at mastery. Vision is to nonvisual experience as words are to affects.

Theory and Observation

I have preferred to use the term *adaptation* rather than *learning*, since it is firmly rooted in Darwin's theory of evolution, ethology, and psychoanalytic ego psychology (Hartmann, 1939). Thus the concept *adaptation* provides a broader conceptual framework from which to make observations, test hypotheses, and intuit and interpret the meaning of data that *do not* seem to correspond to a more narrowly defined conceptual base.[1] This leads me to state something that I have come to include as a principle in my own research orientation, namely, there is no such thing as a naïve observer. Observers are more or less or not at all aware of the substructure of theory, affects, and conflict that underlies the observations they choose to record and interpret. Our scientific literature is dry and somewhat sterile because the use of the first person singular *I* is forbidden (except in this volume), and because most researchers who have survived very long have learned to be very parsimonious in expressing the theory, affect, or conflicts that motivate them.[2] My own experience convinces me that observational skills and methods are strengthened by a clear explication of theory and that theory building, particularly the very necessary small-scale theory building that leads to testable hypotheses, is sharpened and clarified by observation.

Clinical Work and Systematic Research

When the clinician turns his energies to systematic research, he has many things to overcome other than internal inertia, external conflict, and educational deficits in research methodology. Following the initial excitement of engaging in research, the clinician may experience a sense of being involved in something trivial compared to the life-and-death issues involved in patient care. He (or she) may experience overt and covert criticism from colleagues who have remained committed to healing people.

The child psychiatrist and psychoanalyst does bring with him to investigative work two very important assets. He knows the difference between a fundamentally important question and a trivial one, and he usually is sophisticated enough in his thinking to acknowledge the complexity of interacting

[1] Observation in the natural setting requires a broader conceptual base than does manipulation of behavior in an experimentally controlled setting.
[2] Science fiction is one outlet for the expression of this side of the research enterprise.

variables in producing any symptom, character trait, or treatment outcome. Both of these assets, however, can become liabilities when the clinician is faced with the sharpening of focus required in the development of systematic research design and methodology.

Brief Summary

This odyssey then began with clinical work that led me to doubt that the newborn infant's behavior was inherently random and purely reflexive in nature. Ethological studies and psychoanalytic investigations of the "snout" and its role in maintaining poise in interpersonal relations had led to the formulation of a "snout hypothesis," which guided observations of infant approach behavior. In making these observations we discovered that the newborn infant is, within certain parameters, capable of showing "anticipatory approach behavior" and making a specific adaptation to his mother's method of holding him and introducing the nipple. This discovery led to a formulation of theory concerning the early adaptive processes in the infant, i.e., a theory of nuclear ego formation, which poses additional questions on the relationship between visual and nonvisual experience.

The Relatively Conflict-Free Sphere

I was aware that such a theory did not take fully into account the relatively conflict-free sphere of early ego development. After additional observational work, it became clear that a study of mother–infant interaction in the postfeeding period promised to reveal additional clues to the mechanism of ego formation within the relatively conflict-free sphere, that is, when drive tensions were low.

Most infants make a transition from a calm, relaxed, drowsy state at the end of a successful feeding experience to a higher state of arousal as soon as the breast or the bottle is actually withdrawn. They become awake and visually attentive, with minimal physical activity, or awake and physically active, without visual attentiveness. The more awake state persists for 2 to 10 minutes prior to postfeeding sleep. Maternal responsiveness to such changes in state vary. Some mothers orient themselves exclusively to the infant's hunger needs, and others maintain eye contact while talking gently to the infant, playing gently with the baby's hands, and responding to the infant's movement patterns, thus setting up the basis for reciprocity. In the latter instance the mother becomes both a need-satisfying object, around which libidinal drive and affects are differentiated and organized, and a source of stimulus nutriment and cognitive complexity. Such stimulus nutriment offered by the mother may be viewed in the context of Piaget's theory of cognitive development, more especially as novel stimulation during the sensorimotor stage of development. The mother may provide an external stimulus configuration, including elements of rhythmicity, intensity, and variety of intersensory experience, around which the apparatuses of primary autonomy in the ego function and become integrated. The result is further adaptive fitting-in of the infant to the environment. Sullivan (1948) has spoken of this lack of reciprocity of the mother in supporting the development of autonomous ego structures in the infant as providing the basis for "disjunctive anxiety." He postulated that this particular form of anxiety led to "insulating" behavior.

Style, Play, and Games

It soon became clear to us in making observations of the interaction of mother and infant during the nonhunger state that such behavior became institutionalized into larger units identified as style. As noted previously (Call and Marschak, 1966), *style*, a concept elaborated by Max Weber (1921) for a theory of society and adapted by Erikson (1950) to psychoanalytic theory, refers to modes of action or the manner in which an act is performed. We may first think of a motor act, then of processes of communication, and finally of ways of thinking. We may speak eventually of a life style of an individual apart from the style of his culture or his historical period. Style, as applied to the mother's care, characterizes not what is done to, for, or with the infant but rather how this process takes place. Other institutionalized structures in this interaction could be identified as games.

The main distinction between play and games lies in the fact that games proceed according to rules. These rules impose a sequence of interrelated events and also presuppose an end point, which gives games the quality of being more decisive than play. However, when humans play games the rules grow and change. Thus new games are constantly being *invented*. This is nowhere more true than it is during infancy. The games are repeated when the context is familiar and the mood is right. Some repetitive sequences of interaction between mother and infant have the meaning of a game for the mother but not for the infant.

The game as an invention was clearly shown by a 13-month-old infant after lunch one day. His mother had given his some juice in a cup. When the meal was finished, she playfully put the cup over her infant's foot while it was swinging slightly. Following the first such exchange experienced, the baby repeated the experience himself by placing the cup on his own foot. He and his mother had *invented* a new game. I believe it was Einstein who said, "Science is constantly invented while Scientists are playing at it."

As noted previously (Call, 1968), most games occur on the mother's lap. The lap is a place of support and comfort. It is formed by the mother's body, arms, and hands. From the infant's viewpoint the mother's body is something warm, stable, and dependably there; her arms provide head support and allow for, and adapt to, the infant's spontaneous movements, and her hands provide objects and relations with objects that meet the infant's needs and wishes. The lap and its components provide an opportunity for the creation of an illusion (Winnicott, 1953). Winnicott (1963) has compared the psychoanalytic situation with the holding mother concerned with the care of her infant. How holding, analytic or maternal, takes place is crucial for the development of the individual. Psychoanalytic material is rich in many illustrations of how the meaning of the lap shows up in the tranference. Many cultural variations of holding exist (Wachsman, 1966).

Integration of Orientation and Anchorage Systems

While rooting behavior, the hand–mouth system, maternal holding, and vision each function as systems to orient and anchor the infant to the mother in a particular way, the play and games of infancy involve all of these systems in consistent sequences and thus serve to integrate them, one with another, thus providing the basis for synthetic processes in mental functioning. All of these systems operate to bring about the satisfaction of oral needs and their mental representation, wishes. Factors responsible for oral fixation in psychological development may be as much related to integrative deficiencies in these orientation and anchorage systems as in frustrations or over indulgence of the oral drive.

Sexual Differences

In the course of any research odyssey many interesting questions and topics must be left to the side. The investigator hopes that it will be possible to return to such questions later. In the next chapter of this research odyssey I returned in a more systematic way to some general impressions made from 1959 through 1962 and reported in 1963 by Constas (Constas and Call, 1963) on spontaneous hand–mouth activity, rooting, and the hand–mouth reflex as related to states in the newborn. It appeared in that study that boys demonstrated more hand–face contacting while in awake states than girls, and that girls, while making fewer hand–face contacts per unit of time, made more of such contacts to the snout area.[3] Statistical analysis of the data, however,

[3] *Snout* is defined as the area of the face from the tip of the nose to the chin and between the right and left nasolabial folds.

was not convincing, and we were not happy with the way in which the original sample was chosen, nor were we satisfied that all of the relevant variables, including feeding, had been controlled. We therefore designed a new study.

Four separate groups of infants—10 breast-fed boys, 12 bottle-fed boys, 8 breast-fed girls, and 9 bottle-fed girls—were compared with each other on each of the first four days of life, both before and after feeding. The infants were all normal at birth, and their mothers had been well during pregnancy, had received minimal medication during labor, and were willing to cooperate in the study. This study has been reported in part elsewhere (Call, 1971), but it can be summarized briefly as follows:

1. During the first three days of life (before breast milk has come in), it is apparent that calories count. The bottle-fed babies spent more time sleeping after feeding than the breast-fed babies, and intensity of rooting, sucking, and hand–face contacting all diminished in relation to the calories provided by the feeding. Thus there is confirmation of hunger as a primary motivation for behavior in the newborn.

2. Girls of equivalent birth weight were more significantly quieted by caloric feeding than were boys. Their caloric needs were more easily met.

3. In states of hunger before feeding and both before and after breast feeding, the girls tended to spend relatively more awake time in the awake attentive states than did the boys, whose awake time was spent either crying or in the awake active state. The capacity of girls to remain visually attentive to the environment in the presence of hunger and the greater disorganization of behavior in boys, as shown by crying and activity, suggest that boys may be more motivated in their behavior by appetitive internal forces than girls and that girls may be more influenced by external visual stimuli. Thus the behavior of boys may become more drive-dependent and thus more drive-organized, while that of girls may be less drive-dependent and more environmentally cued and visually organized at an earlier period in development.

4. The girls were found to be capable of targeting more of their hand–face contacts to the snout area when the level of arousal was controlled as a variable. The girls could even target hand–face contacts to the snout area when crying, while the boys could not. This observation suggests a higher degree of neural organization in girls than boys.

All of these data supplement other studies that show a higher degree of vulnerability in boys to disruptions in object relations and to almost all other kinds of disruptions in normal development, including illness. Perhaps these differences may underlie the higher incidence of psychotic reactions and other psychopathology in boys during infancy and childhood and the much higher incidence of reading difficulty in boys than in girls. Recent studies by Richard Bell and his associates (1971) have shown that very active, hyperresponsive boys are more likely to be those with social difficulties and disruptive play at nursery-school age.

Despite these differences, one should be careful in suggesting any degree of higher or lower biological advantage in boys or girls. I would favor Weston La Barre's (1954) concept of mutual complementarity in male and female roles during evolutionary hominization as a basis for viewing these apparent biological differences.

The Natural Environment

It should be noted that even in the systematically organized research projects outlined above, the research design and study were molded around the naturally occurring behavior of mother and infant and served to maintain rather than distort these naturally occurring events. The decision I made early in the work was to take an observational position, *vis-à-vis* the research subject, that would maintain rather than distort the naturally occurring behavior of mother and infant and would not remove them from the setting and expectancies operating throughout the time of the observations. This procedure had the advantage of supporting the ongoing expectancies of the mother rather than introducing the complex, distorting influences of the experimentally controlled laboratory experiment. The mother's participation as an observer was invited. The effect was to increase her self-observing and infant-observing capacities without directing them. This approach in itself seemed to involve many of the mothers in a positive way. Certainly it enlivened and made more meaningful their capacity to observe their own infants and, hence, enhanced the possibilities of reciprocity with them. While such an approach lacks the superimposed "rigor" of method that is so often equated with anything "scientific," it has the advantage of interpreting data in context and leading the investigator to contiguous clinical phenomena.

Transference and Countertransference Reactions

Observing the mother–infant relationship usually arouses strong countertransference reactions in the observer. Most often this involves the identification of the observer with the infant rather than the mother, as is seen in the early development of the child psychiatrist in helping the disturbed child within the family. In these studies it has also been possible to trace the evolution of the mother's transference feelings toward the observer. If we asked the mother to participate in the study either before or while she was in labor, she was very much more ready to say yes than if we asked her after the baby was delivered. Anticipation of labor or ongoing labor may serve to mobilize the mother's object cathexes. She prepares herself to accept the baby as a new object in the outer environment. The research observers were in the some ways an extension of the infant. Mothers who breast-fed their infants were very much more ready to participate in the study than those who bottle-fed, probably because the breast-feeding mother had accepted the biological functioning of her body and was thus less conflicted about exhibitionistic–scoptophilic activity than was the mother who bottle-fed. A third way in which the mothers revealed their feelings toward the observers was found in the fact that mothers who positively accepted their infants positively accepted the observers; those who felt ambivalent or negative toward the infants also felt ambivalent or negative toward the observers.

Clinical Articulations of Research Findings

This project began with clinical observations and has, for the investigator, been a source of continuing clinical insight in the treatment of children and families and in formal psychoanalytic treatment. Reference has already been made to an understanding of autism and learning disorders and the, increased vulnerability of boys to psychopathology, anxiety, and early symptom formation in infancy (Call, 1965). In addition, approach, attachment, and disattachment provide an interesting tripart model for teachers and educators and for the evolution of transference during analysis. Mention has been made of Winnicott's analogy between the holding mother and holding during the analytic process. The latter holding, I believe, refers to the dosage, timing, and tact of the interpretive process, and to appropriate shifts of analytic attention from the depth to the surface and *vice versa* in keeping with the patient's level of ego functioning. In this manner reciprocity can take place within the framework of classical psychoanalytic technique.

It would be tempting to list all the loose ends, all the questions that should be pursued further, and all the ways in which this kind of research endeavor interdigitates with the literature on early development. This has, to some extent, been done in papers already published.

Influence of the Research Project on Colleagues, Student Participants, and Others

A "by-product" of the research enterprise is the development of people involved in the research effort, such as a few colleagues and the many students

who have participated in the research. I am convinced that participation in research by medical students, residents, and fellows in child psychiatry has provided an important locus around which much of their learning has been organized and provides a counterpoint to a deepening understanding of clinical
phenomena. I am convinced that the participation of students in this project,
involving as it has the early mother–infant interaction, has increased their
sensitivity to subtle phenomena in the doctor–patient relation.

Many colleagues and students who have read my papers and seen the
films that illustrate the findings have developed a long-term memory of specific
film sequences demonstrating the early adaptive and deviant behavior of the
infant.[4] The films illustrating the findings from this series of studies have
proved useful in initiating discussion among groups of widely varying backgrounds, from low-income parent groups to psychoanalytic candidates.

Members of one's family, fellow students, or colleagues wonder why a researcher spends so much of his time, usually uncompensated, in pursuing any
of the esoteric questions in the general category of research. "Is it worth it?"
they will ask openly and to themselves. The answer to that question in my
own case has always been yes, but I can't give a really satisfactory explanation
of why. Perhaps, like Darwin, I was never fully satisfied with the story of
creation.

Funding and Other Support

I must include at least a note on the funding and other support for this
project. The project probably would not have been possible without National
Institute of Mental Health Psychiatry Fellowship monies available to medical
students. Initially a grant request was submitted to the California Department
of Mental Hygiene (in 1960), which turned it down as inappropriate because
it was not related to the mental health care administered to patients in
California institutions. The NIMH approved a small grant to start the
project. This was of considerable help in purchasing a camera and in covering
the cost of filming. The UCLA Medical Center Auxiliary provided an additional fund for the purchase of special lenses, and the Los Angeles
Psychoanalytic Society and Institute provided an additional sum to support the
study on sex differences. The Foundations Fund for Research in Psychiatry
supported the study. A rather ambitiously designed follow-up study was
turned down recently by the NIMH. My own experience has been that

---

[4] Deviant behavior (of someone else's baby) is apparently registered in long-term memory more
than adaptive, average, expectable behavior.

funding is not always predictable, nor can it be relied upon as a major source of motivation for initiating and carrying through research activity. The major source of support for this research came from the University of California, mainly in terms of secretarial help, student help, support for my own salary, etc.

Summary

The human infant is no less resourceful than other mammals in making use of what it has to survive and actively determine the nature of the attachment formed to the mother who protects it, feeds it, and stimulates its development.

The earliest attachment of infant to mother and mother to infant is centered around the feeding situation and rapidly becomes *specific* for each mother–infant unit. While the human infant is born with the capacity to suck and swallow, to orient his head and mouth to a nipple when the nipple touches the snout area, and to incorporate and suck effectively thereon, he cannot exercise this adaptive capacity unless the mothering person can provide firm, close, bodily support, head support without restriction of head movement, and sensitive timing in introducing the nipple during optimal states of arousal in association with hunger needs. The mechanism for specific attachment—i.e., the process of adaptation—begins with the use of snout reflexes, including rooting behavior, which rapidly undergo adaptive modifications and are integrated with hand and head movement patterns that facilitate oral attachment to the breast or bottle nipple.

The capacity of the infant to show anticipatory approach behavior by the fourth day of life has prompted me to formulate a nuclear theory of ego formation based upon the infant's capacity to integrate a series of memory traces in relation to feeding and the experience of satisfaction associated with it.

The nonvisual nature of this early specific adaptation has led to a consideration of the relationship between nonvisual and visual experience. It is postulated that vision becomes prepotent over other sensory modalities in organizing the individual's experience with the outside world, and that the visual mode of perception provides a template on which the mental representation of objects and later of concepts takes place, notwithstanding the fact that the essence of one's experience with an object is found in its nonvisual qualities. Further research and theory is required for an understanding of the way in which visual bonding between mother and infant takes place.

An examination of the reciprocity between mother and infant that occurs in the relatively conflict-free situation after feeding while the infant is in a state

of alert attentiveness, and particularly the casual, playful sequences of behavior observed during this period, including lap and finger games and the
visually organized game of peek-a-boo, has suggested to this investigator that
these activities determine the matrix for the development of the relatively conflict-free sphere of ego functions in the infant.

A systematic study of sexual differences in relation to the behavior of the
infant before and after feeding during the first four days of life has suggested a
biological basis for the higher degree of vulnerability of boys to disruption of
object relations and for the increased incidence of various forms of deviant
development so commonly observed in males throughout childhood. The data
suggest that boys may be more influenced by appetitive internal forces than
girls, while girls may be more influenced by external visual stimuli, even in the
presence of physiological need states. Thus, the behavior of boys may become
more drive-organized, while that of girls may be more environmentally cued
and visually organized at an earlier period in development. This difference
could explain the higher predisposition to anxiety found in boys and the more
obvious distress shown by male infants to disruptions in the relationship with
the need-satisfying object, i.e., the mother. The relationship of a boy to his
mother is thus closer to the gut than that of a girl to the mother.

Some comments have been offered on why this particular research design
was molded around naturally occurring events in the natural environment,
around transference and countertransference relationships between the observer and the observed, around the influence of this project on the students
who participated in it, and around the problems of funding such research.

Conclusion

My research odyssey, like Homer's, has included a series of explorations
and adventures in relatively uncharted waters. As with Ulysses, each expe-
dition has provided just enough satisfaction to make it worthwhile but has
presented new possibilities that in their elusive quality have contined to recruit
a significant portion of this investigator's resources and energies.

This research odyssey has taken place alongside other commitments, some
grossly distracting and some broadening and deepening the exploration so that
more relevant and precise questions could be posed.

The interplay of theory and observation of clinical work with research
and of phenomena of infancy with those of "maturity" have provided the kind
of paradox and ambiguity that keeps me committed to this project as a continuing center around which thoughtfulness about human development at all
phases of the life cycle can be organized.

References

BABKIN, P. S. The establishment of reflex activity in early postnatal life. *Sechenov Physiol. J. USSR*, **44** (No. 10), 1958, 922–927.

BELL, R. Q., WELLER, G. M., & WALDROP, M. F. Newborn and preschooler: organization of behavior and relations between periods. In *Monographs of the Society for Research in Child Development*, Series No. 142. Chicago: University of Chicago Press, 1971.

CALL, J. D. Newborn approach behaviour and early ego development. *International Journal of Psychoanalysis*, 1964, **45**, 286–294.

CALL, J. D. On the psychic development of the newborn infant. Published in Spanish in *Cuaernos de Psicoanalisis*, 1965, **1**, 237–256.

CALL, J. D., & MARSCHAK, M. Styles and games in infancy. *Journal of the American Academy of Child Psychiatry*, 1966, **5**, 193–210.

CALL, J. D. Lap and finger play in infancy, implications for ego development. *International Journal of Psychoanalysis*, 1968, **49**, 375–378.

CALL, J. D. Emotional-social factors. *Journal of Special Education*, 1971, **4**, 349–359.

CONSTAS, R., & CALL, J. Spontaneous hand-mouth activity, rooting and hand-mouth reflexes as related to state in the newborn infant. Presented to the Society for Research in Child Development, University of California, Berkeley, 1963.

FRAIBERG, S. Libidinal object constancy and mental representation. *Psychoanalytic Study of the Child*, 1969, **24**, 9–47.

GLOVER, E. The concept of dissociation. In *On the early development of mind*. New York: International University Press, 1943.

HARTMANN, H. *Ego psychology and the problem of adaptation*. New York: International University Press, 1939; London: Imago, 1958.

LA BARRE, W. *The human animal*. Chicago: University of Chicago Press, 1954.

LORENZ, K., TINBERGEN, N., & VON FRISCH, K. The 1973 Nobel Prize for Physiology or Medicine. *Science*, 1973, **182**, 464–466.

RANGELL, L. On the psychology of poise: With special elaboration on the psychic significance of the snout or perioral region. *International Journal of Psychoanalysis*, 1954, **35**, 313–332.

SPITZ, R. A. (1945). Diacritic and coenesthetic organizations. *Psychoanalytic Review*, 1945, **32**, 146–162.

SULLIVAN, H. S. The meaning of anxiety in psychiatry and in life. *Psychiatry*, 1948, **11**, 1–13.

WACHSMAN, F. Implications from the content of music in Africa. In Edward L. Margetts (Ed.), *The mind of man in Africa*. Oxford: Pergamon, 1966.

WOLFF, P. Observations on newborn infants. *Psychosomatic Medicine*, 1959, **21**, 110–118.

WOLFF, P. H., & WHITE, B. L. Visual pursuit and attention in young infants. *Journal of Am. Acad. of Child Psychiatry*, 1965, **4**, 473–484.

THE CONCEPTION, BIRTH, AND CHILDHOOD OF A BEHAVIORAL RESEARCH

THE NEW YORK LONGITUDINAL STUDY

STELLA CHESS

On the Olympus of any science, the researcher stands at the pinnacle and the clinician at its base. From this lofty vantage point the researcher engages in "investigation or experimentation aimed at the discovery and interpretation of facts, revision of accepted theories or laws in the light of new facts, or practical application of such new or revised theories or laws [*Webster's*, p. 730]." Indeed, when I began my career as a clinician, this definition, together with reports in the literature, led me to assume that all researchers started their investigations with elegant, unbiased designs, carried them through with single-mindedness of purpose, and finished with clear, unequivocal, meaningful results.

The clinician, on the other hand, is a practical person, defined by what he is *not*—namely, a researcher. To him falls the task of matching theory to actuality. When the fit is a poor one, he may ignore the research, place the facts of the case on the Procrustean bed of psychiatric theory, or follow a clinical hunch.

When the clinician decides on the latter course, he may not realize at first that he has embarked on a long, hazardous trek up the mountain. The journey is full of pitfalls; the erstwhile "clinical investigator" will skid and slide, get caught in the crevices of his own data, give up, start again, and change course many times before he arrives, years later, at his destination.

STELLA CHESS, Department of Psychiatry, New York University Medical Center, New York.

Now, with my own status as a researcher clearly established, I can look back with some indulgence at my earlier conceptions of research methodology. During the day I was a clinician. In the evening—in my free time—I searched my records in an attempt to find answers to the questions that arose out of my clinical practice. Since I was clearly not in the Arrowsmith arena, replete with laboratories and test tubes, I adopted a trial-and-error approach to research, with Pavlov as my model. If I X'd a group of patients, did they Y? Why did this patient react, and not that one? No thought then of statistics and long-term studies!

However, over the years I have found that clinical impressions are not to be demeaned in any way. For the clinician they provide a valid starting point for any research—no more and no less. The original hunch, or theory, will undergo a constant metamorphosis as new data come to light. Basic to the transformation of a clinician into a researcher is the realization that data analysis is of primary importance, definitely not to be done in the evening after a full day's work plus everything else that happened up to the moment of putting the children to bed!

The methodology and results of the New York Longitudinal Study of Temperament have been reported in depth elsewhere (Thomas et al., 1963). Here I intend to relate the story of how it all came about—the story of my own dissatisfaction with the clinical applicability of certain theories, the steps through which that dissatisfaction was transformed first into an idea, then into a test of that idea, and finally into a workable research design.

Initially two people were involved: Dr. Alexander Thomas and myself. We shared, in our personal lives, four children, all of whom seemed to have different personalities from the day they were born. Professionally, we shared an increasing awareness of the gap between the clinical situations that confronted us daily and psychiatric theory, which, when applied, failed to alleviate our patients' distress. Often no apparent relationship existed between our patients' behavioral difficulties and their early environments.

As a child psychiatrist I had the opportunity of comparing the theoretical and the actual effects of certain childhood trauma. For instance, I observed that separation was fraught with fear for one child, and clinging became a behavioral characteristic. However, another child, lost in a large department store, had such a delightful time with the strangers who entertained him that getting lost became a desirable end in itself. Similarly, the child with insatiable demands had not necessarily been rejected, unless one postulated a symbolic need so well covered up on the part of the mother that it could only be inferred from the child's reactions.

The list of unexplained behavior was indeed very long. Unless one assumed that the child's reactions were so subtle as to be unobservable or that counterphobic or repressive mechanisms were in operation, there simply had to be other explanations for the variety of reactions that appeared in early childhood. Gradually I came to the opinion that the child was an important and active agent in the creation of his own environment.

In adult behavior a similar elusive element appeared to be at work. In the reported quarrels of a couple coming for psychiatric help, there was a component beyond the neurotic issues of the moment. He would end a name-calling match by going into a prolonged sulk, while she would go off on the crest of a rage, only to return cheerful and friendly half an hour later. He would then insist that they talk it out, refusing to believe her statements that she hadn't meant most of what she had said. Aside from the psychodynamic element in the sensitivities that had originally evoked the quarrel, there appeared to be other individual differences in reactivity that determined the *style* of quarreling and postargument behavior.

Here I should state that instead of immediately producing a research design Dr. Thomas and I thought and talked about these observations for a good 10 years. Initially we thought we must be wrong in giving these reactive styles so much importance. However, in our clinical practices with children and adults we had noticed that it seemed more helpful to recognize this aspect of behavior than to ignore it. We found that, both in the informing interview with parents and in psychotherapeutic discussions with adult patients, clarification of the individual style of reactivity was useful to both ourselves and the parent or other adult in understanding the interplay between the patient and the significant people in his life.

Finally, in 1952, after years of observation and discussion with each other and our patients, we began our first systematic explorations into the nature and effects of individual reactive patterns. Still taking Pavlov as our model, we thought primarily in terms of conditioned behavior, or more correctly, conditional responses. Our first approach arose out of a personal experience with our first child, born in July—a hot month in a hot city apartment. Although I have great difficulty waking up, I did not like to disturb the neighbors, and therefore it was of some importance to discover that on some nights our baby stopped crying almost as soon as I got up to warm the bottle, while on other nights the crying continued until she could taste the milk. Sleepy though I was, I soon discovered that the baby stopped crying almost immediately whenever I pushed open our squeaky bedroom door. Thinking only in practical terms, I had incorporated this knowledge into my child-care practices. The baby cried. I stumbled out of bed and squeaked the door. Then, with a clear conscience about waking the neighbors, I took time to wash my face and proceeded without urgency to the business at hand.

Out of this experience arose our first experiments with babies' individual adaptability to conditioning. We assembled a list of expectant mothers, assured them that their babies would not be subjected to any unpleasant stimulus, provided them each with a stopwatch, a tinkly elephant bell, and a chart, and explained our procedure to them. When the baby cried at feeding time, the stopwatch was pressed and the bell tinkled. The parent then went about his or her usual business of feeding—first diapering, if so desired, picking up or not, in advance—in short, simply acting naturally. When bottle or breast went into the baby's mouth, the stopwatch was pressed again. At the end of the feeding the trial was numbered on the chart, the time interval entered, and a zero entered in the column "Stopped Crying in Response to Bell." The first time the baby did stop crying at the sound of the bell, the time interval was to be noted and entered. This was indeed a most ingenious design and we are still quite proud of it. Unfortunately, it was a complete failure. Only later did we realize that, even in Hanuš Papoušek's interesting work on conditioning infants, one could not expect integrated stimulus–response reactions in the first two weeks of life. At a later age some children did stop crying when placed in the feeding position or when their bibs were tucked in. Others, including my second child, appeared completely disinterested in any stimulus other than the milk itself.

As it turned out though, this first trial, albeit a failure, inadvertently set us on the right track. At first our conversations with parents seemed to contain primarily irrelevant material—irrelevant, that is, to the study as designed. However, as Dr. Thomas and I discussed these conversations, we began to realize that much of this material, dealing with the babies' moment-to-moment activities and the handling that evoked these responses, pointed to individual styles of behavior. By refining our interviews with the parents, we were able to determine precisely which stimuli gave rise to a given response. Fortunately, we were able to modify our study early enough to do a six-week-old behavior protocol with this group of infants.

After further experimentation with ages and time intervals, we finally decided that two to three months was the optimum time for an initial interview, taking in behavior from birth to this point. This plan led to another obstacle—namely, determining the maximum time lapse possible for accurate parental recall. We checked reports on anterospective recall in the literature, took histories at different intervals, and refined the nature of our questions to ensure objective descriptive data. Sometimes our methods were very obvious. On one occasion, for example, when a mother was explaining her son's behavior, her husband said, "You can skip that. She'll start writing again when you tell her *what* he did, not why he did it."

Before we committed ourselves to a major research project, we had to answer certain basic questions: Precisely what did we wish to study? How did we propose to carry out that study? And what methods were we going to use to ensure the accuracy of our data? We were only too familiar with unfocused studies in which the researchers had indiscriminately assembled quantities of data only to discover that many of them were irrelevant and that truly significant information was missing altogether. We were also aware of studies in which the method of data collection and analysis had changed from year to year, resulting in virtually unintelligible results. It was essential, therefore, to plan ahead.

The first question was certainly the most difficult to answer. From my clinical work I had theorized that children reacted differently to the same situation. From our first test we had discovered that these different reactive styles were present in early infancy. We wanted to investigate more precisely the different characteristics that made up a given "style of reactivity," which characteristics were likely to endure into adulthood, and, most importantly, the significance of the various characteristics in overall personality development.

It was obvious from the nature of our inquiry that a longitudinal approach was necessary. In order to reduce the hazard of overlooking significant information, we had to make an educated guess as to which characteristics were most likely to endure. Therefore we conducted a pretest, using as our sample a group of children ranging in age from 5 to 15. In order to minimize the variability of parental handling, we chose our sample from professional families with similar approaches to child rearing. We conducted innumerable interviews, identifying current behaviors and tracing them back to their apparent antecedents. Some of these youngsters were tempestuous from the beginning, other serene. Some would forget semipromises, other would remember forever. The sedentary ones had been so as toddlers, the energetic ones were the early daredevils. It appeared, then, that the behaviors described by the parents of our infant group had enough continuity with those of the older group to warrant further study along the same line.

We also gave the older children standard intelligence tests, later using a separate observer to make notes on the children's individual responses to the test situation. This procedure proved to be a valuable source of data, providing us with both a record of individual scoring on a standardized instrument and an individual style of response to a standardized set of demands.

Up to this point Dr. Thomas and I had been almost the full research team. We had written the questionnaire, organizing our inquiry around activity areas such as eating, sleeping, and dressing. We had developed the interview technique, probing for complete answers to each question. We had interviewed and observed parents and children. By this time we had interviews on each of 20 children four times. Now we needed an experienced researcher to go over our material and help us prepare a proper research design to verify our theory of early differences in style of reactivity.

The first researchers we consulted were hardly encouraging. They agreed that this was indeed a most important area of investigation but wanted none of it. At this point we exploited our friendship with Dr. Birch. Undaunted by our mass of anecdotal records, he proceeded to do an inductive analysis of the data, divided them into categories, worked out definitions, and developed a system of item scoring that became the basis of our future work. This analytical approach shed new light on our study. We found that many categories confirmed our original ideas, some categories had escaped our notice completely, and others were debatable. In fact the next phase of our study might be politely termed "debatable." Arguments raged, categories were redefined, their relevance, frequency, and degree were questioned. By the time we finished this phase, labor had been vigorous, but a viable infant research was born.

Our baby was born but was not in fact named for a good year thereafter. At first we used the phrase "individual patterns of reactivity." Later we adopted the word *temperament*, which seemed equally correct and much less clumsy. There still remained one major hurdle in our study. We had pages of descriptive reports but no way of verifying their accuracy. We had considered placing an observer in the home for extended periods, or using recording devices. However, aside from the prohibitive cost of home observers or tape analysis, we couldn't guarantee that the interactions observed would be identical with those occurring when the family was alone. If, on the other hand, our interview technique could generate accurate data using the family as observer, we would have the advantage of continuous round-the-clock reportage with no distortion of behavior. Direct observation could be used at intervals to cross-check the histories obtained from the interviews.

Thus a sample of children were seen by two trained observers for a two-hour period, arranged to include awakening from sleep, a feeding, and whatever other events took place in this time. The observer, a stranger, was also able to assess the child's reaction to new and unfamiliar people. These observations, together with a scheduled history from the parents, all took place within a two-week period to ensure that differences in behavior didn't arise out of maturation and newly achieved activity levels. When these data were all scored according to our standardized procedure, we found that each observation was in closer agreement with the history than with the other observations. Let us say, for example, that there were 100 items scored for each observation and the parent interview. If each observation disagreed with the history on one score, the item might not be the same for each; thus there would be 98 items of agreement and 2 items of disagreement between the two observations, as opposed to 99 and 1 between each observation and the parent interview.

We had now developed a method of obtaining reliable data, using the family as observers. But we soon realized that there was yet another problem: How accurate was our scoring?

For example, if a normally docile child reacted in an uncharacteristically vigorous fashion—though in fact only of moderate intensity when compared to an absolute standard—would our scorers be influenced by the halo effect of this child's unusual behavior and overscore the stronger reaction? Would his behavior in one area influence the scorer to anticipate behavior in another area? Once again Dr. Birch outlined the proper statistical procedures to check for bias. Each protocol was submitted to interscorer and scorer–rescorer reliability tests. Finally, a snip analysis was done on each protocol. To Dr. Birch, who remained with us until his death in February 1973, we owe a debt of gratitude for bringing to this study not only his expertise in data analysis but also his extraordinary ability to interpret and conceptualize the results of these analyses.[1]

Once we had solved these problems, which are basic to a good research design, we were able to proceed with our longitudinal study, add to our sample, and enlarge the scope of our questions as our study population moved from infancy to chilhood and on up into work and college, as some of our 17-year-olds are now doing. At each new stage we have done pretests with a small section of our total sample to determine which were the best sources and methods of obtaining the necessary data. For example, when our children started school, we arranged interviews with the teacher and added information on school performance and peer-group relations to our study. Our older group of 16- and 17-year-olds are now able to provide us with reliable observations of their own behavior, although this was not possible at an earlier stage of development.

Eventually a researcher must submit his results to the comments and criticism of his colleagues. Essentially the early reports of our study were greeted with three different reactions, which could be roughly classified as: "So what?" "Horrors!" and "Yes, but . . ."

In the first category I am reminded of a story about George Bernard Shaw. On learning of Pavlov's experiments in conditioning dogs to salivate to the sound of a bell, Shaw reportedly commented that Pavlov had finally learned as much about dogs as a London bobby had known all his life. The initial response to our reports on temperament was of the same order.

These ideas were not new, merely a statement of the obvious, that individuals had individuality. Of course this simple statement was true as far as it went, but we felt that current theories of personality development placed unidimensional emphasis on environmental influences. To date there had been very little organized exploration into the nature of that individuality and its impact on the environment. There is, after all, some merit in going beyond the observation that a falling apple will hit the ground to the exploration of the laws of falling objects.

---

[1] Colleagues who, throughout the research, worked most closely with us were Dr. Sam Korn and Dr. Margaret Hertzig. In addition there was an unusual group of competent and dedicated people who worked on various other research projects.

Our reports were viewed with alarm by a second group of critics who felt that we were simply returning to the constitutionalism of an earlier period—the "bad seed" concept of behavioral causality. These critics assumed that we were postulating an unalterable, constitutionally predetermined personality and denying the modifying effects of the environment on the child.

Strict proponents of psychoanalytic theory offered a third type of criticism. This is perhaps best shown by an incident that took place at a meeting where I presented our data on the occurrence of behavior disorders from birth to preadolescence. Under the impression that the clinical questions, study design, and case illustrations were extremely clear, I was startled by the first questioner, who asked: "Since the purpose of your research is to disprove the developmental theories of Anna Freud, why didn't you . . . ?" He then proceeded to outline a totally different research project. I explained that our study was not attempting to align itself in an adversary position against Anna Freud but was, as I had stated initially, an inductive analysis of behavioral manifestations in infancy and childhood. However, my questioner was so locked into the paradigm of psychoanalytic theory that he could not conceive of any research that was not based on this one, presumably universally accepted, theoretical position.

While such criticisms were distortions of the main thrust of our reports, to some extent they did influence the way we examined the data. As our study progressed and our children grew, we began to see that it was not enough to examine the nature of temperament itself. It became increasingly evident that the child's temperament had as great a potential for interactional impact as did his environment. Thus a baby's style of reactivity did indeed influence the way in which his parents handled him, and as a result did determine, to some degree, the quality of his day-to-day experiences. Similarly, the quality of the experiences provided by the parents differed according to the child's type of temperament. Detailing the interactional nature of temperament and environment has been no small task, though clearly of overriding importance.

We launched our first longitudinal study of temperament in normal, middle-class children years ago. Since that time we have studied the effects of temperament on Puerto Rican (Chess et al., 1967), mentally retarded (Chess, 1970), and currently, rubella children (Chess et al., 1971). However, perhaps because we have invested so much of our time, our energy, and our intellectual curiosity in it, this first study will always be our first love. We have watched as each child gained mastery over the physical and social environment, each in his or her own individual way. We have observed the gradual transition from action to ideation in both normal and abnormal development. As the children were faced with new challenges from the schools and their peer groups, we expanded the scope of our study. We noted the changing nature of symptom formation from actions and reactions at earlier ages to the development of psychodynamic patterns of defense at later ages. Our research subjects are now almost young adults and the data are still coming in.

Thus far the results of all our studies have been remarkably consistent. Certainly no one would deny the importance of other factors of heredity and environment; however, throughout our research we have found temperament to be a remarkably important variable in overall behavioral development. Temperament can be isolated and classified. To some extent its effects are predictable. For instance, we know that those who are temperamentally "difficult" are at greater risk for the development of behavior disorders than any other group of children. We know that "slow-to-warm-up" children will always have difficulty making transitions. Even the "easy" child can be too malleable for his own good. Certain temperamental characteristics can potentiate the effect of other hereditary or environmental variables, such as mental defect or the death of a parent. Similarly, the potentially negative effects of certain temperamental characteristics such as persistence or high intensity can be alleviated if parents and teachers are made aware of these characteristics and the best way of dealing with them.

When we began our investigation of styles of reactivity so many years ago, we had no idea then of the scope that such a research project would encompass. Little did we know that we would some day be instructing project supervisors, wrestling with data, and booking computer time. We merely wanted to explore an area that we felt had been largely ignored by other researchers. We began with Pavlov and tinkling bells. His method proved wrong for our purposes, but his advice to scientists still holds true today:

> Firstly, gradualness. About this most important condition of fruitful scientific work I never can speak without emotion. Gradualness, gradualness and gradualness. From the very beginning of your work, school yourselves to severe gradualness in the accumulation of knowledge.
>
> Secondly, modesty. Never think that you already know all. However highly you are appraised, always have the courage to say to yourself—I am ignorant.
>
> Thirdly, passion. Remember that science claims a man's whole life. Had he two lives they would not suffice. Science demands an undivided allegiance from its followers. In your work and in your research there must always be passion [1936, quoted in Bartlett's, 1968].

References

CHESS, S. Temperament and behavior disorders in mentally retarded children. *Archives of General Psychiatry*, 1970, **23**, 122–130.

CHESS, S., KORN, S., & FERNANDEZ, P. *Psychiatric disorders of children with congenital rubella.* New York: Brunner/Mazel, 1971.

CHESS, S., SARLIN, M. B., MENDEZ, A., & THOMAS, A. Social class and child rearing practices. paper presented at the American Psychiatric Association Divisional Meeting, Nov. 17, 1967.

PAVLOV, I. P. Bequest to the academic youth of Soviet Russia by Ivan Petrovich Pavlov (1936) (as quoted in Bartlett's 14th edition, 1968).
THOMAS, A., BIRCH, H. G., CHESS, S., MERTZIG, M. E., & KORN, S. *Behavioral individuality in early childhood.* New York: New York University Press, 1963.
THOMAS, A., CHESS, S., & BIRCH, H. G. *Temperament and behavior disorders in children.* New York: New York University Press, 1968.
Webster's Seventh New Collegiate Dictionary. Springfield, Mass.: Merriam, 1961.

PSYCHOSOMATIC RESEARCH

INTRODUCTION

Cohen draws attention to the advantages of being a child psychiatric investigator: not only is he present at the beginning of individual development, but his background and experience enable him to assess data correlating body, mind, and environment. Furthermore, his comprehensive medicopsychological education gives him the freedom to range from genetics to sociology, taking in psychology, psychoanalysis, child development, and pediatrics on the way. However, he points out that this "linguistic versatility" has some dangers attached to it in that there is a certain risk of becoming a somewhat confused polyglot. The chapter is remarkable in several different ways. It displays a scholarship and a philosophical understanding of epistemological issues that is well beyond the knowledge of the average clinical investigator, who is unlikely to have read Descartes, let alone to have written a thesis on him. In such hands, the analysis of models becomes a highly sophisticated exercise, which could be of little more than academic interest were it not for the important fact that it is made operational through a study of eczematous children. To use a model deriving from Wittgenstein is an extraordinary thing and puts to shame those of us still grappling with hydrostatic structures designed for a simpler age.

The clinical setting in its wide variety of forms has not only provided Fischhoff with many research opportunities but has also permitted him to bring together the often-segregated spheres of research, service, and teaching so that each can profit from the other. This is truly a rare concatenation in child psychiatric centers. One must therefore regard Fischhoff as a clinical organizer as well as a clinical investigator, since he undoubtedly has a facility for making diverse environments work for him in his projects. His empirical approach is tied to the "good" question rather than to the "good" theory, and he is more interested in what is likely to work than in glamorous technology. He is prepared to make use of any method of examination without prejudice, from questionnaire to intensive case study. His preference is to attack on a broad front, covering such aspects as fantasy, physiology, and family. A sound clinical background coupled with psychoanalytic training have helped to give breadth and depth to his observations without apparently confusing his research orientation. As we have seen with others, a stronger physical approach might have created a real "conflict of interests." Like every good investigator, he is prepared to "drop everything" when an "experiment of nature" comes along to illuminate the research scene. His type of steady work is needed to fill the many gaps in our clinical knowledge.

Mattsson is basically interested in the coping process in response to stress, particularly that deriving from physical illness and handicap. His background in pediatrics has made it possible for him to bring the physical and the psychological together in the same context. This background also gave him entry to the pediatric wards and the opportunity to use crisis techniques to deal with hemophiliac patients. The idea of looking at serious childhood ill-nesses in the special context of adaptation transformed what might have turned out in other hands to be no more than a straightforward empirical study of a most intriguing question, each step of which opened up new possibilities of investigation. Thus endocrine studies became a logical step within the adaptation framework. This is a good example of how fruitfully theory and investigation work together in bringing the practicalities involved in the care of sick children into line with psychological thought. Here we can remind ourselves constantly of Lewin's well-known aphorism that there is nothing so practical as a good theory and that a researcher has no need to feel ashamed of his preconceptions.

Bruch's name has become so inextricably linked with a particular area of psychosomatic research that the very sound of it conjures up images of very fat or very thin children. Her presentation reveals just how much background and experience is needed to make original contributions to the field. It has always seemed to me that Bruch's research strength lay in her capacity to cut through a great deal of clinical complexity and come up with some very direct and pertinent findings. A part of this capacity could be attributed to her impatience with clichés and well-worn, threadbare clinical beliefs. She is one of those rare individuals who knows what she knows and, more importantly, knows what she does not know. This has led her to make giant strides in an area in which far too much had previously been taken for granted. She has brought a breath of fresh research air into a very stale clinical environment.

PSYCHOSOMATIC
MODELS OF
DEVELOPMENT

Donald J. Cohen

An investigator's conception of mind, body, and human behavior will determine his selection of problems and methods. Long before he finishes collecting data, the form of his explanations may be shaped by his philosophical viewpoint. This essay illustrates some aspects of the relationship between philosophical themes and empirical studies in child psychiatry.

Philosophical Themes

My initial interest in child development research was related to the possibility of finding new directions in the resolution of classical philosophical dilemmas surrounding the explanation of human behavior and the limits of behaviorism. Reviewing these will introduce the historical context for the empirical studies.

There are two main traditions of scientific explanation. The teleological or finalistic tradition considers natural processes in relation to their aims. In physics this tradition is associated with the interpretation of concepts as referring to "real" things (as in Aristotle's natural philosophy), and in psychology with explanation of action in terms of reasons, justifications, intentions, and motives. In contrast, the causal or mechanistic tradition offers a positivistic interpretation of scientific theory in which concepts are considered useful conventions for summarizing and predicting, and in which there are only prior causes, not goals. In physics this viewpoint is associated with the naturalism and mathematical models of Galileo; in psychology with the explication of the causes and determinants of behavior.

DONALD J. COHEN, Departments of Pediatrics, Psychiatry, and Psychology, and the Child Study Center, Yale University School of Medicine, New Haven.

Both traditions of explanation have pre-Socratic and pre-Platonic roots, and, as suggested by Piaget (1950), they may be part of every man's development. Over the centuries, their boundaries have at times been blurred. Yet their main trunks can be traced to issues in contemporary philosophy of science (e.g., see Colodny, 1970; Hesse, 1961; Taylor, 1970; Toulmin, 1970; von Wright, 1971).

The two traditions of explanation are of special interest to historians of psychology because they have interwoven with another, equally venerable dichotomy: the two-worlds conception of mind and body (e.g. see Passmore, 1961, pp. 38–57; Ryle, 1949). The lineage of the two-worlds conception also has pre-Socratic, Stoic roots, and proceeds through Philo, the Church Fathers, Maimonides, and Thomas of Aquino to the schoolmen (see Descartes, 1947; Gilson, 1951; Wolfson, 1947, 1956). Thus, the simple, compelling differences between body and soul were well-defined, almost crystallized doctrine centuries before being taught to Descartes as an adolescent in the academy of La Flèche. Yet his radicalism and the special tensions of the seventeenth century brought the two-worlds conception and the two traditions of explanation into clearer juxtaposition and distinctive focus. Descartes recast the arguments in forms and terms that have endured as our own.

Descartes's century was a period of dramatic scientific change distinguished by empirical and conceptual discoveries in mathematics, physics, and biology. This new science coexisted with an unbroken tradition of philosophical and theological discourse. To be an active intellectual in Descartes's circle was to participate in both the new science and this philosophical discourse—a style of mind that later ceased to be possible or, perhaps, valued (Buchdahl, 1969). Thus Descartes contributed to optics, physiology, and geometry and, at the same time, wished to write a textbook on metaphysics, in the scholastic style, which would be acceptable to the Jesuit faculty of the Sorbonne. The intellectual stage was set, then, for conflict: between Descartes's basic theological and metaphysical language, which defined his identity in a long history, and his enthusiasm for extending the limits of science to all of nature.

Easy resolutions for this conflict were at hand. An almost classical resolution would have been to maintain a teleological explanation for all mental processes and a causal explanation for physical events. But Descartes questioned the validity of this bisection. In the process, he confronted major dilemmas: How universal is universal physics? How does the soul cause the body to move? Does the body cause the soul to feel? How separate are the concepts applicable to mind and body? What is human about the human mind, and what does a man's behavior share with that of animals?

What emerged was a conception of human reasoning, imagination, and language that separated these uniquely human capacities from basic passions of the soul, reflexive behavior, and the movements of objects (including animal behavior). This conception set limits on physics and causal explanation. However, these limits easily could be overlooked in some texts—e.g., *Le Traité de l'Homme* (Descartes, 1897–1913), in which Descartes elaborated an apparently unreserved, causal mode of behavior. And thus Descartes was followed by two disputatious camps, each claiming to be his true descendants: those who saw him as a philosopher who invigorated classical metaphysics with a new phenomenology and a modern, critical spirit (e.g., see Husserl, 1960) and those who saw in his causal explanations of behavior and models of automata the origins of reflex psychology and the end to Thomistic psychology (Canguilhem, 1955; Keele, 1957; Vartanian, 1960).

The results of Descartes's meditations and ambivalence have left their imprint on our own thinking. Questions similar to his motivate contemporary philosophy of mind (e.g., see Wittgenstein, 1958, and those who have developed from him: e.g., Anscombe, 1957; Hacker, 1972, Kenny, 1973; Peters, 1958; Winch, 1958). Now, we may see ramifications of Descartes's dilemmas in questions about intention, action, purpose, and meaning and about whether these, and concepts of a similar type, should be found in a "truly" scientific theory of human behavior. We wonder what the explanation of such a science should most resemble—those of physiology or those of history (e.g., see Dray, 1966; Lakatos, 1970; Nagel, 1961). And we are concerned, more parochially, about whether psychoanalysis is a science in search of laws like any other (see Hook, 1960); a hermeneutic method to uncover meanings (Ricoeur, 1970); or a "successful pseudoscience" resembling the art of numerology (Cioffi, 1970).

This essay describes studies done under the influence of two models of mind and two different conceptions of the explanation of human action. The last section addresses the subject of a psychosomatic model of development and suggests how child psychiatry might contribute to the philosophy of mind.

Causal Explanation: Laboratory Paradigms

Ogden Lindsley (1956, 1960, 1963a) working in an inconspicuous laboratory in a state mental hospital, was the first scientist to use the advanced technology of operant conditioning to study chronic psychosis. His basic instrument was a six-foot square room, bare except for a plunger and a trinket dispenser and monitored by a periscope and cumulative recorders. Using this laboratory setup, Lindsley examined what he conceptualized as the psychotic symptoms (pacing and vocalizing) and adaptive behaviors (pulling the plunger for candy and cigarettes) of regressed, destructive, and often nonverbal men and women. His goal was to demonstrate that schizophrenic behavior could be understood and manipulated by the use of operant paradigms.

While writing a thesis on Descartes, I visited the hospital to learn more about behavior and chanced on the Behavior Research Laboratory. The model of human action it embodied seemed elegant, precise, and not very distant from what I then understood, wrongly, as Wittgenstein's behaviorism. Lindsley's invitation to spend time in the laboratory led to several years of that type of collaboration, fundamental to the history of laboratory science, in which a student learns to imitate his teacher's attack on problems and to extend his concepts.

I was drawn to issues concerning the operational definition, measurement, and control of social behavior (Cohen, 1962; Lindsley, 1963b, 1966; Nathan, 1964). Could relations between human beings be confined within operant paradigms?

The laboratory instrument for the social studies doubled the basic, six-foot square chamber. Two school-age children were seated in adjacent rooms, separated by a screen in which plungers and trinket dispensers were mounted. When a child pulled his plunger immediately after a signal light flashed, his room dimmed, a tone sounded, and a penny was delivered. The signal light flashed when the child in the adjacent room pulled his plunger. Social behavior was thus defined as the coordination of plunger-pulling operants involving two individuals who worked to optimize the frequency of reinforcement. And we studied how children learned to pull together ("cooperation"), which child initiated the team responses ("leadership"), and how the children acted when only one was rewarded for a team effort ("competition"). (For a review of this approach, see Hake and Vukelich, 1972.)

The most intriguing findings related not to simple learning but to a chance observation: that it was easier for children to learn to coordinate their operant responses when they could see each other through the opened window than when they relied on the signal light; and that it was much easier to use the signal light after they knew it was controlled by another person—after it "acquired social connotation"—than before.

But why should behavior change when a person learns that a signal light is controlled by another human rather than by a machine? What are the dimensions of this phenomenon and how can it be manipulated? We explored these questions by having college students and school-age children enter the experimental setup without being told that there was a partner next door. Suddenly the window was opened and each "subject" could observe the other for brief periods of 30 to 60 seconds. These brief "presentations of human stimulation" often led to dramatic improvement in the acquisition of team responses (Cohen and Lindsley, 1964). It was thus surprising when a young "schizophrenic" girl, teamed with a normal college volunteer, had precisely the opposite reaction to "human stimulation." Even after many hours of experimental sessions, the presentation of human stimulation led to her acute disorganization and to disruption of team behavior. For the patient, we hypothesized, human stimulation led to "overarousal" and the elicitation of "psychosis-specific emotional interference."

The study of social behavior in the context of operant conditioning theory—which we were the first to explore systematically—articulated well with classical social-psychology observations: increased arousal by human stimulation facilitated healthy individuals in learning socially relevant tasks; it created competitive responses ("anxiety") and behavioral deterioration in less well-integrated people (see Allport, 1924; Zajonc, 1965).

This account gives the flavor of the model and the language that evolved. They bear a family resemblance to Descartes's automata model, in which he likened human actions to those of fountain figures triggered to move when a visitor to a grotto depresses a tile in the floor and initiates a hydraulic mechanism (Descartes, 1897–1913). There would be much to say today about the meaning of observing "normal" and "psychotic" people in six-foot rooms and the "control" of social behavior by pennies (see, e.g., Friedman, 1967). Our data suggest discussion in terms of intention, object relations, and the participants' understanding of the situation, as well as in terms of compliance, methodological constraints, and validity of extrapolation. Then, however, the paradigms seemed essentially valid descriptions of the major facets of social behavior.

Let one more example stand for many. In a study of pain healthy individuals were seated in chairs and small electrodes were attached to their arms and legs. The sharp, pinlike shocks delivered through these electrodes could be reduced by the volunteer's pressing a button. In addition the subject could press a foot switch to maintain a television picture on the screen and still another to earn rewards at the sound of a tone. Thus, we believed, this experimental situation simultaneously assessed pain (responding to avoid shock); interest (the television-viewing operant); and attention (vigilance for the tone). Typically, an adult volunteer was given a placebo, a mild analgesic, or a potent analgesic at some point during an experimental session. An ideal analgesic, it was hypothesized, would affect only pain-avoidance behavior; a soporific would affect all three operants.

Marked individual (or "idiosyncratic") differences were more prominent, and interesting, than differences in the efficacy of medication. Without medication some individuals accepted high-intensity shocks with little discomfort or avoidance responding; others responded maximally even with very potent medication. As a frequent "volunteer," I knew to which group I belonged.

Complex behavior, it seemed to me then, was the unfolding of various operants controlled by environmental discriminative stimuli (which were occasions for responding) and by environmental reinforcing stimuli (which were signals that the response was acceptable or not). In this model, development involves the movement of stimuli from outside to inside, and social interactions can be understood in terms of simple learning theory, equally applicable to man and pigeon. Over the course of the years, in response to the demands of his environment, a child develops by coming under the control of new discriminative stimuli and new rewards, which are generated by and for himself as well as by others (see, e.g., Ulrich and Mountjoy, 1972).

In this formulation, *development* and *learning* are synonyms. Individual progress is possible because most humans are endowed with the equivalent of Kantian categories: the ability to associate stimuli, respond to different types of reinforcement, and form discriminations. Those individuals who are not well endowed with these behavioral givens are, thus, "patients" of one sort or another. Retarded people have innate defects involving functioning within one or more categorical areas; psychotic patients suffer from short circuits and odd stimulus–operant or operant–operant chained connections; and neurotic patients have milder disturbances in their behavioral repertoire resulting from a history of bad conditioning.

Given this type of model, the goals of psychology (and of psychological therapy, in particular) are to understand the normal organization of the basic processes of learning; to elucidate the various kinds of distortions and breakdowns to which this organization is vulnerable; and to create environmental techniques for reshaping and reorganizing behavior or, failing in this, to design environments in which behaviorally defective people can behave well (see Lindsley, 1964; Ulrich, Stachnik, and Mabry, 1966). Underlying this viewpoint is a philosophy of mind based on causal explanation: that there are no limits to the concept of the reflex and the learning theory associated with it. If a behavior is inborn and spontaneous, it is an unconditioned operant, if congenital and elicited by the environment, it is an unconditioned Pavlovian reflex. If a behavior is learned and controlled by its consequences, it is a conditioned operant; if controlled by its antecedents, a conditioned classical reflex.

These concepts would appear to exhaust the universe of behaviors, which have to be either learned or unlearned and controlled by consequences or by antecedents (Skinner, 1938, 1959). Thus actions for which people usually offer justification, reasons, or explanations in terms of intentions and those for which they normally do not can be handled conceptually with equal ease.

This framework has guided the most important advances in behavioral therapy. Along with most investigators concerned about understanding and modifying the behavior of developmentally disabled children, I remain convinced of its utility. My move from the exclusively operant viewpoint was not the result of experiments nor based on a clear sense that the theory had been superceded by a broader, more useful one. The approach was made less compelling because of increasing interest in questions—which arose in part from observing and talking with "subjects"—that could not be studied when confined by the paradigms of the operant laboratory (Kuhn, 1970). These questions centered on the inborn organization of behavior and the basis for disturbances that did not seem caused, or remediable, by environmental manipulations alone. An additional, powerful source of discontent was more personal: the need for a philosophy of mind concerned not only with the behavior of objectified others but with feelings.

Clinical Studies: The Formation of Character

My observation of newborn infants led to a model of the behavioral equipment with which a child is born (Cohen, 1967, 1974a, especially Chapter 2). This was its blueprint: the child is endowed with behavioral functions (such as the ability to deploy attention, to suck, and to swallow); with the capacity to change states in an orderly way (for example, to awaken gently from sleep); and with feedback mechanisms to modulate arousal and physiological overactivity in order to maintain homeostasis while slowly learning to sort out regularities in perception and environmental consequences. When all goes well for an infant, his various functions—e.g., sucking, swallowing, crying, moving, looking, hearing, and feeling—are optimally stimulated but are not excessively or unevenly called upon. His basic, biologically determined rhythms are not unduly constricted or blocked (see Wolff, 1966). And his parents become stable figures in his world by virtue of their shielding, comforting, and stimulating.

Perhaps in reaction to the emphasis on operant conditioning and the limitation of my data to newborns, environmental forces in this conception were dwarfed by biological ones. I was most impressed by the child's capacity to limit environmental impact and by the power of genetic determination. How environmental stress could interfere with smooth functioning seemed more impressive than how parental provision could facilitate it. Thus the studies of newborns, which focused on sucking, led to a change in vocabulary and manner of organizing what were taken to be the relevant data (Hanson, 1958). The givens of the operant model—e.g., the ability to form associations—seemed epiphenomenal, while others—e.g., the capacity to modulate arousal while deploying attention—appeared more basic.

In this transition from an operant to a more psychobiological theory the basic epistemological question persisted: What are the elements from which mind is constructed? How does the newborn, with his physiologically given behavioral endowment, become an adult with a complex, unique personality?

Following common practice, I looked for models in which this process of growth seemed most vulnerable to disturbance (e.g., in children with oral–facial defects and those with central nervous system damage) and selected children with severe eczema as a model (Cohen and Nadelson, 1971). The care and study of about 80 children afflicted with eczema resulted in a new language, new paradigms, and a new quality of theoretical understanding. As a clinical researcher, it was no longer tenable for me to remain separate from the researched, to exclude "confounding" variables, or to ignore "subjects" for whom data were "contaminated" or "incomplete."

In most children who suffer from eczema a mild rash appears during the first year of life, intermittently reappears, and then mysteriously vanishes at school age. For a small group of children eczema is a profound disturbance marked by months and years of unremitting, oozing, crusting, and itchy eruption from which there is no escape. During these years of torment, scratching creates more rash, and the rash creates more itchiness. While the proximal causes of the scratching (or itchiness) can sometimes be identified in the physical environment, the initiation and sustenance of the scratch–rash cycle are more often based in arousal, anxiety, and emotional stress.

What happens to a child who is constantly irritable, scratching, and ugly? To a child who turns away from parents and turns inward to attend to his own body? What is the impact on character formation of being driven, thousands of times, in secret and alone at night, to acts of self-destructive scraping, rubbing, clawing, scratching, and gouging at one's own skin?

Evidence about these questions came from observations, interviews, and play; from being with the child, his parents, and important people in their lives; and from impressions and feelings, gathered with empathy and growing affection, without concern for a specific research protocol. Each child and family was historically unique, and to the extent that my work was successful, I became part of their lives, especially at times of crisis, thus confounding the observational field even more.

The child with severe eczema is locked, from the first months of life, in insoluble conflicts. He is impelled to scratch but wishes to avoid the pain his own scratching creates after he has succeeded in destroying the peripheral itch receptors. He is driven to find relief through his own ministrations and against the restraints imposed by his parents, who attempt, in their own way, to provide comfort. He is motivated, like all children, to express himself through physical action in space and yet may experience pain from his cracking skin with every vigorous movement.

Given good enough care, the psychic wounds caused by such conflicts may heal without obvious scarring. But providing such care for a child with severe eczema may be beyond the power of ordinary mothers and fathers. It is not hard to understand the frustration, rage, and projection of rage that may be felt by parents who wish to love their infant but find him ugly and who attempt to console him but often find him irritable beyond their capacity to comfort. A child with severe eczema learns to sense the hesitation, the momentary but telling holding-back that characterizes the way his parents, and other adults, reach to pick him up. He learns what is is to have people look at him and make contact not with his eyes but with his rash. The child learns, through the mirror that is his mother's face (as Winnicott describes this situation), that he is not fully acceptable and is certainly not beautiful.

These observations reveal the thrust of the inquiry, its scope and motivating themes, and the types of paradigms demanded by clinical research. In outline this is the explanatory model that emerged.

Eczema is a disease with a physiological basis, probably a vasculitis that reflects a diffuse instability of the autonomic nervous system. Perhaps for reasons associated with the same underlying physiological disturbance, children with eczema may tend to have a lower threshold for the elicitation of scratching as well as to be more irritable, more difficult to console, and more easily overaroused. When the tendency to vasculitis and the disturbance in the modulation of stimulation (i.e., the lowered threshold and ease of disorganization) are not too extreme, the eczema tends to be localized and of limited severity. When the child's biological and associated behavioral endowment are, however, less fortunate, or when his environment adds its challenge to his ability to modulate anxiety, the pernicious scratch–rash cycle can be initiated. Once this channel is established, the child's tensions are discharged through scratching, and the scratching leads to more rash and itchiness. Scratching may displace other, more adaptive, externally directed displays of anger and aggression. This pattern becomes crystallized and self-perpetuating.

The child's irritability and difficult disposition create strains on parenting. The rash adds additional burdens, arousing fantasies, concerns about adequacy, and often profound anxiety in his parents. Unable to comfort or to love their child unambivalently, perceiving his rash and behavior as barriers to the expression of their own, psychobiological motivation to be able parents, mothers and fathers find it difficult to remain available, comforting, and supportive.

In his turn the child who is unable to be comforted and fully accepted by his parents does not develop trust in his own body nor trust in the outside world (Provence and Rivto, 1961). He turns his attention away from the external world of objects and people, whom he may begin to see as persecutory; directs his attention inward to his bodily sensations and their control; and, finally, attempts to detach himself from his body and to treat it as if it were a separate, foreign object. At this point his skin, and by extension his body as a whole, may also become a "thing"—to be observed, to be medicated, and to be hated. In addition, the redeployment of attention may itself have important physiological consequences. The brief rejection of external sensory input and the inward focusing of attention induce epinephrinelike cardio-vascular responses (decreased forearm vascular resistance, increased forearm blood flow, and increased heart rate). That this pattern may be more than transient is indicated by the finding that it characterizes people who are sensory "augmenters"—those individuals who habitually reject external sensory input and who may be more sensitive to it (Williams, 1974).

For a child with severe eczema a variety of forces thus conspire: cracking skin; active and passive social isolation; almost ceaseless discomfort; and redeployment of attention from the external world to the internal. These forces may result in social distancing and uninvolvement; difficulties in the experiencing of pleasure; chronic anxiety; and lagging intellectual and motor development. A child's character, built upon such a foundation, may display motifs of disordered aggression and narcissism: depression, sadomasochism, and paranoia. At best a child with a lifelong history of severe eczema may be-come unusually sobered and blocked in the healthy expression of his ag-gression and imagination. At the expense of mastering the normal develop-mental tasks, by age five years the severely afflicted child may have his energies dissipated in the care of his body; in his fantasies (flavored with attack and being attacked); and in controlling, and being controlled by, his anger and unrequited need for tenderness. In the myriad of interactions that shape a child's emergent identity, he learns that he is not a fully worthwhile person. And his parents, unsupported by their own families or physician, find themselves isolated, guilty, chronically fatigued, and angry.

This model arose in the course of several years of work, mainly with children suffering from the most severe, full-body eczema. When a child is not extremely disposed to vasculitis or anxious, behavioral disorganization, or when his parents, in spite of the child's disposition, can remain available, the life of a child with eczema may be relatively undisturbed by his skin disease and the consequent alterations in his inner life. The short-term outcome is, thus, the resultant of three main vectors: biological disposition to vasculitis; psychobiological endowment, particularly relating to modulation of anxiety and the stimulation–stress continuum; and environmental facilitation.

Two observations will complete the set for the final model. The first is that some children with mild eczema seem remarkably sensitive and alert. One wonders if this enrichment results from increased parental attention and concern; from the children's increased experience of tension and subsequently greater capacity for recognizing and coping with anxiety (as suggested by Zetzel, 1970, to be important developmental achievements); or from an association, on a biological basis, between the disposition to develop the au-tonomic vascular instability and the metabolic vulnerability to anxiety and the subsequent elaboration of defenses. (See Cohen, 1974a.) These three hypotheses are not exclusive, of course, but each has a distinctive theoretical thrust: learning theory; psychoanalytic ego psychology; and the neurochemical unity of autonomic responses and central nervous system neurotransmission.

The second observation is that eczema tends to "run in families," and one may speculate if some parents of children with severe eczema may also have the disposition to vascular instability and the tendency to heightened arousal and the experience of anxiety. Such adults, even without the manifest skin disease, may be more sensitive, with all the potential benefits as well as the increased burdens of their physiological disposition.

An advantage of a model for eczema, as for other conditions, is that potential points of entering the system are suggested. Concern only with the most obvious symptom, the rash, is often doomed to therapeutic failure. In caring for severely afflicted children, I aimed at the following in the treatment: reducing the child's anxiety (through the use of medication and by restructuring the environment); redirecting attention to the outside world (planned activities leading to reinforcement); soothing the skin (steroids and lubricants); reestablishing pleasant relations with parents (beginning with soothing baths and leading to shared activities); and allowing the child to sleep comfortably, sometimes for the first time (sedatives). In caring for the parents, I aimed at helping to reestablish the sense of parental self-esteem (understanding their child's predicament, and their own, and knowing how to respond to the child's problems in a medically sanctioned way) and equanimity (time off, sleep, and medication).

This process of care can proceed only if there is a physician who is willing to become involved and take responsibility, perhaps even with authoritarian control at the start; able to remain available and uncritical, especially at times of exacerbation; and ready to accept (with the goal of helping to modulate) the anger and dependency that families and children who have felt overwhelmed and hopeless will bring to their relationship with a care giver.

Psychosomatic Models in Clinical Research

As clinicians we are interested in models that are broad enough to give coherence to the many kinds of observations that interest us and that we must use in doing our work; as researchers we are interested in models that are sufficiently explicit to generate hypotheses capable of refutation. Thus we are often caught between theories that are overly ambitious (as in the model outlined for the pathophysiology of eczema) and laboratory paradigms that are overly restricted (as were those that emerged in the operant studies of social behavior). Fortunately, involvement in clinical care is a fine antidote for theoretical despair.

In this essay I have tried to illustrate the relation between models and research. The operant studies were characterized by causal explanations and a limited domain of variables; the newborn observations by increasing appreciation of the subtle organization of innate behavior; and the studies of eczema by an attempt to remain aware of biology, congenitally organized behavior, endowment, and environmental provision through a model closer to Aristotelian than Galilean explanation. Each stage in this development was characterized by a different style of setting questions or problems; by different methods; and by a different theoretical stance, which shaped observations and set criteria for accepting explanatory statements. This process was influenced by many forces: new teachers; personal development; experience with social planning for poor children and families (Cohen, 1972, 1974b; Cohen, Parker, et al., 1972); and research with behavior genetics and twins (Cohen, Allen, et al., 1972; Cohen et al., 1973; Dibble and Cohen, 1974).

However, as Hegel taught, what is overthrown becomes integrated into what is new. Development is dialectical. The stages in the development of the model for eczema are reflected in the most recent formulation. Operant concepts are used to describe how eczematous children learn about themselves and their place in the family, and how they fail to learn about objects and the world when their attention and energies are directed to their bodies. The themes of the newborn studies are integrated in the emphasis on a child's capacities to attend, modulate arousal, and organize his perceptions of external and internal stimuli, and in the concern with disturbances in development that are created when some functions are overtaxed. Behavioral genetics and interest in the family as a whole unit are reflected in the concern with the interrelations between parents and children and with a family's need for support from important people in their lives, often including a physician.

When the world is divided into separate domains—heaven and earth; feelings and thoughts; body and soul—there is a need to bring the realms into communication. In a dualistic conception not only psychosomatic disease but intentional acts as simple as saying hello raise dilemmas about what makes the "mysterious leap" across the undefinable gap between mind and body. To serve in this role, special entities or modes are created: "interaction" in psychology, "angels" in theology, and "animal spirits" in Descartes's physiology. These entities or "forces" have a share in the qualities of both domains and thus can serve as metaphysical diplomats carrying messages between the two. Yet their existence raises a more fundamental question: Why have a radical separation at all?

Wittgenstein's (1958) analysis of action, and the forms of language that are inextricably embedded in patterns of human action can provide a foundation for a psychosomatic model of development in which children are not divided into growing minds and growing bodies. In elaborating such a model we are in need of a rich enough array of concepts that pertain to children as whole people and a sufficient flexibility to use different types of explanation. Many components for a psychosomatic model of development have been explicated already, and they are familiar to any physician who has cared for sick children and families. In summary they need only be mentioned: genetic endowment; congenitally organized patterns of behavior; the enduring impact of early experiences; the power of environmental shaping through contingent reinforcement; the modulation of arousal and stress; the developmental functions of anxiety; the deployment of attention; the ordering of perception and regularities; the crystallization of behavior; the vicissitudes of aggression and narcissism, and the formation of character; the origin and development of language and the capacity for complex, intentional actions; the shaping of parents by children and of children by parents; and the social context in which physiology and experience are expressed in the unfolding of personality. A multivariate, psychosomatic model of development not only provides such conceptual bridges as these between mind and body but reduces the temptation to view human life in terms of this dichotomy.

The discussion of eczema sketched one way these various components of a model can be organized. Other clinical studies will reveal different patterns and sites of accent or emphasis. But it may be possible that the sets of important variables, developmental lines and patterns, and patterns of reaction are not only finite but relatively small. If so, it can be expected that we will find similar models useful in understanding diverse clinical situations, ranging from the development of twins (Cohen, Allen, et al., 1972) to childhood psychosis (Cohen, Shaywitz, et al., 1974; see also Cohen, 1974a, an essay that is complementary to this one).

Thus the two-worlds conception of mind and body with which we started has, in a certain sense, exploded. Development, we have seen, occurs in many worlds, not two. The child psychiatrist has a unique vantage point from which to investigate these. Present at the very beginning of individual development, he may study newborn infants as psychosomatic wholes (see, e.g., Winnicott, 1958, pp. 243–254). Later he is in a position to consider data that reveal the dynamic relations among mind, body, family, and community and that demonstrate that these concepts cannot be understood outside of a system that includes them all.

That conditions for observation from the child psychiatric vantage point often have been marginal may result from obscurity introduced by our own basic concepts and unanalyzed clinical epistemology. Explanation in the clinic has a different style—if not a different logic—from explanation in the laboratory. In contrast with the disciplines from which child psychiatry may borrow concepts and paradigms, the child psychiatrist is always in need of shifting between domains (e.g., genetics, physiology, psychoanalysis, biochemistry, cognitive psychology, child development, general psychiatry, pediatrics, and sociology) and of weighing the relations between domains. In the clinic it is obvious that changes in one domain are linked with changes in many others (Cohen and Frank, 1973). There are thus a variety of languages, and forms of explanation, necessary for understanding a particular child, as a whole person, living in a whole family in a complicated society. As clinicians who *must* understand, we become adept at borrowing phrases and paradigms and switching between types and levels of explanation in mid sentence.

However, such linguistic versatility has its dangers. How are the various languages systematically related, and how sound are the fundamental concepts? Difficulties in the use of such "theory-laden" concepts as anxiety, vulnerability, and competence—difficulties that this essay has in large part ignored—are immediately apparent. But even stock-in-trade clinical concepts—autism, psychosis, mental retardation, learning disability, minimal cerebral dysfunction, to cite but a few of those that interest me—seem entangled, elusive, and in need of analysis (Cohen, Granger, *et al.*, 1974). Thus conceptual, as well as empirical, investigation will be required for the evolution of appropriately broad models of normal and atypical development that can be productive of research as well as of understanding.

ACKNOWLEDGMENTS

I am indebted to a number of investigators who have encouraged my work and have allowed me to participate in theirs: Dr. Spyridon Alivisatos, Dr. Ogden Lindsley, Dr. Peter Wolff, Dr. William Kessen, Dr. Robert Griesemer, Dr. Daniel X. Freedman, and Dr. William Pollin. I am very grateful to Dr. Albert Solnit, professor of pediatrics and psychiatry, and to Dr. Edward Zigler, professor of psychology, Yale University, for their guidance and friendship.

The research was supported, in part, by Public Health Service Research Grant HD-03008 and the Grant Foundation.

References

ALLPORT, F. *Social psychology.* Boston: Houghton Mifflin, 1924.
ANSCOMBE, G. E. M. *Intention.* Ithaca, N.Y.: Cornell University Press, 1957.
BUCHDAHL, G. *Metaphysics and the philosophy of science.* Oxford: Basil Blackwell, 1969.
CANGUILHEM, G. *La formation du concept de réflexe aux XVIIe and XVIIIe siècles.* Paris: Presses Universitaires de France, 1955.
CAVELL, S. *Must we mean what we say?* New York: Scribner, 1969.
CIOFFI, F. Freud and the idea of a pseudo-science. In R. Borger and F. Cioffi (Eds.), *Explanation in the behavioural sciences.* Cambridge: Cambridge University Press, 1970.

COHEN, D. J. Justin and his peers: An experimental analysis of a child's social world. *Child Development*, 1962, **33**, 697–717.

COHEN, D. J. The crying newborn's accommodation to the nipple. *Child Development*, 1967, **38**, 89–100.

COHEN, D. J. Viewpoint: meeting adolescents' needs. *Children Today*, 1972, **2**, 28f.

COHEN, D. J. Competence and biology: Methodology in studies of infants, twins, psychosomatic disease, and psychosis. In E. J. Anthony (Ed.), *The child at psychiatric risk.* (Volume 3 of the *Yearbook of the International Association for Child Psychiatry and Allied Professions.*) New York: Wiley, 1974.(a)

COHEN, D. J. *Serving preschool children in day care.* Washington, D.C.: Government Printing Office, 1974.(b)

COHEN, D. J., ALLEN, M. G., POLLIN, W., INOFF, G., WERNER, M., & DIBBLE, E. Personality development in twins: Competence in the newborn and preschool periods. *Journal of the American Academy of Child Psychiatry*, 1972, **11**, 625–644.

COHEN, D. J., DIBBLE, E., GRAWE, J., & POLLIN, W. Separating identical from fraternal twins. *Archives of General Psychiatry*, 1973, **29**, 465–469.

COHEN, D. J., & FRANK, R. Between childhood and adolescence: Growth, tasks, and problems in the preadolescent phase of development. Technical Report submitted to the Office of Child Development, DHEW, 1973. Yale University School of Medicine.

COHEN, D. J., GRANGER, R., PROVENCE, S., & SOLNIT, A. Classification and mental health services for children. In Nicholas Hobbs (Ed.), *Issues in the classification of children.* San Francisco: Jossey-Bass, in press, 1974.

COHEN, D. J., & LINDSLEY, O. R. Catalysis of controlled leadership in cooperation by human stimulation. *Journal of Child Psychology and Psychiatry*, 1964, **5**, 119–137.

COHEN, D. J., & NADELSON, T. The impact of skin disease on the person. In Thomas Fitzpatrick (Ed.), *Dermatology in general medicine.* New York: McGraw-Hill, 1971.

COHEN, D. J., PARKER, R., HOST, M., & RICHARDS, C. (Eds.). *Serving schoolage children.* Washington, D.C.: Government Printing Office, 1972.

COHEN, D. J., SHAYWITZ, B., JOHNSON, W., & BOWERS, M. Biogenic amines in autistic and atypical children: CSF measures of HVA and 5HIAA. *Archives of General Psychiatry*, 1974, **31**, 845–853.

COLODNY, R. G. *The nature and function of scientific theories.* Pittsburgh: University of Pittsburgh Press, 1970.

DESCARTES, R. *Oeuvres de Descartes.* Charles Adam and Paul Tannery (Eds.). Paris: Léopold Cerf, 1897–1913. Traité de l'Homme, Vol. 11, p. 131.

DESCARTES, R. *Discours de la Méthode.* Text and commentary by É. Gilson. Paris: Librairie Philosophique J. Vrin, 1947.

DIBBLE, E., & COHEN, D. J. Companion instruments for measuring children's competence and parental style. *Archives of General Psychiatry*, 1974, **30**, 805–815.

DRAY, W. H. (Ed.). *Philosophical analysis and history.* New York: Harper & Row, 1966.

FRIEDMAN, N. *The social nature of psychological research: The psychological experiment as a social interaction.* New York: Basic Books, 1967.

GILSON, É. *Études sur le rôle de la pensée médiévale dans la formation du système cartésien.* Paris: Librairie Philosophique J. Vrin, 1951.

HACKER, P. M. S. *Insight and illusion.* Oxford: Clarendon Press, 1972.

HAKE, D., & VUKELICH, R. A classification and review of cooperation procedures. *Journal of the Experimental Analysis of Behavior*, 1972, **18**, 333–343.

HANSON, N. R. *Patterns of discovery.* Cambridge: Cambridge University Press, 1958.

HESSE, M. B. *Forces and fields.* London: Thomas Nelson, 1961.

HOOK, S. (Ed.). *Psychoanalysis, scientific method, and philosophy.* New York: New York University Press, 1959.

HUSSERL, E. *Cartesian meditations.* The Hague: Martinus Nijhoff, 1960.

KEELE, K. D. *Anatomies of pain.* Oxford: Blackwell Scientific Publications, 1957.

KENNY, A. *Wittgenstein.* Cambridge, Mass: Harvard University Press, 1973.

KUHN, T. *The structure of scientific revolutions. International encyclopedia of unified science.* Vol. 2, No. 2. Chicago: University of Chicago Press, 1970. Second edition, enlarged.

LUKATOS, I., & MUSGRAVE, A. (Eds.). *Criticism and the growth of knowledge.* Cambridge: Cambridge University Press, 1970.

LINDSLEY, O. R. Operant conditioning methods applied to research in chronic schizophrenia. *Psychiatric research reports* 5. American Psychiatric Association, June 1956, 118–139.

LINDSLEY, O. R. Characteristics of the behavior of chronic psychotics as revealed by free-operant conditioning methods. *Diseases of the nervous system.* Monograph Supplement, Vol. 31, No. 2, February 1960, 66–78.

LINDSLEY, O. R. Direct measurement and functional definition of vocal hallucinatory symptoms. *Journal of Nervous and Mental Disease,* 1963, **136,** 293–297.(a)

LINDSLEY, O. R. Experimental analysis of social reinforcement. *American Journal of Orthopsychiatry,* 1963, **33,** 624–633.(b)

LINDSLEY, O. R. Direct measurement and prosthesis of retarded behavior. *Journal of Education,* 1964, **147,** 62–81.

LINDSLEY, O. R. Experimental analysis of cooperation and competition. In Thom Verhave (Ed.), *The experimental analysis of behavior.* New York: Appleton-Century-Crofts, 1966.

NAGEL, E. *The structure of science.* New York: Harcourt, Brace, and World, 1961.

NATHAN, P. E., SCHNELLER, P., & LINDSLEY, O. R. Direct measurement of communication during psychiatric admission interviews. *Behavior Research and Therapy,* 1964, **2,** 49–57.

PASSMORE, J. *Philosophical reasoning.* London: Duckworth, 1961.

PETERS, R. S. *The concept of motivation.* London: Routledge, 1958.

PIAGET, J. *Introduction à L'Épistémologie Génétique.* 3 volumes. Paris: Presses Universitaires de France, 1950.

PROVENCE, S., & RITVO, S. Effects of deprivation on institutionalized infants: Disturbances in development of relationship to inanimate objects. *The Psychoanalytic Study of the Child,* 1961, **16,** 189–205.

RICOEUR, P. *Freud and philosophy: An essay on interpretation.* New Haven, Conn.: Yale University Press, 1970.

RYLE, G. *The concept of mind.* London: Hutchinson University Library, 1949.

SKINNER, B. F. *The behavior of organisms.* New York: Appleton-Century-Crofts, 1938.

SKINNER, B. F. *Cumulative record.* New York: Appleton-Century-Crofts, 1959.

TAYLOR, C. The explanation of purposive behaviour. In R. Borger and F. Cioffi (Eds.), *Explanation in the behavioural sciences.* Cambridge: Cambridge University Press, 1970.

TOULMIN, S. Reasons and causes. In R. Borger and F. Cioffi (Eds.), *Explanation in the behavioural sciences.* Cambridge: Cambridge University Press, 1970.

ULRICH, E., & MOUNTJOY, P. T. *The experimental analysis of social behavior.* New York: Appleton-Century-Crofts, 1972.

ULRICH, R., STACHNIK, T., & MABRY, J. *Control of human behavior.* Glenview, Ill.: Scott, Foresman, 1966.

VARTANIAN, A. *La mettrie's l'homme machine.* Princeton, N.J.: Princeton University Press, 1960.

VON WRIGHT, G. H. *Explanation and understanding.* Ithaca, N.Y.: Cornell University Press, 1971.

WILLIAMS, R., BITTKER, T., BUCHSBAUM, M., & WYNNE, L. Cardiovascular and neurophysiologic correlates of sensory intake and rejection. *Psychophysiology.* In press, 1975.

WINCH, P. *The idea of a social science.* London: Routledge, 1958.

WINNICOTT, D. W. *Collected papers.* London: Tavistock Publications, 1958.

WITTGENSTEIN, L. *Philosophical investigations.* Translated by G. E. M. Anscombe. Oxford: Basil Blackwell, 1958.

WOLFF, P. H. The causes, controls, and organization of behavior in the neonate. *Psychological Issues,* 1967, Monograph #17, V (1).

WOLFSON, H. A. *Philo.* Cambridge, Mass.: Harvard University Press, 1947.

WOLFSON, H. A. *The philosophy of the church fathers.* Cambridge, Mass.: Harvard University Press, 1956.

ZAJONC, R. Social facilitation. *Science,* 1965, **149,** 269–274.

ZETZEL, E. R. *The capacity for emotional growth.* New York: International Universities Press, 1970.

FAILURE TO THRIVE
AND MATERNAL
DEPRIVATION

Joseph Fischhoff

A children's hospital in a large metropolitan center offers a child psychiatrist unlimited opportunities for research. Depending on his interests, he can study infant and child development, psychosomatic illnesses, reactions to illness, hospitalization and surgical procedures, the effects of chronic illness in children and families, learning disabilities, disturbances in gender identity, congenital amputations and body image, death and dying, child abuse, suicide, family organization and disorganization, and social and environmental deprivation. The preceding list is not exhaustive and in fact is small when contrasted with the opportunities for research in a setting such as the Children's Hospital of Michigan with 320 inpatient beds and approximately 140,000 outpatient visits per year. The limitations in research activities are limitations common to other settings: teaching and service obligations, financing, space and personnel requirements, and last but not least the child psychiatrist's personal inclination and interests. Notwithstanding these factors, the opportunities for individual or interdisciplinary clinical research are great. In addition, laboratory studies are readily available as is the expertise of investigators in the basic sciences.

Knowledge of growth and development is fundamental to the specialty of pediatrics, and frequently infants and young children pose complex diagnostic problems because of failure to grow or failure to thrive. Of this group of infants and children a number have physiological causes for the failure to thrive. However, a substantial number do not have a physiological etiology for the failure to thrive, and we must look elsewhere for the cause of their difficulty, which is in the emotional and social environment of the child.

A number of years ago our clinical experience suggested that the majority of mothers whose infants failed to thrive without demonstrable organic cause had severe personality disorders, and studies were initiated in the 1960s to as-

---

JOSEPH FISCHHOFF, Professor of Child Psychiatry, Wayne State University, Detroit, Michigan.

certain, by systematic investigation, the validity of this observation. Other factors that play a role in the pathogenesis of the failure to thrive or "maternal deprivation syndrome," such as the role of the father, mother–father interactions, and social, economic, and environmental conditions, were also investigated, but emphasis in this instance is on mothers' personalities and their infants.

Review of the Literature

Several contributions to the literature are summarized in the following section.

Failure to thrive or the "maternal deprivation syndrome" was first recognized in institutionalized infants, and Spitz (1945) focused the profession's attention on this condition in his pioneering report. In the ensuing years it was recognized that infants living in their own homes, not in institutions, failed to thrive and exhibited signs and symptoms of failure of physical growth, malnutrition, and motor retardation, in addition to affective and cognitive deficits. In the majority of cases the infants were being cared for by their mothers, and observers recognized that it was the inability to be an adequate mother for the infant that caused the failure to thrive. However, little was published concerning the reasons these mothers were not able to care for the infants, and virtually no data were available concerning the mothers' personality structures.

Barbaro and his associates (1963) stated that the mothers were depressed, angry, helpless, and desperate and had problems in maintaining self-esteem. They said, "In those instances where the malidentification is part of a more pervasive and structured pathology, it becomes obvious to all concerned that these parents should be referred to the appropriate psychiatric and social agencies." Later Barbaro and Shaheen (1967) reported that depriving mothers had lived under significant environmental and psychosocial disruption, such as alcoholism, childhood deprivation, physical abuse between parents, and considerable strain between the parents and their own families. One mother felt isolated from early childhood, had very little relationship with her mother, constantly felt criticized by her, and never felt competent. Another mother was severely deprived and abused as a child. She disliked her child from the time of his birth and was angry with him. Some time after his first admission, he again was losing weight and was found to be a "battered child."

Leonard *et al.* (1966) described some characteristics of 13 mothers of infants who failed to thrive. Tension, anger, anxiety, depression, and inappropriate behavior were present. The mothers were lacking in self-esteem and were unable to assess their babies' needs and their own worth realistically.

"Not a single mother reported sustained supportive nurturing in her own childhood," and the mothers were lonely and isolated. Elmer (1960) described five cases of failure to thrive and presented highlights of the mothers' psychological state. One mother had "excessively strong needs to be cared for" and appeared to dislike males. Another mother appeared anxious and depressed. In another case the mother had been "nervous" since age 10. She had not wanted her pregnancy, was depressed, and was remote from her infant. In these cases there is reference to severe personality difficulties, anxiety, and depression but not sufficient data to draw conclusions about personality structure.

Bullard et al. (1967) reported some aspects of the mothers' personality and behavior in three cases. One mother resented her two children and was "openly abusive with the boy during the interview." Ultimately she left her child with a neighbor and moved to another city. In the second case, when the child was ready to be discharged, the psychiatrist noted, "Child to be discharged, recognizing that mother has not recognized Linda's trouble and is not willing to be under psychiatric care." In the third case the mother had many "neurasthenic" complaints: "She was hyperactive, overtalkative and extremely anxious. Her thoughts shifted from topic to topic, her feelings varied quickly from forced gaiety, and thence to emotions clearly depressive in nature. Her history and reports from other sources confirmed a long-standing condition. The "impression was of a severe and chronic disorder of character in which depressive, compensatory euphoric and hysterical elements were prominent.: Coleman and Provence (1957) gave some pertinent information about two mothers. In one case, when the infant was seven months old, the mother was three months pregnant and the father committed suicide. The mother developed a prolonged period of grief, depression, and anger. The second mother was isolated and detached from her infant. She stopped breast feeding on the fourth day because she was afraid she would smother the baby and spanked the infant because the crying drove her "wild." She alternated between depression and hopelessness over the baby's developmental lag and wondered whether or not she should "start over with a new baby." Later she denied that she was concerned. Glaser et al. (1968) reported in a follow-up study that "no specific psychological configuration was found consistently in the mothers."

In a study of 45 mothers Evans et al. (1972) found that they fell into three groups. In general, the 14 mothers in group 1 were extremely depressed, had sustained a severe recent object loss, and had a good prognosis. The 15 mothers in group 2 were extremely depressed, had very deprived living conditions, had been poorly mothered themselves, had sustained chronic losses, and had a guarded prognosis "unless there was a dramatic change in the home environment." The 11 mothers in group 3 were extremely hostile, antagonistic, and belittling. They perceived their children as "bad." They gave bizarre, distorted histories and "gave fleeting glimpses of poor mothering in their own childhoods," and each appeared never to have had a "meaningful relationship throughout her life." The prognosis was poor unless the child was placed out of the home. Of 40 mothers, 26, or two-thirds, were considered to have a severe emotional disturbance, and the prognosis for the children was guarded or poor.

The Study

Certain criteria were established for the infants to be studied: (1) age, 3 to 24 months; (2) gestation, at least 9 months; (3) birth weight, more than the premature level of 5 pounds 8 ounces, or 2500 grams; (4) current height and weight, below the third percentile on the Stuart growth grids; (5) no evidence of an organic cause for failure to thrive by history, physical examination, or laboratory analysis; (6) presence of at least one of the following: autoerotic behavior, watchfulness, apathy, developmental lags, or irritability; and (7) historical data indicating that the infant had had little physical handling by and social contact with the mother. In all the infants the diagnosis of maternal deprivation was subsequently established by the demonstration of marked improvement following a period of adequate mothering (which included the provision of adequate food). When a decision was reached that the infants were to be studied, extensive interviews were held with the mothers.

The Mothers

Dynamic and genetic assessments of the mothers' personalities, in addition to a cross-sectional study, were the goals of the psychiatric evaluation. The assessments emphasized how each mother had developed into the individual she was and how she came to express herself both verbally and nonverbally in relation to her infant and in relation to her total environment. We were interested in identifying the forces that entered into the organization of her particular personality and in determining how these forces influenced the child-rearing function of the mother. What the mother was able to relate about her past and present was important. However, equally important was her nonverbal behavior.

The interviews were unstructured, and we attempted to explore as many facets of the mother's personality development as possible. Her early childhood development and significant personal relationships were discussed, e.g., significant relatives, illegitimate births, important illnesses or handicaps, methods of discipline, parental dissension, care and concern, and placement in a foster home or institution. Childhood and adolescent memories were discussed: Was she passive, assertive, frustrated, or defiant? What were her daydreams? Did she recall dreams, nightmares, thumb sucking, enuresis, lying, or stealing? Further details were elicited concerning school and occupational, medical, and sexual history, in addition to general activities and interests, emotionally disturbing experiences, and psychiatric illnesses and difficulties. The assessment of ego functions was organized along the following lines: intellectual ability, mode of association, perception, memory, predominant defenses, fund of information, judgment, and insight. We attempted to elicit important experiences at any time during her life, to discover areas of conflict and how they were handled, and to determine what defense mechanisms were primary. Since the mother might not recognize the significance of her own past history or the importance of the infant's nonverbal behavior, the psychiatric evaluation included assessments of the mother's social and emotional development. Interviews were conducted with the mother alone and with the mother and her infant together so that we could observe the mother's interaction with her infant. Frequently the interviews were videotaped for later review. The mother's comments about her children and observations, if possible, of her interaction with her other children were noted. The material for each mother was summarized under the following headings: age and marital status, initial appearance and manner, affect and mood, past history, past memories, self-image and ego functions, present mode of behavior, object relationships, defenses, fantasies, hopes, and daydreams. Table 1 summarizes highlights of the assessment of the mothers.

The three following illustrative vignettes are condensations of a number of interviews, observations, and informal contacts with each mother.

Case 1. Mrs. A. was 25 years old and had four children at the time of the initial interview in 1966. She was appropriately dressed. Her 11-month-old daughter was the youngest child and failing to thrive. Mrs. A. smiled frequently to hide her tears. She was distressed because her husband drank excessively and had been fired "again" from a well-paying job. Mrs. A. said she was aware of being depressed and often was unable to sleep. She kept "busy" at home, otherwise "the kids get on my nerves."

Mrs. A remembered that her mother was incapable for caring for her and her four siblings. Her mother left the family, and her father cared for the children until he died when Mrs. A. was 11 years old. Her mother did not remarry, but she did not return to the children and is still living. She remembered her mother as a disturbed woman and her father as affectionate but strict. After her father's death she and two sisters lived with foster parents until she was age 17. She married when she was 17 and in the eleventh grade. She completed high school while her husband was in college. Mrs. A. could not say why she married at 17, but she was not pregnant at that time. She soon discovered that Mr. A. drank excessively. She attempted to save some money when he worked so that the family would have

TABLE 1

Summary of Assessment of 20 Mothers

1. Age at time of first pregnancy		8. Concrete thought patterns	
<18	15	Yes	18
>18	5	No	2
2. Behavior on initial contact		9. Poor self-image	
Indicative of psychopathology		Yes	18
Yes	13	No	2
No	7	10. Poor object relationships	
3. Inappropriate affect		Yes	18
Yes	16	No	2
No	4	11. Predominantly pregenital defense	
4. Evidence of depression		Yes	18
Yes	15	No	2
No	5	12. Fantasies reflecting hope	
5. Abnormal past history		Yes	4
Yes	17	No	14
No	3	Unknown	2
6. Predisposition to acting out		13. Diagnosis	
Yes	16	Personality	18
No	4	disorder	
7. Poor performance in day-to-day		Psychoneurosis	2
activities			
Yes	17		
No	3		

money when he did not work. She begged him to stop drinking to no avail. She maintained that they had not gone out together since before the marriage. Mr. A. did not help her in the house or with the children. She felt that he did not want her to be pregnant, but he wanted a boy and she submitted to having intercourse although she derived no pleasure from it. She had begun taking the "pill" recently but had been afraid to before. She now was determined not to become pregnant. Mrs. A. believed that there was no hope that her situation would change but did not see how she could divorce her husband. She was, in a vague way, still hoping that her husband would change. She remembered that her father and foster parents had cared for her and wished to have a home and family herself.

When her baby was four months old Mrs. A. was worried because the baby was listless, did not laugh or smile, and "did not seem to care." She did not know why but spontaneously said, "My husband needed as much or more attention than any of the children. He would not get up to get an ashtray but would tell me to hand it to him." She was very aware of feeling isolated and lonely, though she had two women friends close by. The three older siblings were observed to be well fed and outgoing and related well to Mrs. A. She quickly understood the explanation that her daughter's growth failure was due to Mrs. A.'s inability to care for her because of her depressed, hopeless state. She was assured that help was available, and within three months there was a dramatic change in the child's weight and affective and developmental state. Mrs. A. was able to function much better at home though her husband had not changed.

Seven years later the daughter was an outgoing child of average intelligence and doing well in school. Mrs. A. had not divorced her husband but now was in the process of doing so. She recalled that once she was assured that her daughter had no physical cause for failure to thrive, she was able to care for her without fear and she felt that supportive counseling was helpful. Mr. A. continued to drink and in addition began to abuse Mrs. A. physically. She would not tolerate this, obtained training as a beautician, and worked part time, preparing for her future without her husband. A friend was her babysitter. She had a hopeful view of the future and had taken the initiative in a number of areas.

Mrs. A. had the capacity for questioning her own behavior and actions. She did not use pregenital defenses predominately, and her capacity for object relationships was good. There was little acting out of her difficulties and she had the capacity for thinking in abstractions. Her personality was in marked contrast to the majority of the mothers.

Case 2.. Mrs. B. was 21 years old when first seen. At the time of her first pregnancy she was 18 years old and was pregnant when she married. She had a "little girl" manner and was overly compliant and eager to please. She wore very tight-fitting clothes and used makeup excessively, and her tension was apparent as she smoked and spoke rapidly and constantly. Mrs. B. spoke about everything with ease, except that she was somewhat tearful about her father's death. At times she had an air of forced gaiety, and at other times she seemed very "bland" and expressionless.

Her father had been very strict, but she felt she was his favorite. Her mother allowed her to date without her father's knowledge. At age 15 she left school in the ninth grade, and she worked until she was 18 years old. Her father died when she was 17, and her mother became suicidal and was hospitalized. Since that time her mother had had recurrent depressions.

When asked to talk about her past, Mrs. B. said she had had a pleasant childhood and then told about her father's rigidity. She also felt she was discriminated against by other children because she was from a white minority group. She had been "bothered since my marriage," but she could not say why she was anxious, though she had married a man diagnosed as a chronic paranoid schizophrenic, whose decompensation more than once had led to hospitalization. She saw herself as a "good little girl" who was unable to alter her circumstances. She had little awareness of her relationships to adults or children. Mrs. B. thought in concrete terms, had poor judgment, and expressed herself in action rather than thought. She was consistent in her behavior, but it was constricted and repetitious. She said, in a not unhappy manner, "It doesn't look like we are going to have anything; life will continue as it is." She rarely went out of her house. Eight months after the initial contact she was content because her mother was living with her, and she denied the severity of her infant son's earlier failure to thrive.

Mrs. B.'s object relationships were of the anaclitic type, and she never felt herself to be in a mothering role. Denial was a predominant defense. She denied that she had had difficulties before marriage and that her children had any difficulties, yet one of the other children was retarded in growth and displayed a flat affect. She denied that she was depressed and helpless.

When she and her children were seen several years later, she was content because her mother was living with her, her husband was working, and they were buying a home. In terms of character structure and daily behavior, she had not changed. She was very dependent on her mother, she rarely went out, and she was content with the children's behavior and performance. They rarely played outside, their performance in school was marginal, and they appeared to be understimulated in history, reports, and observation. Growth failure was not present.

Case 3. Mrs. C., referred by protective services, was age 23 when first interviewed. She attempted to appear at ease but intermittently was angry or reserved about specific questions. When talking about how she felt used and abused by her family, she appeared depressed. She said that from ages 2 to 5 she had lived with an aunt but did not know why and was not curious. At 5 she was returned to her mother, and she could not give a reason except that she may have been "homesick." When asked if her life would have been better if she had stayed with her aunt, she became angry and said she might have finished school, she would not have had three children, and life would have been good.

Her father left her mother when Mrs. C. was age 10, but she did not know the reason. Mrs. C. felt her mother and siblings took advantage of her and that her mother approved of this. Mrs. C. cleaned house and cared for some of the younger siblings. She first became pregnant at age 16 in the tenth grade and left school. She worked part time, life was unpleasant and "hopeless," and subsequently she had two more children by different men. Again she said she was not sure why. She was on drugs at age 20 and became angry when asked how was paid for the drugs because she felt that the question implied she was prostituting. Drug usage ceased because she was afraid that during pregnancy the drugs would cause the fetus to be deformed. At that time she went on a methadone maintenance regime.

Mrs. C. hoped to move to another state with her boy friend because nothing hopeful was happening where she was. She had hoped to be a nurse when she was younger but now was going to raise her children. She had little hope for herself but wished to marry her boy friend and give her children opportunities that she had not had. The severity of her infant daughter's growth failure did not impress her. The severity of her own rage and depression, which were readily apparent, were minimized, and she acted out her conflicts repeatedly. Her dependency needs were denied. Repeated attempts at very active social-service intervention were unsuccessful, and protective service and court intervention did not materialize. Approximately one year later information was received that the infant daughter had died of malnutrition.

The Infants

Gross distortions in development and maturation were manifested by the infants in various ways. On infant testing they were frequently retarded, and developmental lags in motor development were evident in the majority of babies (Whitten *et al.*, 1969). Autoerotic behavior was present in many forms: nodding spasms, head banging, sucking of fingers or fists, rocking, rumination, and bizarre, rhythmic hand movements. More than half of the infants exhibited infantile posturing and moved their hands up and parallel to their heads when approached. Sometimes this movement was accompanied by crying and screaming, as if the sight of an adult approaching were a distressing experience. Watchfulness or hyperalert staring was frequent, as were a withdrawn apathetic response and anorexia. These babies appeared "frozen" in terms of affective responses, and smiling was minimal. Speech and language development were often severely retarded.

Though a large group of infants who failed to thrive were studied, we observed a certain group of infants to determine whether infants with failure to thrive, receiving a paucity of mothering, would gain weight at an accelerated rate when adequately fed (Whitten et al., 1969). Thirteen infants were hospitalized, given basic physical care, visited infrequently by their parents, monitored constantly with a television camera, and offered a generous diet of at least 140 calories per kilogram of ideal weight for ideal height for two weeks. Ten of the 13 showed an accelerated weight gain. Two of the 3 who did not gain at an accelerated rate had grossly inadequate caloric intakes. The third gained at an accelerated rate in the third week. During the two-week study period the infants behaved as though they were accustomed to this type of handling, which would be considered relative understimulation normally. However, 5 infants became progressively more active and less withdrawn. Five of 6 infants showed no change in scores on the Cattell infant intelligence scale administered before and after two weeks; one gained from 90 to 100.

After two weeks 6 of the infants continued in the hospital and were given a gread deal of "mothering"—fondling, social contact, and physical handling—plus the same quantity of calories as in the previous two weeks. The 4 infants who had gained weight before continued to do so. The two who had not gained weight earlier did not gain with the high level of mothering. However, continued contact with the mothers of these two infants revealed that they had repeatedly attempted to force-feed them. Also, one of the fathers had attempted to "ram a hamburger down the infant's throat," after which the baby virtually refused to eat for several days.

Following discharge from the hospital the effect of adequate calories on weight gain at home was evaluated in 4 infants. For a two-week period a measured diet was carried to the home for each mealtime. The mother fed the infant, but the worker did not offer advice or instructions to her. The worker returned the uneaten food to the hospital for measurement. Also added to this group of 4 infants were 3 infants who were fed at home under the same regime prior to parental awareness of the diagnosis. With one exception the 7 mothers whose infants were fed a diet brought to their homes subsequently said that the quantity of food eaten during the two-week period was greater than the quantities usually eaten by the baby. Yet these diets were duplicates of those the mothers had originally claimed they fed the infants. All 7 of the infants gained weight at home on adequate diets being fed by their mothers during a period when we believed the infant was still being "maternally deprived," since this was during the early period of work with each mother. The mothers almost always gave inaccurate histories concerning the infants' food intake because their severe emotional difficulties distorted their observations. Rarely was it a conscious distortion.

Of the group of 13 infants 3 were placed in foster homes and 10 were discharged to their mothers. Despite efforts to enable the mothers to improve their mothering, only 4 of the 10 babies who were returned to their mothers continued to gain at a satisfactory rate. The remaining mothers claimed that the infant's daily intake was adequate. However, 4 of 4 who had not gained satisfactorily at home gained at an accelerated rate when fed the diet sent to the home. The weight gain far exceeded the weight gain of the interim period during which the mother claimed an adequate intake.

Discussion

In a review of the literature the impression gained is that the infants' failure to gain weight is secondary to apathy, depression, or some other affective state. Another hypothesis in the literature is that the failure to gain weight may be due to endocrine dysfunction after prolonged starvation. However, no other study monitored the feeding process and the food intake as closely as the one described above. In this study, when the babies received sufficient food, they gained weight quickly. This weight gain was not due to a change in the mother–child relationship, since it occurred rapidly and in the face of clear evidence that the mother had not changed in relationship to the infant. Optimism should be tempered with a great deal of caution when the baby begins to gain weight. In the majority of instances the distortion and/or deprivation in the mothering process continues. In all areas of development, e.g., emotional, cognitive, and object relations, the risk for the infant is still great. If anything, the study demonstrated that the mothers gave grossly inaccurate histories about the babies' food intake and their relationship to the babies in all areas. Rarely were the inaccuracies due to conscious distortion.

The mothers and infants described, in addition to many other mothers and infants who failed to thrive, were involved in vigorous, dedicated efforts directed toward intervention, treatment, and remediation. The clinical descriptions, observations, and material for any one mother–infant pair is voluminous, and illustrative anecdotes are limitless but are not relevant to the purpose of this presentation, which is to describe two aspects of a larger project. Table 1 is an illustration of a number of observations concerning the mothers. From extensive clinical experience, before the initiation of the research project, we were impressed by certain characteristics of the mothers that appeared repeatedly. Attempts were made to define these characteristics and to determine if our earlier impressions were valid and significant for mothers whose babies failed to thrive. The clinical data in ongoing interviews were rich in descriptive details, but the object was to determine which observations, if any, were significant for this group of mothers. From Table 1 there emerges a composite picture of the mothers, who, with rare exception, had severe personality disorders. The individual observations for 12 of the mothers have been reported previously (Fischhoff et al., 1971). Whether the mother was married was not significant. The sex of the baby was not significant. As a group the siblings of the infants manifested emotional, intellectual, and behavioral deviations to a disporportionate degree. Perhaps in families with infants who fail to thrive attention is focused on the baby because of the serious illness and because he is identified as the youngest in the sibship. In those families that had an older child who had failed to thrive as an infant, we noted that he had been the "youngest" child in the family at that time. This fact deserves emphasis, since recovery from growth failure does not mean that there is necessarily improvement in the mother or the mother–child relationship, increased appropriate stimulation in the home, or greater optimism for the child's future positive psychological growth. Observations of the siblings indicates that the families are multiple-problem families. Anna Freud used the phrase "unwilling mothers" in elaborating a picture of mothers who did not mean to be pregnant at a certain time or who felt that the role of motherhood had been forced upon them. The phrase "unwilling mothers" could extend to the mothering of other children in these families who were not thriving in other ways. The mothering of these mothers had been sufficiently deficient or distorted to make it difficult to identify with or conceptualize what an "average" or adequate mother should be.

Recently Cravioto (1973) reported an ongoing study, now in its seventh year, of 300 children in a Mexican village, where malnutrition of some degree is prevalant among all the children because of "low socioeconomic and cultural backgrounds," but severe malnutrition is a "seemingly random occurrence." The investigators concluded that the "development of severe 'third degree' malnutrition is strongly associated with the lack of social, emotional, and cognitive stimulation within the home." In this study the psychologist making the observations on all aspects of the families' functioning was unaware of the infants' and children's nutritional histories.

One Style of Research

My base of operations has been the clinical setting, whether in private practice, consultation, residential treatment homes, children's psychiatric hospitals, schools, agencies, or, for a number of years, a children's hospital. Consequently, research, service, and teaching have inevitably been intertwined. At any one time in a clinical setting there are a number of intriguing questions that arise, to which there are a number of possible solutions or for which there is no present answer. A clinical judgment and decision is made on the basis of available knowledge. However, the unanswered questions remain. At times the personnel and resources are available to study the problem without much delay, but frequently the clinical problem is one of several that are being studied, and information is slowly being gathered and recorded, ultimately to be analyzed. Impressions are influenced in one direction or another as the research proceeds. Sometimes a situation occurs in which it is possible to initiate research at the time the question arises. Some years ago several preschool boys were in treatment simultaneously because they definitely preferred to be girls. It was possible to have the boys in intensive psychotherapy, to work with their families, and to conduct ongoing research on the problem for an extended period (Fischhoff, 1964). Such a set of circumstances does not occur as often as one would desire.

Leonardo da Vinci said, "He who appeals to authority when there is a difference of opinion, works with his memory rather than with his reason." The formulation of a question implies that one has to wait before one knows. During the period of waiting we hope that investigation can be carried out. Sometimes the questions are of the survey type. Other times they can be more specific. A "good" question, if capable of solution, would alter our previous assumptions and perspectives, therefore broadening our horizons and leading to more questions. In child psychiatry there are many vistas to be explored, and we are often in the process of mapping the terrain. For this reason my personal preference or bias is to include as many aspects or factors as possible in any one investigation, e.g., the child's inner life, physiology, physical development, cognitive development, environment, family, and cultural setting. At this point in child psychiatry each child is an "experiment in nature," and the more information we have on a longitudinal basis the better we might be able to understand this experiment. Some studies are suited to a cross-sectional approach and others to a longitudinal approach. However, whichever method is used, my predilection is for a holistic approach.

Even when a "single" phenomenon is being studied, multiple factors are involved. My interest is not only in a list of these factors but in how and to what degree they are integrated and influence and complement one another. The phenomenon being studied is not treated in isolation. It is one factor among many, and highlighted, but all other parameters are observed, recorded, and studied. Clinical experience and psychoanalytic training have been influential in evolving this philosophy of research, and it is a stimulating and enriching experience.

References

BARBARO, G. J., MORRIS, M. G., & REDFORD, M. T. Malidentification of mother-baby-father relationships expressed in infant failure to thrive. *Child Welfare*, 1963, **42**, 13.

BARBARO, G. J., & SHAHEEN, E. Environmental failure to thrive. *Journal of Pediatrics*, 1967, **71**, 639.

BULLARD, D. M., GLASSER, H. H., HEAGARTY, M. C., & PIVCHIK, E. C. Failure to thrive in the neglected child. *American Journal of Orthopsychiatry*, 1967, **37**, 680.

COLEMAN, R. W., & PROVENCE, S. Environmental retardation (hospitalism) in infants living in families. *Pediatrics*, 1957, **19**, 285.

CRAVIOTO, J. Paper in symposium. Nutrition and its contributions to mental functions. Kitty Scientific Foundation, 1973. Reported in *Hospital Tribune*, May 21, 1973.

ELMER, E. Failure to thrive: Role of the mother. *Pediatrics*, 1960, **25**, 717.

EVANS, S. L., REINHART, J. B., & SUCCOP, R. A. Failure to thrive: A study of 45 children and their families. *Journal of the American Academy of Child Psychiatry*, 1972, **11**, 440.

FISCHHOFF, J. Preoedipal influences in a boy's determination to be "feminine" during the oedipal period. *Journal of the American Academy of Child Psychiatry*, 1964, **3**, 273–286.

FISCHHOFF, J., WHITTEN, C. F., & PETTIT, M. G. A psychiatric study of mothers of infants with growth failure secondary to maternal deprivation. *Journal of Pediatrics*, 1971, **79**, 209–215.

GLASER, H. H., HEAGARTY, M. C., BULLARD, D. M., & PIVCHIK, E. C. Physical and psychological development of children with early failure to thrive. *Journal of Pediatrics*, 1968, **73**, 690.

LEONARD, M. F., RHYMES, J. P., & SOLNIT, A. J. Failure to thrive in infants: A family problem. *American Journal of Disabled Children*, 1966, **3**, 600.

SPITZ, R. A. Hospitalism: An inquiry into the genesis of psychiatric conditions in early childhood. *Psychoanalytic Study of the Child*, 1945, **1**, 53.

WHITTEN, C. F., PETTIT, M. G., & FISCHHOFF, J. Evidence that growth failure from maternal deprivation is secondary to undereating. *Journal of the American Medical Association*, 1969, **209**, 1675–1682.

PSYCHOPHYSIOLOGICAL STUDY OF BLEEDING AND ADAPTATION IN YOUNG HEMOPHILIACS

AKE MATTSSON

Introduction

Robert Louis Stevenson, a victim of pulmonary tuberculosis, once wrote, "Life is not a matter of holding good cards, but of playing a poor hand well." Children with a chronic physical disorder, such as hemophilia, who have mastered the physical, social, and emotional hardships associated with their illness, well illustrate this point. This chapter describes a six-year study of the psychophysiological aspects of hemophilia that began with an investigation of the common forms of emotional stress experienced by the hemophilic child and his family and the major coping techniques enabling them to achieve a satisfactory psychosocial adaptation. This investigation was followed by a group therapy project with the parents of young hemophiliacs that provided further information about parental adjustment to chronic childhood illness. The study ended with a long-term psychoendocrine study aimed at examining the possible correlation between the urinary excretion of stress hormones and the degree of adaptation in hemophilic boys. From its beginning our project was of a naturalistic nature and was service-oriented. Many short-term psychotherapeutic interventions took place involving both the boys and their parents. The longitudinal scope of the study allowed for certain conclusions regarding children's coping with long-term physical illness in general.

Hemophilia is a lifelong serious illness almost exclusively of males, characterized primarily by bleeding into the soft tissues and joints. The bleeding tendency is due to clotting defects transmitted as sex-linked recessive traits by the carrier mother to the recipient son. Consequently half of a car-

AKE MATTSSON, Professor of Psychiatry and Pediatrics, University of Virginia Medical Center, Charlottesville, Virginia.

rier's sons are hemophiliacs and half of her daughters are carriers. The defects in clotting are caused by a deficiency in the plasma antihemophilic factor (factor VIII) in classic hemophilia or in the Christmas factor (factor IX) in Christmas disease. Clinically the two types of hemophilia are practically indistinguishable. Most patients with hemophilia show an onset of symptoms in early childhood and are subjected to repeated bleeding episodes, often causing severe pain and requiring immobilization, hospital admissions, and various treatment procedures. Despite recent improvements in the treatment of acute hemorrhages with concentrated plasma-fractions and greatly increased chances for a normal life span, the constant threat of a bleeding episode that might prove fatal looms over the young hemophiliac and his family. The parents have to cope with such hardships as constant precautions against physical trauma and attendance to their son's bleeding episodes, the need to raise him as normally as possible and not to ignore their healthy children's demands, the necessity to inform the daughters of their possible carrier states, and often staggering medical expenses.

How did we become interested in examining the psychological aspects of hemophilia? Two reasons stand out. First, my former background in pediatrics prompted me, as a child psychiatry resident, to choose a long elective in consultation and liaison work with the pediatric department. From the beginning of my pediatric training I had been intrigued by my common observation that children and adolescents with serious physical disorders showed a remarkably good adaptation. I was curious to learn more about how children "play a poor hand well" in coping with physical illness and handicaps. The second reason was that such an examination offered an opportunity to pursue a study attractively in line with my curiosity.

The leading hematologist at our university medical center asked the psychiatric department if we had an interest in studying the possible influence of emotional factors on the clinical course of bleeding disorders such as hemophilia. For a number of years he and his associates had observed a seeming relationship between stress factors in the environment of some hemophiliacs and the occurrence of so-called "spontaneous bleeding episodes," i.e., hemorrhages that cannot be accounted for by physical trauma. These observations suggested that psychophysiological factors might at times be superimposed upon the clotting deficiency in hemophilia and be responsible for some bleeding episodes. Earlier studies had shown that the vascularity of the lining of some internal organs, as well as of the skin, was subject to change under certain emotional states. Furthermore, some dentists had demonstrated the value of hypnosis in promoting hemostasis in the control of bleeding during dental surgery in hemophiliacs. These observations supported the view that the integrity of the vascular wall is influenced by factors in the upper central nervous system.

When a colleague and I gladly agreed to collaborate in a psychosomatic investigation of hemophilia, the hematologists also told us about signs of psychological maladjustment among some of their hemophilic patients, such as the occurrence of repeated risk-taking behavior that exposed the patients to physical trauma, often followed by bleeding. Other hemophiliacs were overly careful regarding physical activity and utterly dependent on their families, which led to poor psychosocial and vocational adjustment in their adult years.

We concluded that the hematologists were as interested as we in learning more about why so many severe hemophiliacs, along with their parents, seemed to adjust well to their illness, whereas others, at times showing less clinical severity, coped with their illness in ways that were socially detrimental to them.

Investigation of Emotional Stress and Coping Behavior in Young Hemophiliacs

The few previous reports on psychosocial factors in hemophilia had utilized cross-sectional examination of small samples. We felt that only a long-term study (Mattsson and Gross, 1966a, 1966b) of a sample as large as possible could provide some answers to the questions related to hemophilic patients' adaptation to their serious disease. In addition a longitudinal approach was necessary if we were to investigate the likely effect of emotional factors on the number and trend of bleeding episodes.

The late 1950s and early 1960s had seen a series of reports in the area of stress research that described the behavioral and hormonal reactions of normal individuals to various contingencies of life, such as major illness, severe injuries, cancer, the threat of death, and naturally occurring disasters. In 1962 Lois Murphy had remarked, "there are thousands of studies of maladjustment for each one that deals directly with the ways of managing life's problems with personal strength and adequacy." These early papers on coping and adaptation in normal persons, aptly summarized by Murphy (1962), Chodoff et al. (1964), Friedman et al. (1963) and Lazarus (1966), provided us with helpful theoretical constructs that we adapted to build our own framework, within which we could analyze our observations on hemophiliac boys and their parents. Many writers on human stress had adopted the term *coping behavior* to denote all the adaptational techniques and defensive activities that a person uses to deal with major life threats in order to function effectively. Coping behavior, as we conceived it, includes the use of cognitive functions, motor activity, emotional expression, and certain psychic defenses. Guided by the approach of Friedman et al. (1963) to the study of adaptation to stress, we planned to make a broad assessment of the coping behavior of hemophilic boys in these areas: (1) Does the behavior observed in the hemophiliac allow him to achieve his personal and socially defined goals despite his illness? (2) Is the boy able to tolerate stressful situations, particularly associated with acute hemorrhages, without disruptive affects' interfering with his cognitive functioning and cooperation?

It is of interest to compare our framework of 1964 for describing coping behavior to Lazarus's delineation of human responses to stress, part of his work, "Psychological Stress and the Coping Process," published in 1966. Lazarus outlined four main classes of reaction to psychological stress: (1) Disturbed affects. (2) Motor-behavioral reactions. (3) Changes in the adequacy of cognitive functioning, such as perception, memory, thought, judgment, and problem solving. Lazarus added that "evidence of defensive thought processes may be included in the above category because these processes can be regarded as a form of adaptive functioning. They are usually inferred from cognitive behaviors, especially from certain styles of thinking and perceiving, and from discrepancies between the interpretation the individual makes and some consensual estimate of the objective circumstances. . . . As misinterpretations of reality, they reflect impairment of cognitive activity in the effort to cope [pp. 7–8]." (4) Physiological changes, including reactions of both the autonomic nervous system and the adrenal glands.

Lazarus's main classes of stress reactions seemed to overlap with our and others' conception of actual techniques for dealing with stress. We noted, however, that we had separated defenses from other cognitive coping mechanisms of hemophiliacs and their parents in our desire to emphasize the essential role of certain psychological defenses in influencing the final outcome of the coping process, i.e., good or poor adaptation. Lazarus's view of defenses as psychological maneuvers, inferred from observed behavior and aimed at reappraisals and distortions of a threatening reality—"to take the sting out of it, to make it bearable [Murphy, 1962, p. 282]"—was completely in line with our thinking. This view of psychological defenses as potentially supporting good coping and adaptation had already been emphasized by Murphy, Friedman et al., (1963), and Chodoff et al. (1964). The use of defense mechanisms ought not to carry with it the common negative implication of always leading to maladaptation. To quote Chodoff et al., "there is an intermediate range of defensive strength which allows for optimum coping, while extreme deviations at either end of this scale have adverse effects on coping." Defenses might be ineffectual, resulting in overpowering anxiety, or they might become "so obtrusive as to dominate the individual's attention" and seriously limit his ability to deal with outer and inner threats.

Thus we had a tentative conceptual framework for analyzing the ongoing coping behavior of hemophilic boys and their families. Next we had to approach the two pediatric hematologists to gain their interest and cooperation regarding our study of adaptation in hemophiliacs.

Many child psychiatrists have established good working relationships with their pediatric colleagues regarding teaching about and caring for children with somatopsychic, psychosomatic, and psychological problems. The situation often differs, however, when a child psychiatrist wishes to study an organically well-defined patient group that is closely followed by a pediatric subspecialist. The latter frequently sees no rationale for psychological investigation of "my patients and families." In our setting the pediatric hematologists at first were lukewarm about a collaborative study of the hemophilic population. One reason was a sense of rivalry between the pediatric and general hematologists; as mentioned, we had initially been approached by the head of the latter group. Another, more important reason, which we soon could counter, was an understandable ignorance on the part of the pediatricians about the value of biopsychosocial approach to a study of chronically ill children. However, like many medical subspecialists, the pediatric hematologists had combined their attention to their patients' clinical course with well-documented concern about their social situation. They were always available for emergency consultations regarding the 35 hemophilic boys followed by the pediatric services.

How could I prove that my psychiatric colleague and I had something worthwhile to offer in terms of improved patient care and educational value? I followed the "old" approach of the pediatric psychiatrist who, by his regular, tactfully interfering presence on the pediatric wards, makes himself known to the medical staff as well as to many of the chronically ill children frequently admitted to the wards. Over a period of four to five months this "backdoor approach" paid off: I became sufficiently knowledgeable about the eventual study group of 35 hemophilic boys and their parents, representing 22 families, to be able to compile demographic and clinical data that aroused the interest of the hematologists. Our careful study of often-bulky hospital records and the many family interviews yielded fresh, composite pictures of the long-term clinical courses of the 35 boys, whose illness usually had been identified around age one.

In addition I soon could provide psychotherapeutic support in those situations on the wards in which a hemophilic boy or his parents gave clear indications of acute anxiety states, depressive reactions, or other management problems. These crisis interventions often included school personnel and vocational issues. My stepping in as a therapist of families participating in our project represented a contamination of the methodology that is difficult to avoid in this type of a naturalistic long-term study. It is awkward if not unethical for the main investigator to refrain from assisting a troubled family well known to him and to refer them to a mental health colleague with less knowledge about the specific problems of an illness such as hemophilia.

Over a period of two years I followed the 35 hemophilic boys, their parents, and many of their healthy siblings by interviews and close observations during hospital admissions as well as during periods of clinical remission. The interaction on the wards among patients, staff, and visiting families was also studied. The interviews and observations were aimed at gaining information relative to: (1) the understanding of hemophilia by the child and the parent; (2) the clinical course in the individual patient and his reactions to bleeding episodes, hospitalizations, and treatment procedures; (3) the child's ongoing adaptive process as manifested at home, in school, and with peers; and (4) the parents' means of dealing with the problems of raising their hemophilic child.

Twenty-two patients fell into the 1–11 age groups, the remainder being adolescents and young adults. There were no only children among the 35 hemophiliacs, which provided opportunities to observe the relationships between a young bleeder and his healthy and hemophilic siblings. Nine families had more than one hemophilic child; of these, one family had successfully raised four boys with hemophilia.

Among the findings related to the clinical picture of juvenile hemophilia, we noted an average of four to six annual major bleeding episodes in the preadolescent boys, necessitating hospital admission and often lengthy orthopedic treatment. Many instances of intracranial hemorrhage took place, frequently associated with coma and transient seizures. Another serious consequence of bleeding occurred in three boys, who hemorrhaged into the soft tissues of the floor of the mouth, the neck, and the mediastinum following pharyngeal infections. One of these boys died at age 8, despite tracheotomy and repeated exchange transfusions. During their first 12 years of life most of the patients had recurrent long periods of freedom from major bleeding, alternating with periods of increased bleeding tendency, which were characterized by many hemorrhages seemingly unrelated to known physical trauma. No discernible changes in their activities had taken place that could explain the cycles of increased bleeding. Another type of "spontaneous" bleeding was observed in eight boys under age 14, four of whom were brothers. They often began to bleed, without previous trauma, just prior to a highly anticipated event, such as a holiday, a birthday, or a camp meeting. Their parents described the boys as "overenthusiastic" and "excited" in looking forward to such events.

Three bleeders, about 20 years of age at the time of our study, had early in adolescence shown a change in their behavior and activity pattern, which preceded or coincided with clinical improvement. Having been overprotected, inactive, and fearful since early childhood, they developed over a short period of time into more active, independent, at times daring teen-agers, despite maternal protests. Their marked increase in physical activities was accompanied by a decrease in bleeding episodes.

The findings mentioned so far confirmed the impression of many hematologists that emotional stress might be related to episodes of spontaneous bleeding. Because of the lack of evidence of changes in levels of the antihemophilic factor at times of stress, some authors have suggested that variations in the integrity of the capillary wall as an autonomic response to stress may be responsible for certain periods of increased bleeding, such as seen among our subjects (Agle, 1964).

As we analyzed our findings regarding the coping behavior and the psychosocial adaptation in the 35 hemophilic boys, we found that the majority of them—27—had for at least the past two years shown a satisfactory adaptation to their illness, i.e., they were functioning effectively at home, in school, at work, and with their peers and with few or no limitations other than those imposed by the disease and its complications. Our long-term observations gave evidence of a brighter outlook for the hemophiliac's personality development than had generally been expected.

Some characteristic coping devices and psychic defenses appeared essential for a successful adaptation. Regarding some aspects of cognitive functioning, a majority of the boys had from age four to five begun to relate memories of past bleeding episodes, associating them with bumps or falls. From the age of six to seven the well-adjusted patients showed an increasing comprehension of the relationship between trauma, bleeding, and common treatment procedures. Their better understanding of the necessary physical restrictions together with wider acceptance of compensatory activities helped these boys to cope with repeated hemorrhagic episodes. This appropriate appearance of a sense of self-protection and of assuming some responsibility for the care of their bodies served the vital function of self-preservation and precluded the development of the helpless, inactive dependence noted in other reports on hemophiliacs.

The use of compensatory motor activity and intellectual pursuits became increasingly evident in the adolescent boys in our study. The range of physical activities that the well-adjusted patients took part in, often under their fathers' direction, was an unexpected finding. Their participation in play and sports, appropriate for their ages, seldom resulted in major bleeding. The boys would often imagine themselves as taking part in hazardous sports, such as horseback riding, ice hockey, and car racing, knowing, however, that they had to settle for less risk-filled pursuits. There was no evidence of repeated, dangerous activities in the large group of well-adapted hemophiliacs.

In addition to cognitive flexibility and compensatory motor activity, the appropriate release of emotions and the employment of certain psychological defenses were essential parts of the coping process of the well-functioning hemophiliacs. They would express, often in succession, anxiety, sadness, anger, hope, and confidence at times of critical bleeding episodes. Murphy (1962) in particular has described how emotional and cognitive flexibility helps children cope with stressful situations, provided the adult environment accepts the release of various feelings, encourages verbalization, and provides for substitute gratification.

The observations of our patients' use of some psychic defense mechanisms contributed to an understanding of the different outcomes of their coping efforts. Among the well-adapted hemophiliacs defenses such as denial, isolation of affect, intellectualization or "control through thinking," identification with other bleeders and the physicians, and occasional projections of resentful feelings seemed to protect the children from disruptive degrees of anxiety and despair. The optimum employment of these defenses also enabled them to maintain hope and develop a positive self-image as future competent and productive individuals.

From the age of 9–10 the well-adjusted hemophiliacs began to show a certain pride and confidence in themselves when discussing their disease. As they experienced repeated successful attempts at mastering bleeding crises, they consolidated their individual coping styles along the lines previously described. These older boys denied the possibility of a premature death, stating, for example, that "plasma can always get us over the hump." They felt confident that they would find gainful jobs as adults and lead reasonably normal lives. Many of the adolescent bleeders related their positive outlook to their parents' early and consistent efforts to raise them with minimal restrictions. As one 16-year-old boy put it, "Don't worry about the kids, Doc, but help the parents with their worries, so they can treat us like normal children."

Turning to the eight poorly adapted hemophiliacs in our group of 35 patients, we found illustrations of Hartmann's (1958) statement that "A 'successful' defense may amount to a 'failure' in achievement [p. 12]." Five of these patients were making extreme use of denial in order to master fears of their illness. They repeatedly engaged in risk-taking activities, challenging the risk of injury in a counterphobic manner. These five daring patients had been raised by oversolicitous and guilt-laden mothers. As preadolescents they rebelled against maternal interference and turned into active, defiant boys.

The remaining three poorly adapted hemophiliacs showed an opposite reaction in that they had acquiesced to maternal demands and led a fearful, inactive life. They were passive-dependent young teen-agers who displayed a strong reluctance to participate in any physical activities because of fears of trauma. They readily accepted treatment procedures and were viewed as ideal patients on the ward. The mothers of these patients spoke about their guilty feelings over being carriers and saw themselves as the only effective protectors of their children. Their fathers played little or no role in their rearing.

The results of the two-year study had illuminated the intimate relationship between the adaptation of the 35 boys and their parents' adjustment to their disease. A crucial factor determining the common positive adaptive outcome seemed to be the mother's ability to master her guilt over having transmitted the illness. Many mothers told us about the importance of having been able to express fears, guilt, sadness, and hopeless feelings to the pediatrician, the father, and other close adults in order for the mother to achieve gradual mastery of her initial strong, conflicting emotions. These were particularly strengthened in those mothers who had witnessed earlier, fatal outcomes of hemophilia or other congenital illnesses among their siblings and children. It is noteworthy that there were as many mothers with a family history of hemophilia or other congenital disorders in the group of well-adapted hemophiliacs as in the group of poorly adjusted ones. We concluded that the successful adaptation to the task of raising a hemophiliac did not appear to be influenced by such variables as the presence of another son with the same illness, parental knowledge of the genetic risk before marriage, the child's age at diagnosis, or the clinical severity of hemophilia.

The mothers of the eight poorly adjusted hemophiliacs had never mastered their guilt and anxiety. They provided an illustrative example of one important, predisposing factor for the development of a "vulnerable child syndrome," first described by Green and Solnit (1964). Each of these mothers had identified her hemophilic boy with a deceased relative (usually a hemophiliac) and saw her son as unrealistically vulnerable at all times. The boy sensed his mother's expectations of his vulnerability and premature death, and he either accepted these expectations, developing into a fearful, passive teen-ager, or challenged the maternal expectation and the risk of injury in the counterphobic manner previously described.

Our observations of the 22 sets of parents, who were part of the original project, made it possible to delineate some major psychological defenses used by the parents in coping with the many stress factors related to their children's illness. These observations of the parents were the main reason for the next phase of our hemophilia study, a group therapy project with 10 parents of young hemophiliacs. In addition my associate and I wanted to learn more about the problems of the siblings of hemophilic boys, as the initial study indicated few unfavorable reactions among the healthy brothers and sisters. The restraints placed on the latter by the parents were sensible in most instances. The older siblings often assisted in the care of the hemophiliacs and assumed a protective role toward them both at home and away. Expressions of resentment among siblings about the parental attention their sick brothers received usually were accepted by the parents as natural and unavoidable. A few sisters had shown pronounced anxious or jealous attitudes toward their hemophilic brothers, for instance, pretending that they were ill and insisting that they stay home from school when their brothers were confined in bed.

Several adolescent girls, in addition to showing an increasing responsibility for the care of their hemophilic brothers, spoke about their future education in terms of nurses' or teachers' training so "I can help my brother and my parents if needed".

Group Therapy Projects with Parents of Hemophiliacs

For this study (Mattsson and Agle, 1972) we had no problems collecting a group of parents of hemophiliacs interested in a series of weekly meetings, whose purpose was twofold: (1) to promote the parents' understanding and mastery of distressing emotions related to their sons' disease, hence improving the parent–child relationship, and (2) to provide us with more information about methods of parental coping with the problems of raising a chronically ill child. The local chapter of the National Hemophilia Foundation had already included me and my psychiatric colleague among their medical advisers, and they were more than willing to obtain volunteers for our group project from among the many parents of hemophiliacs in our geographic area.

The study group of 10 parents consisted of 4 married couples and 2 mothers. This group was not representative of the population at large of parents of hemophiliacs but contained motivated and verbal parents of the middle socioeconomic class. A series of 25 weekly meetings, each meeting lasting 1½ hours, was conducted in a nondirective manner with all sessions tape-recorded. After each meeting the co-leader and I independently wrote down its major contents and dynamics. A two-year follow-up was provided by further group meetings and interviews with individual group members.

Based on our previous experience with the conceptual model of coping behavior, my colleague and I were hopeful that the wealth of material that emerged during the group sessions could be examined and described within a similar framework, i.e., including the parental use of cognitive functions, motor activity, emotional expression, and some psychological defenses. These hopes were largely fulfilled, thanks to the work of the parents, whose emotional and intellectual involvement resulted in the development of a strong group cohesiveness after the first six weeks. The initial sessions had been characterized by an intense sharing of common hardships and emotional distress among the parents, at times sounding like abreacting "horror stories" about raising a hemophiliac. The universality of the parents' experience was probably the key factor in binding the group together and maintaining its cohesiveness. The parents accepted one another and came to view the co-therapists as nonjudgmental and helpful in calling attention to both adaptive and maladaptive ways of parental coping with a stressful life situation. The initial sessions also were important in exposing the frustration of the group's wishes to obtain psychological advice and medical information from the leaders. In addition we were presumed to have healthy children and hence to be unable to understand the plight of parents of chronically ill boys.

Thus, after the initial two months, the parents began to recognize and describe their habitual modes of coping with the many problems related to raising a hemophiliac. The parents described, in nontechnical language, their essential tension-relieving mechanisms, which we, in turn, could present by way of some well-known cognitive, defensive process. In our task to delineate these we received considerable guidance from "Glossary of Defenses" by Bibring *et al.* (1961).

The parents provided striking examples of the use of such defenses as isolation of painful affect, especially during bleeding crises, and denial of frightening realities associated with hemophilia and the common sense of guilt and helplessness. During several group sessions the parents gave evidence of using rationalization in their attempt to hide from themselves and their children sad, angry, and despairing states related to their unique burden. Examples were, "What a wonderful thing it is to have a hemophilic child—it has emotionally sharpened me and my husband—it has made our whole family life spiritually richer."

Like many of their hemophilic boys the group members continually relied on the use of intellectual processes to defend against distressing emotions, i.e., on the cognitive strategy of "control through thinking" (Bibring *et al.*, 1961). In listening to the parents' emphasis on learning as much as possible about the medical, physiological, and psychological aspects of hemophilia, we as group leaders became aware of the important distinction made by Bibring *et al.* (1961) between the defensive mechanisms of control through thinking and of intellectualization. These authors suggested that through the use of the former, "the content of the frightening situation is not primarily drained of anxieties, but through extended anticipatory familiarization with the danger, an attempt is made to prepare oneself and thus lessen the anxiety." The parental reliance on control through thinking confirmed our common observations on the pediatric wards that repeated dosages of factual information regarding a child's disease and treatment procedures engage the parents in a "therapeutic alliance" with the medical staff and prepare the family for changes in their child's condition.

The group readily acknowledged how easily parents of chronically ill children develop martyrlike attitudes and direct their whole life to caring for their "sufferers." In other words, the parents were describing an extreme use of reaction formation, which, when optimally employed, may be quite helpful for parents who harbor affects of anger, guilt, and sadness about their ill child.

All members of our group reported periods during which they had felt like martyrs, isolated from friends and social life. At these times bitterness and resentment about their fate had been close to the surface. As group leaders we wondered if the behavior of a devoted parent-martyr was not an effort to block a negative wish toward the chronically ill child, that is, the wish to be completely free of parental responsibilities. No parent in the group, however, vented or acknowledged such wishes. In this regard it was of interest to note that the fathers were better able to verbalize their anger and disappointment about their boys' disease. These fathers would at times "furiously look for some reason to blame" their sons for hemorrhages and would also admit impatience and resentment toward the pediatricians in charge. The same fathers, however, claimed no negative feelings toward their wives for being carriers of the hemophilic trait.

Obviously identification with other parents of hemophiliacs was an essential adaptational mechanism of our group members. Through many years of affiliation with other hemophilic families they had adopted more realistic and relaxed attitudes toward supervising their sons' activities and had become more open in discussing genetic and other factors of hemophilia within their families. In addition to identification among the group members the parents of the older hemophiliacs at times gained strength by identifying with their sons' stoic and hopeful attitudes in the face of repeated bleeding episodes. An illustrative comment is "Now when we feel frustrated, we can learn from him; he accepts setbacks and interrupted plans better than we do." The son's effective adaptation to his illness had become a helpful source of strength for his parents to imitate and identify with. Behind this recognition was the awareness that the parents had "done a good job" in raising their hemophilic son. Their long-standing ordeal had "paid off."

The two-year follow-up of the group of 10 parents showed a continued improvement in their self-confidence as parents of chronically ill children. They seemed to be effectively promoting their sons' acceptance of realistic limitations and pursuit of healthful physical and intellectual activities. Some group members had become engaged in counseling younger parents regarding the practical aspects of raising a hemophiliac. In this role the parents received supervision by me or other mental health workers.

The 25 weekly group meetings with the 10 parents had proved to be an effective vehicle for promoting parental understanding and mastery of the distressing emotions related to their sons' disease. In addition our experience pointed to the feasibility of training certain parents to serve as "lay counselors" to less-experienced parents of handicapped children. Finally, the project had provided rich data about common methods of psychological adjustment used by parents of chronically ill children.

We were ready for the third and final phase of the by now four-year-old hemophilia study: the psychoendocrine study of adaptation (Mattsson *et al.*, 1971).

Psychoendocrine Study of Adaptation in Young Hemophiliacs

The conceptual model of coping behavior had been useful in enabling us to explain and communicate our observations on the adaptation of hemophilic boys and their parents. Like any theoretical construct of proven value, this model suggested further testable hypotheses regarding the interaction between biological and psychological factors in hemophilia. As noted before, among the four main classes of stress reaction Lazarus (1966) had included responses of a physiological nature including the autonomic nervous system and the adrenal glands. So far our research team had neglected measurements of physiological reactive manifestations in the hemophiliacs and had assessed stress responses and coping techniques only in the areas of affects, motor activity, and cognitive and defensive processes.

A major reason for including physiological measurements in our ongoing study was the early finding of spontaneous, anticipatory bleeding in many of the boys before exciting events. The hematologists and we had confirmed that some bleeding episodes in hemophiliacs appeared to be triggered by emotional arousal. This clinical impression posed the question: How could be objectively assess evidence of emotional arousal in the hemophiliacs preceding or coinciding with seemingly spontaneous hemorrhages?

A novel approach to the investigation of both the psychophysiological aspects of bleeding in hemophilic boys and their coping effectiveness suggested itself as we became aware of the impressive body of data on the responsiveness of the pituitary–adrenal-cortical system to psychological influences. In 1968 John Mason the leading American neuroendocrinologist, summarized a number of studies with animals and human subjects on adrenal cortical activity under normal and stressful conditions. Under ordinary environmental conditions a healthy person shows little day-by-day fluctuations of his adrenal cortical activity as judged by the 24-hour urinary excretion of the major cortisol-cortisone derivatives, the 17-hydroxycorticosteroids (17-OHCS). During exposure to stressful life situations, for instance, basic combat training, final examinations, admission to a "control" research ward, or preoperative periods—situations characterized by novelty, threat, and uncertainty—most persons will show elevations of their 24-hour 17-OHCS excretion. In other words, the latter has proved to be a sensitive index of the adrenal cortical reflection of a person's state of emotional arousal or distress. The corticosteroid responses to such states, which presumably are mediated via the limbic system, the hypothalamus, and the anterior pituitary, correlate significantly with such variables as degree of affective distress, effectiveness of psychological defenses, and body size.

Accordingly there were two objectives for the psychoendocrine study of hemophilic boys:

1. The investigation of the possible relationship between emotional arousal and increased bleeding tendency. It should be noted that increased adrenal cortical activity as a stress response bears no direct relationship to changes in bleeding tendency. If emotional arousal can precipitate hemorrhages in hemophilia and related disorders, the pathway most likely involves the hypothalamic–autonomic-nervous-system axis, with unknown neurohumors causing changes in the permeability of small vessels. We speculated that this hypothetical end-organ response to stress, mediated by the autonomic nervous system, would be paralled by increased adrenal cortical activity, which could be assessed by 17-OHCS measurements.

2. The investigation of the relationship between degree of psychosocial adaptation and adrenal cortical activity under varying conditions, i.e., at home, in a clinical research center, and during acute hospital admission. We hypothesized that the well-adapted hemophiliac would experience less emotional arousal in all settings and therefore show lower mean 17-OHCS excretion.

The families of 10 hemophilic boys agreed to cooperate in our study, whose objectives were explained as an examination of the relationship between urine excretion of certain normal hormonal substances and the clinical course of hemophilia. The local chapter of the National Hemophilia Foundation gave much assistance in the form of funding the position of a technician and collecting many of the 24-hour urine samples at the homes of the subjects. At the beginning of the study period, which lasted 2½ years, the ages of the boys ranged from 6 to 14 years. All of them attended public school and were of at least average intelligence. With one exception the families were in the middle economic class and showed consistently high motivation to participate in our project, which called for many inconveniences to the families because of the numerous urine collections and the completion of weekly questionnaires. Nine of the boys had particularly severe hemophilia, with the diagnosis made during their first year of life.

These boys were studied in three settings in terms of behavioral observations and the collection of 24-hour urine samples for 17-OHCS determinations:

1. At home, urine samples were obtained on weekends in two five-

month periods about a year apart. Our aim was to obtain weekly samples of each boy. This proved to be impossible because of activities away from home as well as the failure of the boys to use the specimen bottles every time they urinated during a 24-hour period. Each of the 10 boys contributed about 20 home urine samples. During the collection periods the parents filled out weekly questionnaires providing information about the child's activities, physical condition, mood changes, and any remarkable events in his environment.

2. The second setting was the Children's Clinical Research Center (CCRC) at our hospital, where the patients were admitted for three consecutive weekend days during a clinically quiescent period. In the CCRC 24-hour urine samples were collected in 8-hour portions. The boys were under continuous observation by the nursing staff, and their time was spent conversing, playing games, reading, and watching television.

3. The third observational setting was our hospital's pediatric ward where the boys stayed for care of acute hemorrhages. The number and length of admissions varied greatly for each boy. The mean number of urine samples during hospital admissions was 17. Daily family visits were the rule, and the boys were allowed as much physical activity as possible. The pediatric hematologist and I observed the boys daily during their admissions to the CCRC and the ward.

We expected the admissions to the CCRC and to the ward to be associated with increased 17-OHCS excretion, reflecting the boys' reaction to the uncertain and distressing experience. Obviously the psychological stress accompanying ward admission was superimposed on the somatic stress caused by bleeding, tissue damage, infusions, and pain.

The 17-OHCS levels were determined by a modification of the Porter–Silber method (1957). All values were expressed as $Mg/24$-hr$/M^2$ because of data showing that 17-OHCS excretion, related to body surface area, does not change significantly during childhood and adolescence. The individual and group mean 17-OHCS excretion levels were calculated for each of the three settings. Urinary creatinine was also measured to estimate the completeness of collection. On the rare occasion that a 24-hour creatinine excretion varied more than the subject's standard deviation, the sample was discounted.

About a year after the beginning of the psychoendocrine project the psychosocial adaptation of the hemophilic boys was evaluated by the pediatric hematologist and by me. Independently we rated each hemophiliac's psychosocial functioning in categories such as relationship with parents, siblings, and peers; range of physical activities; academic performance and avocational interests; and general adaptiveness or coping ability. This last area referred to the boy's ability to cope with the stressful demands associated with the fluctuating course of his illness. In line with our previous studies high adaptiveness implied optimal use of such mechanisms as cognitive functions, motor activity, emotional expression, and psychological defenses. We gave a single adaptation score to each boy by obtaining the mean of ratings over the different categories. The mean scores never differed more than half a point between the pediatrician's and my rating of a given patient, and these numerical differences were adjudicated.

During the admission to the CCRC certain aspects of the behavior of the hemophiliacs were independently rated by three nurses, using a scale similar to the one used by the physicians. The nurses' areas of rating included relations with staff and other patients; degree of cooperation; attention span; mood; and overall adaptiveness based upon the quality of the boy's coping with the demands of the observational setting. We obtained a single CCRC coping score for each hemophiliac by computing the mean of ratings across all scales and all raters. This value was compared with the global adaptation scores based on the physicians' ratings.

Both the nurses' and the physicians' ratings were correlated with the endocrine data, with the expectation that the more well-adapted boys would tend to experience less emotional distress and therefore show lower mean 17-OHCS excretion.

In analyzing our data we first noted the highly significant positive correlation between the physicians' rating of the hemophilic boys and the nurses' rating: the 6 boys that ranked high in terms of satisfactory adjustment at home, in school, and with peers were the same boys that the nurses felt were coping well with the CCRC admission, and in addition they seldom presented management problems during acute ward admissions. The remaining 4 hemophiliacs with low adaptation scores were frequent management problems in the hospital and showed a poor adjustment at home and with peers.

In the endocrine data the group mean corticosteroid excretion level for the 10 subjects varied according to the degree of environmental distress, i.e., the level was lowest at home, higher in the CCRC, and highest during ward admissions. This finding was in line with our expectations. The respective group mean differences were all statistically significant. Each individual hemophiliac showed a rather constant 24-hour 17-OHCS excretion at home over the $2\frac{1}{2}$-year period, and in addition his admissions to the CCRC and the pediatric ward were in almost all instances associated with 17-OHCS elevations that remained characteristic for him. In other words, the patients held their relative 17-OHCS level ranks within the group in the three observational settings, which represented varying degrees of environmental stress.

This rewarding confirmation that a child's adrenal cortical activity under normal and stressful conditions remains characteristic for him, just as for an adult, was followed by a disappointing finding. Our attempt at assessing the relationship between emotional arousal and an increased bleeding tendency at home, utilizing the questionnaire data, failed. Although many of the boys showed 17-OHCS levels above their means at times of minor bleeding at home as well as during periods of anticipation of exciting events, these data were too infrequent to allow for statistical analysis. Long-term, daily 17-OHCS determinations and behavioral observations would be necessary to substantiate the impression that many episodes of bleeding in hemophiliacs seem related to emotional arousal.

The final step of our project was to examine the relationship between the boys' psychosocial adaptation and corticosteroid excretion levels. There was indeed a significant correlation between the ratings of adaptation and the 17-OHCS levels in all three settings. The direction of this correlation, however, was not anticipated. Contrary to our expectations, 5 of the 6 high adapters were consistently high 17-OHCS excretors in all three settings, indicating relatively high chronic physiological arousal. Three of the 4 poorly adapted hemophiliacs were consistently low 17-OHCS excretors, implying low chronic physiological arousal.

In trying to understand these unexpected findings we carefully evaluated the types and effectiveness of the coping techniques employed by the 10 hemophiliacs. The 6 well-adapted subjects all made extensive use of reasonable physical activities, cognitive functions, and appropriate release of distressing emotions. These findings were, or course, in line with our earlier observations on adaptive coping techniques in hemophilia, and they also included repeated evidence of the importance of some psychological defenses in supporting successful coping. We had to conclude that the coping behavior of the well-adapted hemophiliac supported excellent cooperation and good social functioning; yet, as indicated by their high mean 17-OHCS levels during both quiescent and acute stages, their coping behavior did not spare them from chronic physiological arousal. This conclusion illustrates the fact that the effectiveness of psychological defenses in warding off painful affects may have little or no relation to their adaptive value (see, e.g., Hartmann, 1958, and Lazarus, 1966). It might be postulated that certain cognitive defensive maneuvers actually cause and maintain inner arousal and at the same time support social adaptation.

The low 17-OHCS levels of the poorly adapted hemophiliacs indicated low chronic physiological arousal, which was also maintained during bleeding crises and periods of disturbed behavior on the ward. What coping techniques were successful in buffering these boys' affective distress, notwithstanding their frequent maladaptive functioning? The coping behavior of the low adapters was above all characterized by intense, often careless motor activity, much irritability, and occasional periods of uncontrolled emotional expression. During admissions for acute hemorrhages they showed poor cognitive functioning, inability to contain negative affects, and restless, uncooperative states. The highly emotional state of these boys during periods of confinement showed some unique characteristics. They avoided talk about their illness, their current symptoms, and medical procedures. Instead they either lamented their discomfort in a dramatic fashion or complained about the ward environment. This disassociation of their affect from its appropriate ideation—their serious physical state—suggested that the defense of isolation of affect from content had been employed, followed by partial displacement of the affect onto the imperfect environment and denial or repression of the content. The combined use of these basic psychological defenses (Bibring *et al.*, 1961) might explain how the intense affect expression of the poor adapters actually served a defensive purpose, particularly during stressful bleeding, and moderated their state of tension so that they held low 17-OHCS level. These boys' dramatic emotional behavior seemed to spare them from the dreaded recognition of their serious condition.

Our discussion of affective behavior serving defensive functions was facilitated by the work of Bibring *et al.* (1961) and Wolff and his co-workers (1964). The latter had been impressed by their observations of "affect as a defense" in some mothers of fatally ill children. The marked affective behavior of these women, who were chronic low 17-OHCS excretors, appeared to protect them from recognition of the impending death of their children. Wolff *et al.* concluded that "overt emotional responses and adrenal cortical activity do not necessarily vary in the same direction."

Conclusion

The psychoendocrine project became the finale of our six-year investigation of young hemophiliacs. My professional relocation made it impossible to continue the study, which had generated many tentative findings that required duplication on other hemophilic subjects. In addition our results suggested a host of intriguing topics for further investigation. The following are a few of the areas into which our research could be expanded.

Would children with other long-term physical illnesses show coping techniques similar to those observed in the hemophilic boys and would they appear in characteristic developmental stages? It is frequently stated that the nature of a chronic disorder is less influential in a successful adaptation than such factors as the child's developmental level, his adaptive capacity, and the quality of the parent–child relationship (Prugh, 1963). Our observations on hemophiliacs bore out the importance of these factors. However, as to the nature of the chronic illness, our data showed that hemophilia carries with it special meanings because of its unique combination of a characteristic mode of inheritance and the relationship between physical activity and symptomatology. Other serious childhood illnesses have certain characteristics that pose special problems of adaptation and are well worth investigating along the lines of our hemophilia project.

In addition to physically ill children we wished to conduct coping and endocrine studies on physically healthy youngsters suffering from emotional disorders. Would children with neurotic disorders have relatively high chronic 17-OHCS excretion, indicating chronic high physiological arousal, while youngsters with tension-discharge disorders be low 17-OHCS excretors, reflecting low degrees of arousal? In normal childhood subjects would there be a correlation between chronic corticosteroid excretion levels and certain styles of coping, including characteristic cognitive and defensive functioning?

In addition to providing us with much information about developmental and family-interactional aspects of coping behavior in hemophilic children, the long-term study had directly and indirectly improved medical and psychological services to the large population of hemophilic families in our area. The much-appreciated support of the patients' families and the hardworking local chapter of the National Hemophilia Foundation provided important stimulation to us, as well as sorely needed financial and practical help.

Our investigative team had involved pediatric hematologists, psychiatrists, and a research psychologist, who provided much assistance regarding project design and statistical analysis. Through our research activities these individuals, along with the participating nurses and house officers, greatly promoted interdepartmental collaboration and mutual respect. These by-products of multidisciplinary investigative work are most attractive as they inevitably lead to more comprehensive patient care, broader graduate and postgraduate teaching within the medical setting, and highly rewarding professional and social interchange.

References

AGLE, D. P. Psychiatric studies of patients with hemophilia and related states. *Archives of Internal Medicine*, 1964, **114**, 76–82.

BIBRING, G. L. DWYER, T. F., HUNTINGTON, D. S., et al. A study of the psychological processes in pregnancy and of the earliest mother-child relationship. Appendix B: Glossary of defenses. *Psychoanalytic Study of the Child*, 1961, **16**, 62–72.

CHODOFF, P., FRIEDMAN, S. B., & HAMBURG, D. A. Stress, defenses, and coping behavior: Observations in parents of children with malignant disease. *American Journal of Psychiatry*, 1964, **120**, 743–749.

FRIEDMAN, S. B., CHODOFF, P., MASON, J. W., et al. Behavioral observations on parents anticipating the death of a child. *Pediatrics*, 1963, **32**, 610–625.

GREEN, M., & SOLNIT, A. J. Reactions to the threatened loss of a child: A vulnerable child syndrome. *Pediatrics,* 1964, **34,** 58–66.

HARTMANN, H. *Ego psychology and the problem of adaptation.* New York: International Universities Press, 1958.

LAZARUS, R. S. *Psychological stress and the coping process.* New York: McGraw-Hill, 1966.

MASON, J. W. A review of psychoendocrine research on the pituitary-adrenal cortical system. Psychosomatic Medicine, 1968, **30,** 576–607.

MATTSSON, A., & AGLE, D. P. Group therapy with parents of hemophiliacs: Therapeutic process and observations of parental adaptation to chronic illness in children. *Journal of the American Academy of Child Psychiatrists,* 1972, **11,** 558–571.

MATTSSON, A., & GROSS, S. Adaptational and defensive behavior in young hemophiliacs and their parents. *American Journal of Psychiatry,* 1966, **122,** 1349–1356.(a)

MATTSSON, A., & GROSS, S. Social and behavioral studies on hemophilic children and their families. *Journal of Pediatrics,* 1966, **68,** 952–964.(b)

MATTSSON, A., GROSS, S., & HALL, T. W. Psychoendocrine study of adaptation in young hemophiliacs. Psychosomatic Medicine, 1971, **33,** 215–225.

MURPHY, L. B. *The widening world of childhood.* New York: Basic Books, 1962.

PRUGH, D. G. Toward an understanding of psychosomatic concepts in relation to illness in children. In A. J. Solnit and S. Provence (Eds.), *Modern perspectives in child development.* New York: International Universities Press, 1963.

SILBER, R. H., & PORTER, C. C. Determination of 17, 21-dihydroxy-20-ketosteroids in urine and plasma. *Methods of Biochemical Analysis,* 1957, **4,** 139–169.

WOLFF, C. T., HOFER, M. A., & MASON, J. W. Relationship between psychological defenses and mean urinary 17-OHCS excretion rates. II: Methodological and theoretical considerations. *Psychosomatic Medicine,* 1964, **26,** 592–609.

THE CONSTRUCTIVE
USE OF IGNORANCE

HILDE BRUCH

Schädliche Wahrheit, ich ziehe sie vor dem nützlichen Irrtum.
Wahrheit heilet den Schmerz, den sie vielleicht uns erregt.
                                                    —Goethe

Dr. Anthony's suggestion to "introspect on the way your research mind is fashioned and the strategies that it habitually uses to solve problems" sounded to me like an invitation for True Confessions about myself. My first confession is that serendipity has played a great role in my life, that things just happened and I made use of them with little conscious planning. I doubt that I would have pursued a professional career, or would even have known about such a possibility for a girl, if the winter of 1917 had not been so very cold and the German school system so conscientious. Instead of being allowed to freeze in unheated classrooms or stay at home, we were taken to a large lake where students from various schools of the whole district went ice skating. There I noticed some girls with red students' caps, and from them I learned about a school in a nearby larger city where girls could learn Latin and mathematics, obtain the *"Abiturium,"* and go on to the university. This was in February— and six weeks later I was enrolled in this school, which corresponded to the *Realgymnasium* for boys.

It was not accidental that my parents, after consultation with the wider family, agreed to this in spite of the hardship it involved. It offered an escape from an uncomfortable situation in the local high school, where the teachers had been openly uneasy about my many unconventional questions and, to them, embarrassing observations, like those made by the child in "The Emperor's New Clothes." A school where the inquisitiveness would be an asset must have looked like a blessing, though it required commuting early in the morning and late at night by the delapidated trains of the war and postwar period. With all the difficulties of the next six years, revolution and retreat of a defeated army, restrictions by the army of occupation, strikes and political up-

HILDE BRUCH, Baylor College of Medicine, Texas Medical Center, Houston.

heavals, and influenza and dysentery epidemics, these years stand out as intellectually stimulating and broadening in many personal ways. However, I
alone finished the course out of 10 students who had started commuting to that
school at the same time.

As relevant to Dr. Anthony's questions, I wish to mention only two
characteristic attitudes. When in mathematics, after two or three explanations,
a student still did not understand a problem, the teacher would turn to me and
ask, "Hilde, why doesn't so and so understand this?" and I usually could
point to some unstated misunderstanding underlying the questions, usually not
directly related to the problem. I am sure I was not familiar then with the concept of "tacit assumption"; I became knowingly aware of its importance only
much later, when already in the United States. An older colleague asked for
my help in translating an article on icterus neonatorum. He had studied all the
figures and graphs but could not follow the author's conclusion; maybe he had
misunderstood the German text. There had been no error in the translation
nor in his deduction. The problem was that the author had failed to draw the
correct conclusions from his own data. The article had been published in 1913,
and I was still close enough to medical school to recall that there had been an
absolute dictum that *all* icterus was hepatogenic; the possibility of a hemolytic
origin had not been established until 1916. The author had unquestioningly
complied with the accepted explanation and had missed drawing his own,
original conclusions. I have made it a habit, when studying a topic or listening
to a discussion, to try to identify the underlying unstated assumptions and convictions.

To return to my high school experiences: another memory appears relevant. I was about 16 years old when we were asked in our literature class to
select a maxim from a page of aphorisms. I was the first to raise my hand because halfway down the page I had found mine; the teacher agreed, "Yes, it
has your name on it." I have used it as the epigraph for this chapter; translated
it means: "Damaging truth, I prefer it to advantageous error. Truth heals the
pain which perhaps it evokes." It has remained my maxim, though I have
often found that not sharing commonly held, erroneous assumptions leaves one
isolated and exposed to attack.

Medical Student and Thereafter

Even with the huge enrollment of German medical schools, students with
similar interests did find each other and I belonged to a group identified as
"scientifically minded." Many years later I met a former classmate from this
group, himself a professor of biochemistry (another having become a professor
of physiology), who inquired about my experiences with the embarrassed
interest of a German toward a Jewish colleague about whose fate he had

preferred to know nothing. On learning that I had become a psychiatrist, he couldn't restrain himself from exclaiming, "But you were a gifted student!"

Following my internship I spent a year at the Physiological Institute in Kiel, which at that time was leading in the field of physical chemistry. There I learned how to formulate clear and succinct questions, how to design an experiment, and how to evaluate data and the validity of the underlying concepts. The specific work dealt with the behavior of electrolytes in semipermeable membranes. Subsequently, during my training in pediatrics, electrolyte studies remained my specialty. If political events had not interfered I might have developed a career along this line.

The great upheaval that put an end to all such plans was Hitler's coming to power. Unable to blind myself to the gravity of the situation or to accept the status of a second-rate citizen, I decided within a few months to leave Germany. It is hard to reconstruct the amazing sense of confusion, bewilderment, sorrow, and bereavement on becoming a refugee, without any inner preparation for living in another country and even less practical preparation; but there was also an unexpected feeling of freedom and adventure. I spent one year in London and held several fill-in positions. Amongst other things I worked as an observer in Dr. Emanuel Miller's Child Guidance Clinic, where my task was to record what went on between mothers and children; I also sat in on staff conferences and met people from the Tavistock Clinic. All this was an exciting experience and offered a glimpse into a world entirely different from the picture of psychiatry that had been taught in German medical schools.

However, the way medicine was practiced in England was not congenial to me and I immigrated to the United States in October 1934. Because of a number of fortunate circumstances I was introduced to Dr. Rustin McIntosh, who was familiar with my former hospital and permitted me to work at the Babies Hospital in New York. My acquaintance with electrolytes was the other entrance ticket, and I participated in several studies along this line, which I experienced as enjoyable and interesting intellectual exercises, without real significance (Bruch and McCune, 1936). The next project that offered itself aroused not only my imagination and intense personal involvement but has engaged my interest through many years. However, I must confess I did not choose it; it just came along.

Obesity in Childhood

In 1935 I was given the assignment to develop a pediatric endocrine clinic. The majority of the children who were referred to this service were fat because it was generally assumed that obesity was of endocrine origin. Within five years more than 250 obese children were observed; many were followed into adolescence and adulthood. During the same period only 23 children suffering from congenital hypothyroidism were studied. In addition there was a sprinkling of children with skeletal disturbances, dwarfism, precocious puberty, sexual maldevelopment, and similar rare conditions.

In congenital hypothyroidism it was amazingly easy to make an accurate diagnosis and to institute effective treatment. The diagnosis was made on the basis of retarded growth and development, sluggish behavior, and the characteristic cretinoid features. The clinical impression could be confirmed by roentgenograms of the wrist, which showed delay in the appearance of ossification centers. Serum cholesterol levels and creatine excretion were other tests useful for diagnosis and the evaluation of progress.

Administration of thyroid resulted in predictable improvement, with reappearance of symptoms and rise of the cholesterol level when medication was temporarily discontinued. In one particular case, in which cancer had necessitated the surgical removal of the thyroid gland, it was noted three years after the operation that the cholesterol level did not rise, nor did other signs of hypothyroidism develop during a trial interruption of the medication (Bruch and Langmann, 1938). This suggested that there were new foci of thyroid production. This was the case in which radioactive iodine was used for the first time to locate metastases. Higher doses of radioactive iodine were successful in destroying the new cancer cells.

By the separate evaluation of various developmental aspects the relationship between hypothyroidism and intellectual development could be clarified (Bruch and McCune, 1944). Though thyroid was effective in restoring growth and development, its influence on intellectual ability was often disappointing. This had been attributed in the past to delayed and inadequate treatment. In our group it could be shown that little or no correlation existed between the onset and adequacy of medication and subsequent mental development. This lack of correlation suggested that the intellectual deficit might be related to some concomitant defect of cerebral development, which could not be modified by thyroid medication. In the absence of such a defect intellectual development was adequate in spite of proven congenital hypothyroidism or delayed treatment.

It appeared reasonable to expect that similar diagnostic criteria could be established for fat children; in this we were disappointed. It is difficult to reconstruct the air of certainty with which, during the 1930s, endocrine diagnostic labels were attached to fat children. The term *Froehlich syndrome*, implying a pituitary disturbance, was commonly applied; in other cases hypothyroidism was "diagnosed." An atmosphere of gloom and apprehension hung over these children, since it was widely believed that puberty would be delayed or deficient as a result of the hypopituitarism. Such pronouncements

were recorded in the literature so consistently that it was a surprising discovery that systematic observations only not did not lend support to the then-
current ideas of endocrine dysfunction but in many ways contradicted them.
These children did not show signs of retardation in growth and development,
as would have been the case if they suffered from the endocrine deficiencies
that were attributed to them, but there was clear-cut evidence of definite acceleration, including early pubertal development (Bruch, 1939a). Their
growth in stature and skeletal maturation was in excess of the average normal
but in harmony with the development of children with an early onset of puberty. They were large in every respect and of good intelligence, though often
severely handicapped in their personality development. Through follow-up
observations it was definitely established that puberty was adequate and occurred at an average or early age (Bruch, 1941b).

My whole development had left me confident about my ability to make
accurate observations and to draw valid conclusions. The question now was:
Why do the others believe that these children suffer from hypothyroidism or
hypopituitarism if we cannot find any evidence for this? The inquiry changed
toward recognizing the erroneous assumptions on the basis of which these incorrect diagnoses had been made. Two sources were identified, namely, unfamiliarity with Froehlich's original report and misapplication of the basal metabolism test. In 1901 Froehlich had observed a 14-year-old boy with an intracranial tumor, who suffered from severe headache, vomiting, and increasing
visual difficulties eventually resulting in complete blindness in the left eye; in
addition he had gained weight and there were no signs of pubertal
development (Bruch, 1939c). Froehlich concluded that the adiposity and
genital underdevelopment indicated that the tumor originated in the
hypophysis itself. In 1904 Erdheim, a pathologist, took issue with Froehlich's
conclusion; his own observations suggested that only tumors that had grown
beyond the cella turcica were associated with obesity, which he attributed to
hypothalamic stimulation. Subsequent experimental work brought increasing
evidence of the importance of the hypothalamus in weight disturbances, but
clinicians clung to the concept of a pituitary disorder. This erroneous diagnosis, with the implication of a possible brain tumor and of inadequate sexual
development, became a fashionable stereotype. Its use was based on ignorance,
loose reasoning, and a disregard for the damage it did to a child and his
family.

The other source of error was related to some misunderstanding of what
the basal metabolism test measures. Reports on obese individuals would invariably speak of a "low" metabolic rate, erroneously implying that this indicated hypothyroidism. In our evaluation of the elements that go into the calculation of this test it could be demonstrated that the customary procedure was
just a complicated way of describing weight excess; it did not measure

anything related to the thyroid function (Bruch, 1939b, 1957c). The standard calculation was based on the assumption that fat tissue was metabolically inert; the concept of the adipose tissue as "an actively functioning organ" was yet to be formulated. During the late 1930s *in vivo* studies utilizing heavy hydrogen revealed that fat tissue was metabolically active. Our observations of the basal metabolism during reducing indicated the same; oxygen consumption steadily decreased, correlating directly with the weight loss. Cholesterol measurements, which had been so valuable in the assessment of hypothyroidism, failed to give any relevant data in obesity.

While these various physiological studies, with negative evidence about endocrine dysfunction, were being carried out, some unexpected positive findings forced themselves upon us. In retrospect it may sound ludicrous to speak of the discovery that fat children ate too much and were conspicuously inactive as "new" observations. It is difficult to explain why these glaring symptoms had been so completely neglected; it had even been stated that absence of a large appetite was characteristic of glandular obesity. Inactivity, when it was mentioned, was attributed to the malfunctioning glands, and so were other behavior disturbances. During the early part of our study we too heard often that a child had grown fat on practically no food; this reflected some erroneous preconceived notion of a mother about her child's needs, or often simple concealment (Bruch, 1940a). Information about the extreme inactivity, often branded as laziness, was given more frankly (Bruch, 1940b).

It looked as if a simple direct road to treatment had opened up, namely, dietary restriction and increased activity; but in connection with these rational instructions unexpected complex underlying problems came into the open. The mothers often appeared acutely upset when such changes were discussed, and they failed to comply with the treatment plan. This poor cooperation aroused my interest in possible psychological problems and led to an inquiry into the factors underlying the overeating and inactivity. Most symptoms were recognized as related to deep-seated and complex problems, particularly those involved in the severe inactivity. It was also recognized that the large bodily size had an important psychological function; it seemed to act as a defense against manifest mental illness.

Certain peculiarities in the mother–child interaction had been observed quite from the beginning. Though advanced in physical and intellectual development, these children appeared extremely immature and clingingly dependent on their mothers, who seemed to encourage this behavior. The signs of this relationship were not particularly dramatic, but they occurred with great regularity, such as an obese child sitting down on the only chair in the clinic office, or a mother putting clothes on a child, even of 10 years or older, who accepted this service like a wooden puppet. When a question was addressed to the child, the mother would answer for him or would hardly let him say a word without prompting and correcting. This hovering, overanxious attitude of the mother could not possibly be explained by "glandular dysfunction" in the child but suggested some disturbance in the family interaction in which the child held an abnormal emotional position. As the result of a detailed inquiry the factors that caused the overfeeding and the inhibition of motor activity, aggression, and spontaneity were recognized as related to disturbances in the ongoing interpersonal processes.

I turned to the psychiatric and psychoanalytic literature, but I found little that was of help for the continuation of the study; during the 1930s the emphasis was on individual patients and traumatic events that had been reconstructed from their associations. Some direct observations of mothers came from child guidance clinics where certain features of their attitudes had been identified, such as "overprotective," "rejecting," and "ambivalent," and were considered the causal explanation of the child's difficulties. References to the fathers, or the interaction of the whole family, were conspicuous by their absence.

For an understanding of how serious personality problems had become associated with disturbances in nutrition, an inquiry into the patterns of interaction of the whole family appeared essential. Out of 160 families with whom we had contact at that time, 40 were selected for detailed study, including the fathers and the siblings. Many of the parents, particularly the mothers, were obese, but the more serious forms of personality disturbance and obesity were observed in families with nonobese parents. The families were of small size and showed much evidence of severe marital discord, open fighting, and mutual contempt. In such an ambivalent and emotionally insecure setting a child would be treated as a personal possession who was supposed to compensate a parent, usually the mother, for his or her own frustration. Offering of food was endowed with high emotional value, whereas physical exertion and social contacts became associated with the concept of threat and danger. This study (Bruch and Touraine, 1941) was published in 1941 under the title "The Family Frame of Obese Children"; the title was chosen to indicate that a study of the family provided only the dynamic field in which a child grew up in this distorted way, and that it did not explain in and of itself the abnormal weight regulation and the serious inner problems of these children.

The aim of the early study had been to furnish a survey, to uncover possible similarities, and to discuss the prevailing fundamental trends. Follow-up observations of these same children have revealed that this focus, the search for a uniform picture in descriptive terms, was a false lead and that it beclouded the fact that there were different forms of obesity even in childhood (Bruch, 1957a). This study was carried out during the depression years in a clinic population; it was felt that it probably gave a slanted picture of the psychological and social factors in obesity and needed to be supplemented by observations of patients with a higher educational and economic background (Bruch, 1948).

Since this early report family studies have flourished; with increasing understanding decided changes have occurred in the style, focus, and conceptual frame. It is no longer considered sufficient to give a family history in biographical or anecdotal details; the essential aspects of family transactions must be formulated and generalized, even into abstract concepts, which might then serve as a basis of comparison from family to family (Bruch, 1966). How this approach applies to patients with eating disorders will be discussed later.

The intent of the early study had been to deal with the children's responses to environmental pressures and with the inner processes that interfered with their proper psychological growth and maturation. The development of obesity in a child was conceived of as an active process, expressing his efforts to achieve growth and self-realization, though in a distorted way (Bruch, 1941a). In a significant number of cases there was increasing evidence of potential schizophrenic development, and follow-up observations confirmed this suspicion (Bruch, 1958). Psychological testing had revealed marked inner imbalance, with high scores on verbal tests, definitely lower scores on performance tests, and outright poor rating on the Draw-a-Person Test (Bruch, 1957b). These findings corroborated the clinical impression of a disturbed body image and confusion in emotional and bodily self-awareness. The pursuit of these problems was delayed, and then indefinitely postponed, because I felt increasingly handicapped by the lack of formal psychiatric and psychoanalytic training.

Encounter with Psychoanalysis

Training in psychiatry, child psychiatry, and psychoanalysis was a broadening and stimulating experience, adding to my range of knowledge and bringing about changes in my personal attitudes and ways of thinking. But some basic patterns changed relatively little, or became even more definite. Having been a pediatrician for over 10 years and having studied the psychological problems within families influenced how I responded and evaluated the new experience. I became deeply involved with various therapeutic possibilities and was fascinated by the broad optimism expressed in the psychotherapeutic approach to schizophrenics, that they could be helped through corrective experiences that counteracted the distorting early influences. I took my psychiatric training at the Childrens' Psychiatric Service of the Johns Hopkins Hospital (Leo Kanner, M.D.) and the Henry Phipps Psychiatric Clinic (John C. Whitehorn, M.D.). I had my psychoanalytic training at the Washington-Baltimore Psychoanalytic Institute with Dr. Frieda

Fromm-Reichmann as my training analyst and Dr. Harry Stack Sullivan as my most impressive supervisor and teacher.

Yet there were also unexpected and perplexing difficulties. As a pediatrician I had felt no restraint in asking questions or reporting findings that ran counter to prevailing teaching. As a matter of fact there had been many open-minded responses from others; whether they confirmed my observations or disagreed with them, nobody took issue with my right to approach problems in my own way. It did not take me long to discover that psychoanalysts functioned differently and that independent questions, particularly about the validity of underlying theoretical assumptions, were not only not welcomed but were immediately branded as indicating something unfavorable about the individual who asked them. I continue to be puzzled by this paradox, that psychoanalysis supposedly liberates one from inner restraints, leading to more open and creative thinking, but does not permit this greater freedom to be applied to its own teaching. Mere assumptions are taught as basic truths that are passed on as articles of faith. I felt as if I were back in my small-town high school, where independent thinking had been equated with misbehavior. Challenging the validity of some theoretical points in psychoanalysis provoked even more disapproval.

Freud had recognized and described with imaginative daring the significance of psychological, particularly unconscious, processes in mental illness, which had been related to the way they had developed in day-by-day experiences. He drew attention in a dramatic way to the importance of these psychic forces within human nature, forces that were not measureable in the exact terms of the highly esteemed laboratory methods that dominated the medical research of his time. The doubting questions with which I was concerned did not deal with the basic issues, namely, the relatedness of mental illness to fortunate or unfortunate early psychological experiences, but they were concerned with the way outmoded concepts, some of which had become mere meaningless clichés, were repeated and presented as precious possessions. There have been enormous changes in what is taught as psychoanalytic theory and in what is conceived of as essential for healthy personality development and what results in disturbances. However, there has been little change in the climate in which the current state of the Theory is presented as something exclusive, not to be examined or questioned, to be defended as the Truth and as superior to any other efforts to explain personality.

During the following years my patients were mainly children and adolescents suffering from a wide range of emotional and personality disorders, including some with obesity and anorexia nervosa. I became concerned with what we as a profession were doing to parents in the name of better mental health. Whatever their individual problems and uncertainties, these parents had in common that they suffered from guilt for not having followed, or not

having known, the "right method" for rearing their children. These self-re-
proaches appeared to be directly related to the crusading spirit in which parent
education was conducted at that time (Bruch, 1954). It is difficult to reconstruct the atmosphere of naïve and unrealistic optimism with which such
advice was drummed into parents, always with the threat of dire consequences
if the latest panacea was not followed. It did not take me long to become convinced that there was something wrong with this approach and that there were
a number of erroneous assumptions in the very concept that there were definite
"scientific methods," which if applied by any parent to any child would
prevent emotional problems.

This "permissive" child psychology was based on the way early
psychoanalytic teaching had been understood; it was based on the idea that
neurosis was due to the repression of instinctual needs or other inhibitions.
Hence the "modern" teaching never to frustrate a child but to give unlimited
satisfaction to all demands and to permit unrestrained expression of all impulses. Even if the theory about the origin of neurosis had been correct, and by
that time progressive psychoanalysts had recognized the limitations of these
early assumptions, I felt it was fallacious reasoning to expect that *doing the
opposite* of something that was supposed to have a damaging effect would have
a beneficial result, though it was done under entirely different circumstances.
To give just one example: the postwar years had brought into the fore the unfortunate consequences for children of abandonment and severe neglect. In
recognition of the importance of the mother–child relationship efforts were
made to build new mental health programs on the "method" of never
separating a child from his mother, without regard to what this would do to
her as an adult person and her capacity to enjoy life, including her children. In
the families of obese children the overanxious and clingingly possessive tie
between mother and child had been recognized as of outstanding path-
ognomic importance. The recurrent theme of these mothers was "I never
let him out of my sight, not for one minute." According to the principle of
doing the opposite, one might have deducted from these findings that any
contact with a mother was dangerous for a child, pointing out the potential
harm of the "never-separate" philosophy.

Many of the parents who had tried to follow this type of teaching appeared perplexed and confused in their feelings and attitudes about themselves
and were anxious in relation to their children. This negative effect appeared to
be related to several factors that, in the eagerness for new methods, had simply
been overlooked. Often the teaching amounted to nothing more than the
recommendation of psychological tricks, whether they fitted the circumstances
or not. Parents were addressed like mindless automatons who had to carry out
the expert's orders, as if their children existed in an emotional vacuum and the
living reality of the whole family interaction could be disregarded. All these

unrealistic recommendations created new anxieties and added to the burden of uncertainty and confusion of many modern parents. The experts themselves seemed to be wholely unaware that their very existence had created new problems; their own attitudes often expressed the very errors for which they blamed parents. I once summarized it as, "The more permissive the teaching, the more authoritarian the preaching."

Expressing such opinions in conferences, or writing about them, did not make me popular (Bruch, 1952). I was accused of being nihilistic or, worse, antianalytic. Now, more than 20 years later, when there is a general feeling of embarrassment about this simplistic enthusiasm, it is easy to see that I was concerned with issues that have subsequently been widely recognized as important, that "communication" occurs on various levels, and that the impact of a message depends as much on what it implicitly conveys to the listener as on its manifest content. The way child psychology was taught at that time contained a damaging "hidden curriculum," the overall message that child care was akin to illness and that parents were in constant danger of doing harm. Parents do need help and instruction, but instead of accusing exhortations it must be practical and relevant for the individual circumstances.

I also felt disappointed that the newly acquired knowledge was of so little help in my efforts to come to a better understanding of the problems of the obese. The complexity of the interaction between parents and child could not possibly be explained by the vicissitudes of the libidinal drive during the oral phase, and I felt that the concept of "orality" beclouded the issue instead of explaining it. I had the uncomfortable feeling that it and similar terms, invented to identify areas of unresolved problems, were used as causal explanations without truly adding to clarification. I did not stand alone in my concern with such problems; at the time of my training, agreement or disagreement with the libido theory was heatedly discussed, particularly in the Washington area. Sullivan had already formulated his concepts of the importance of interpersonal processes for human development; in many ways this style of thinking was in good agreement with what I had observed in the study of childhood obesity. However, the interpersonal theory did not help in my efforts to understand how bodily functions could misdevelop in such a conspicuous way.

I also felt some dissatisfaction with treatment results. Psychoanalytic training had left me with the naïvely optimistic expectation that "gaining insight" would be a curative step for fat people, helping them toward a better general adjustment and then to lose weight. I became impressed with the ease with which my fat patients, many of them gifted adolescents, grasped psychodynamic relationships and acquired an extensive psychoanalytic vocabulary. However, I soon discovered that they, and many patients seen in consultation who had been previously analyzed, had remained basically untouched in some important aspect of their personality, namely, in their conviction of helplessness. When discussing such difficulties with other analysts, I was often struck in an uncomfortable way by a definite parallel between the medical approach to obesity and the psychoanalytic attitude toward treatment in general. If a drug or diet results in weight loss in some but fails with others, then the failure is blamed on the "poor cooperation" of obese patients. Psychoanalysts display a startingly similar attitude toward the results of treatment. If results fall short of expectations, the patient is branded as "resisting," "engaging in a power struggle," or plainly as "unanalyzable"; or the other therapist is suspected of not having done "real analysis."

In the obesity study this so-called "poor cooperation" had aroused my curiosity. I now made the fact that some patients did not fulfill treatment requirements the object of inquiry, asking whether the assumptions on which traditional therapy was based were valid. Since I had found that many patients who had been little affected by the previous therapy were filled to the brim with useless, though not necessarily incorrect, knowledge of their psychodynamics, I changed the focus of my therapeutic inquiry from being interpretative to becoming purely fact-finding. This new approach implied a close collaboration with the patient, with alertness to the minutest discrepancies and confusion in the way he represented his past history, or to the misperceptions and misinterpretations underlying his reactions to current events. This approach represented for many patients, and most of them had previously been in psychoanalytic treatment, a new type of interpersonal experience: they were not merely told by another person what they "really" or "unconsciously" felt and meant, but they were told that *what they had to say was listened to as important*. It became apparent that the traditional psychoanalytic model, with the patient contributing his associations and the analyst giving meaning to them through interpretation, represented for many the devastating reexperience of the most disturbing aspect of their earliest experiences, namely, what mother said and did was dominant, but their own expressions of needs, feelings, and thoughts had not been valued or acknowledged. The pursuit of these transactional patterns eventually led me to a new formulation of personality development.

New Integration

There is probably no lonelier feeling than "Everybody is out of step but me." At times I openly envied the ease and enthusiasm with which others seemed to be able to follow the teaching and practices of their particular group. I often wished that erroneous assumptions or overinclusive deductions were not quite so obvious to me so that I could disregard them, or that I could feel comfortable with some new expression or concept as "explaining" an issue instead of seeing it as a new cover-up for continued ignorance. Gradually certain marginal observations began to add up to a new positive view, and I finally succeeded in summarizing my own observations in a new and independent theoretical frame.

I had been puzzled for some time about certain paradoxes in the theoretical assumptions about the functional state of the newborn. On the one hand, he was conceived of as fairly competent, something of a homunculus, and less undifferentiated and more organized in his capacities than he could possibly be. Therefore he was conceived of as perfectly capable of developing into some kind of supernormality if only the environment with its damaging influences would not interfere. In psychoanalytic language this interference was explained as libidinal repression, and in Sullivan's interpersonal theory as the all-pervasive and damaging effect of anxiety. That constant interaction with people around him was something positive, essential for the organization of his potential abilities, was quietly overlooked. On the other hand, the infant was conceived of as entirely passive in this process, a helpless receiver of his mother's fortunate or hapless administrations. His behavior was explained in terms of conditioning and responses to environmental stimuli. No real consideration was given to his own active contribution, from birth on, to all developmental processes or to the fact that each individual brings rudiments of his own style of behavior into interactional patterns with his environment. The question was how to conceive of these early interactional processes, how these innate potentials were integrated and organized into effective behavior, and what processes prevented optimal organization (Bruch, 1961b).

My inquiry in this direction stemmed from a series of observations made during my treatment of obese and anorexic individuals. As I have stated before, I felt increasingly dissatisfied with the results of "interpretative" and "insight-giving" psychotherapy; I gradually recognized that these people needed help, in spite of their apparent good intelligence, with developing deficient tools and guideposts for orienting themselves to their own needs and their relationship to others. Traditional psychotherapy had been nearly exclusively preoccupied with feeling states and motivations, and the importance of perceptual and conceptual aspects of mental functioning had been comparatively neglected (Bruch, 1962b).

In obese and anorexic patients the abnormal eating, both voracious intake as well as rigid refusal, had been recognized as carrying an enormous range of motivational and symbolic meanings. For anorexia nervosa it was nearly axiomatic to explain the food refusal as due to an unconscious fear of oral impregnation, though many other motivational connections could easily be established. It was increasingly difficult for me to conceive of these various unconscious conflicts as "causing" these disorders. The enormous diversity in itself suggested that these symbolic misinterpretations were symptomatic of some underlying disturbances. The question offered itself, in addition to the inquiry into the *why* of the disturbed eating patterns, of *how* it had been possible for a body function as basic and essential as food intake to develop in such a way that it could be misused in the service of such a multitude of nonnutritional needs. The precondition for such abuse was the organism's failure to differentiate between hunger and other sensations and feeling states, with the brain continuously making mistakes in identifying bodily and psychological needs.

Pursuit of this question led to the deductions that the awareness of hunger is not innate knowledge but contains elements of learning and that incorrect and confusing early experiences kept an individual from learning to differentiate "hunger," the need to eat, from other signals of discomfort that have nothing to do with "food deprivation," including emotional tension states aroused by the greatest variety of conflicts and problems. The fact that feeding in the human infant always demands the cooperation of another person and is accompanied by emotional-affectional experiences has found ample attention in the clinical and psychoanalytic literature; that the perceptual and conceptual awareness of hunger also has a developmental history, that it is organized only through continuous interaction with another person, has been largely neglected.

Once the question was formulated this way, evidence of deficits in hunger awareness quickly accumulated. When questioned on this point, many fat patients answer with an immediate sense of recognition that all their lives they have suffered from such an inability, that they go on eating as long as there is food, and that they never know when they have had enough. During eating binges they feel driven to eat against their wish not to gain more weight. They may find temporary relief from the anxious and depressive feelings that they mistakenly experience as "need to eat," but this relief is short-lived, and the cycle of "not feeling right" and unsatisfying eating is endlessly repeated. The old charge against obese people of having "no willpower" actually describes their not being clearly aware of their bodily sensations; they cannot exercise control over a function or a need that is not even recognized. Anorexics will defiantly declare, "I do not need to eat" and seem to mean it literally; at other times the urges to eat become overpowering, and they will gorge themselves to the point of spontaneous or induced vomiting.

Abnormal eating is not an isolated symptom but always occurs together with other problems in the area of active or passive self-awareness and is also observed in schizophrenics and other psychiatric patients whose weight is not abnormal (Bruch, 1962a). Passivity has always been considered a characteristic of obese people; it was surprising to discover that underlying their vigor and stubbornness anorexics, too, suffer from a deep-seated fear of losing control, of being helpless under the domination and power of others. One of the more subtle expressions of not feeling self-directed and in control can be found in language patterns that reflect the basic lack of autonomy and initiative (Bruch, 1961; Bruch and Palombo, 1961).

A common deficit was recognized in the background of such patients, namely, absence or paucity of responses to a child's expressions of his needs. Evidence of such disregard and of how parents use a child to bolster their own position can be readily recognized in the ongoing transactions during conjoint family sessions. In anorexic families there is often a shocking discrepancy between the bland and unobservant attitude of the parents and their nearly frantic emphasis on happiness, directly denying the evidence of the serious physical and emotional illness of a patient. In obesity the parents' monotonous repetition that everything would be fine if only their child would not eat so much and were slim crudely disregards the serious inner plight of such a fat youngster.

In an effort to understand the genetic background of this failure in self-differentiation and its association with inaccurate hunger awareness, I constructed a simplified conceptual model of personality development (Bruch, 1973b). Behavior from birth on must be conceived of as differentiated into *two basic forms*, namely, behavior *initiated* in the infant and behavior *in response* to stimuli from the outside, relating to both the biological and the social-emotional fields. The mother's behavior toward the child is either *responsive* or *stimulating*. The interaction between the environment and the infant can be rated as *appropriate* or *inappropriate*, depending on whether it fulfills the need that the signal indicated or disregards or distorts it. These elementary distinctions permit the dynamic analysis, irrespective of the specific area or content of the problem, of an amazingly large variety of clinical situations, and they avoid the traditional dichotomy separating the somatic and psychological aspects of development or contrasting genetic properties with experimental events.

Sufficient *appropriate responses to clues coming from the infant* are necessary for the child to organize the *significant building stones for the development of self-awareness and self-effectiveness*. For healthy development experiences in both modalities are essential: confirmation of clues originating in the child and stimulation from the outside to which he learns to respond. *Insufficient regular and consistent appropriate responses to his needs, deprive* the developing child of the essential groundwork for his "body identity" with perceptual and conceptual awareness of his own functions. If *confirmation and reinforcement* of his own initially rather undifferentiated sensations indicating needs and impulses has been *absent, contradictory,* or *inaccurate,* then a child will grow up perplexed when trying to differentiate between disturbances in his biological field and emotional and interpersonal experiences, and he will be apt to *misinterpret deformities in his self-body concept as externally induced.*

This perplexity can actually be observed in obese and anorexic patients;

they are deficient in their sense of separateness, feel controlled by external forces, and feel helpless under the impact of bodily urges. There is an overall feeling of *not owning their own bodies* and of functioning with their centers of gravity not within themselves but somewhere in other people or in the outside world. Such patients also suffer from an *overriding, all-pervasive sense of ineffectiveness* in their relations to others and from mistrusting as pretense or fraudulence any thought and feeling originating within themselves. They also suffer from great uncertainty and confusion in trying to understand the behavior of others or in expressing their own feelings and needs in a way that is understandable to others. This ineffectiveness is not specific for patients with severe eating disorders; it can be recognized, in an even more intense degree, as a key issue in schizophrenia (Bruch, 1962a).

A child growing up this way may acquire the facade of adequate functioning by robotlike cooperation with environmental demands. The gross deficit in initiative and active self-awareness becomes manifest when he is confronted with new situations and demands for which the distorted early life experiences have left him unprepared; usually the deficits become manifest at the time of puberty. In anorexia nervosa it had always been a puzzle that this very severe disorder develops in children who until then had been outstandingly good, excelling in schoolwork, and precociously dependable. The developmental scheme I have just outlined helps one to understand how in a seemingly well-functioning family a child can develop deficiencies in his sense of separateness under this facade of normality, with "diffuse ego boundaries," and feel helpless under the influence of external forces.

The eating function permits the direct observation, or a fairly accurate reconstruction, of the transactional patterns during infancy. An alert and non-neurotic mother soon learns to recognize signals indicating nutritional need and will offer food accordingly. The child can develop the engram of "hunger" as a sensation distinct from other tensions or needs, and at the same time experiences himself as a participant in this process. If, on the other hand, a mother's reaction is continuously inappropriate, be it neglectful, oversolicitous, inhibiting, or indiscriminately permissive, the outcome for the child will be a perplexing uncertainty. Even more confusing to the child are the actions of a mother who is eternally preoccupied with herself; whatever a child does, it is interpreted as expressing something about the mother. In such a setting noneating may be equated with criticism of the mother and eating with the expression of happiness and love.

This model conceives of personality development as the outcome of a continuous stream of circular and reciprocal transactions between parent and child. This concept is in good agreement with other modern studies of infancy, though, as far as I know, no one has expressed it in quite such simple and general terms. Commonly the transactions resulting in individuation and autonomy are attributed to later stages of infancy or early childhood. In my observations the essential patterns begin to form birth on. Modern observations on animals and other experimental evidence give broad support for this model, including the fact that the establishment of bodily controls requires such ongoing transactions.

The therapeutic implications of this formulation are far-reaching. Though interpretation of symbolic conflicts and clarification of resistance and transference attitudes continue to be part of the therapeutic intervention, the emphasis has shifted toward an assessment of functional capacities (Bruch, 1964, 1973a). For therapy to be effective such patients need assistance in acquiring the until-then-undeveloped tools for orienting themselves to their own "self," body, and competence. Therapy must be directed toward evoking an awareness of impulses and feelings originating within themselves and toward their learning to discriminate between various bodily sensations and emotional states. Thus, by becoming effective participants in the treatment process, they may reach the point of differentiating themselves from others, of discriminating bodily sensations and emotional states, and of growing beyond helpless passivity, hateful submissiveness, and uncritical negativism. I have been asked whether this type of therapy was still analysis. There are few questions that I consider more irrelevant; what matters is that patients who had been considered untreatable before have responded well when they were approached in this way.

Throughout my life the *leit motif* of my work has been the effort to diminish areas of ignorance, however small a step any one individual can take, rather than getting involved in debates over the superiority of one or another theory. On danger of being called an unrenegated rebel, I should like to conclude with a quotation from Maimonides, the great physician–philosopher: "Teach thy tongue to say *I do not know* and thou shalt progress."

References

BRUCH, H. Obesity in Childhood, I. Physical growth and development of obese children, Am. J. Dis. Child., **58**, 457–484, 1939.(a)

BRUCH, H. Obesity in Childhood, II. Basal metabolism and serum cholesterol of obese children, Am. J. Dis. Child, **58**, 1001–1022, 1939.(b)

BRUCH, H. The Froehlich syndrome, Am J. Dis. Child. **58**, 1282–1289, 1939.(c)

BRUCH, H. Obesity in Childhood, III. Physiologic and psychologic aspects of the food intake of obese children, Am. J. Dis. Child, **59**, 739–781, 1940.(a)

BRUCH, H. Obesity in Childhood, IV. Energy expenditure of obese children, Am. J. Dis. Child, **60**, 1082–1109, 1940.(b)

BRUCH, H. Obesity in childhood and personality development, Am. J. Orthopsychiat., **11**, 467–474, 1941.(a)

BRUCH, H. Obesity in relation to puberty, J. Pediat. **19**, 365–375, 1941.(b)

BRUCH, H. *Puberty and Adolescence: Psychological Considerations*, Monograph, Advances in Pediatrics, Vol. 3, Interscience Publ. Inc., New York, p. 219–296, 1948.

BRUCH, H. *Don't Be Afraid of Your Child*, Farrar, Straus and Young, New York, 1952.

BRUCH, H. Parent education or the illusion of omnipotence. Am. J. Orthopsychiat. **24,** 723–732, 1954.

BRUCH, H. Developmental obesity. In *The importance of overweight.* New York: W. W. Norton, 1957.(a)

BRUCH, H. The mental development of obese children. In *The importance of overweight.* New York: W. W. Norton, 1957.(b)

BRUCH, H. Some basic facts on basal metabolism. In *The importance of overweight.* New York: W. W. Norton, 1957.(c)

BRUCH, H. Developmental obesity and schizophrenia. *Psychiatry,* 1958, **21,** 65–70.

BRUCH, H. Some comments on listening and talking in psychotherapy. *Psychiatry,* 1961, **24,** 269–272.(a)

BRUCH, H. Transformation of oral impulses in eating disorders: A conceptual approach. *Psychiatric Quarterly,* 1961, **35,** 458–481.(b)

BRUCH, H. Falsification of bodily needs and body concept in schizophrenia. *Archives of General Psychiatry,* 1962, **6,** 18–24.(a)

BRUCH, H. Perceptual and conceptual disturbances in anorexia nervosa. *Psychosomatic Medicine,* 1962, **24,** 187–194.(b)

BRUCH, H. Psychotherapy with schizophrenics. In *International psychiatry clinics.* Boston: Little, Brown, 1964, Vol. 1.

BRUCH, H. Changing approaches to the study of the family. *Psychiatric Research Report 20.* American Psychiatric Association, 1966, 1–7.

BRUCH, H. Evolution of a psychotherapeutic approach, In *Eating disorders: Obesity, anorexia nervosa and the person within.* New York: Basic Books, Inc., 1973.(a)

BRUCH, H. Hunger awareness and individuation. In *Eating disorders: Obesity, anorexia nervosa and the person within.* New York: Basic Books, 1973.(b)

BRUCH, H., & LANGMANN, A. G. Carcinoma of the thyroid gland in children. *American Journal of Diseases of Children,* 1938, **56,** 616–638.

BRUCH, H., & McCUNE, D. J. Involution of the adrenal glands in newly born infants. *American Journal of Diseases of Children,* 1936, **52,** 863–869.

BRUCH, H., & McCUNE, D. J. Mental development of congenitally hypothyroid children. *American Journal of Diseases of Children,* 1944, **67,** 205–224.

BRUCH, H., & PALOMBO, S. Conceptual problems in schizophrenia. *Journal of Nervous and Mental Diseases,* 1961, **132,** 114–117.

BRUCH, H., & TOURAINE, G. Obesity in childhood. V: The family frame of obese children. *Psychosomatic Medicine,* 1940, **2,** 141–206.

CLINICALLY ORIENTED RESEARCH

INTRODUCTION

Cytryn is not merely a good clinician with sound training in child psychiatry and pediatrics, of whom there are many, nor merely a clinician who, in contact with patient groups, develops interesting ideas, as most clinicians have a tendency to do. What makes him a clinical investigator is his strong and persistent drive to pursue these ideas further while using his background and training as an adjunct. Another factor that differentiates him from the general run of clinicians is his penchant for research environments and the researchers who populate them. One could call him a contact researcher or someone who has become a researcher through contact with researchers. He could as easily, and certainly more rewardingly from a financial point of view, have elected to remain in a clinical environment, but he was obviously swayed by the powerful urge to find out things and this particular "itch" took precedence over other competing attractions. His research environments have, therefore, determined the nature of his research to a large extent. The retarded, the physically ill, and the depressed child have successively engaged his attention to the exclusion, at the time, of almost every other interest. He gives himself over very completely to his investigations. His mode of approach to the problem is fairly patterned: on entering the field, he familiarizes himself with every niche of it through the literature, and there is very little that he misses. His research strategy is equally characteristic and follows the mode of "successive approximation." He gradually works his way into the heart of the problem. Like a good investigator, he is well aware of his weaknesses and his strengths and admits both. He knows that he is not an abstract thinker nor a basic researcher but a sound clinical investigator who deals with issues that bear "an obvious relationship to clinical reality." It is this type of insight that safeguards the worker from the omnipotent strivings that can bog him down in large, amorphous projects. Cytryn always seems to keep within the area of his competence.

In the next contribution Futterman points to the personal equation that is so often the "hidden agenda" in research and is so rarely made explicit. Yet without this knowledge the reasons for carrying out a particular piece of work may seem quite fortuitous. In this case a series of experiences with death during vulnerable periods of his life made his acutely aware of the way in which families adapt themselves to this dreaded crisis or ward off its often devastating effects. Later on, while working in a ghetto, he was able to observe at first hand the techniques used by the grossly disadvantaged in order to survive. The impact of death, disaster, disease, or decay all bring into play the coping mechanisms that appear finely attuned to the requirements of the

267

specific predicament. Being a good investigator, he put his own upset feelings "between brackets," as Husserl would say, and set to work generating data. So well did he succeed that he was then confronted with the most familiar of all research crises—the accumulation of more data than he could reasonably handle, and yet much of it too good to be discarded. The solution was both ingenious and instructive; he turned to "grounded theory."[1] This allowed him to create necessary theory as he went along. The data became susceptible to all kinds of conceptual manipulation and produced a variety of explanatory constructs such as "self-concept," the "Rashomon effect," the idealization of the dying child, and the phenomenon of "anticipatory mourning." Eventually he was able to identify the very processes that participated in the act of adaptation, which provided an elegant demonstration of the use of grounded theory.

Shapiro belongs to that special group of research workers, several of whom will be encountered in this volume: the psychoanalysts who turn to empirical investigation. Some seem well adapted to this development and some mildly maladjusted. Here we have an example of someone who does not seem to recognize that adaptation may constitute a problem! However, whatever the difficulties entailed, the combination, as elsewhere, has appeared to have its usual effect of enlarging and enriching the general framework of any research undertaken. Furthermore, Shapiro is one of the few child psychiatrists and psychoanalysts who has made language behavior a focus of inquiry. It is difficult to understand why so few enter this promising field from psychiatry and psychoanalysis, since these professionals live so completely by the word. The area is still in a stage of rapid growth. Jakobson, Chomsky, and Roger Brown are the major "gurus," and some knowledge of their work is an essential preamble for the clinician on his way to becoming a language researcher. His next requirement is subjects for research. Psychotic children have a sufficient range of language disturbances to constitute an obvious target population, and since Bellevue appears to have a seemingly endless source of psychotic children, this seemed to be the place to undertake the investigation. The coming together of a researcher, an area of research, the research environment, the method of research, and a research sample is a mysterious coincidence that is often left unexplained, but besides the element of magic, there is in most cases a good deal of hard preparatory spadework. Following this one needs energy, enthusiasm, and commitment, and Shapiro has shown that he has an abundance of all three.

The new field of psychoeducation has so far attracted only a dismally few child psychiatrists. Blom is one of the exceptions to the rule that clinicians are

---

[1] See also E. J. Anthony's discussion of grounded theory in "Bridging Two Worlds of Research" in this volume.

rarely enthralled by the educational process, although there are obvious similarities to the dynamic interchanges and internalizations of psychotherapy. He has been associated with the movement from its inception and has pioneered some notable achievements. His model day hospital at Denver has enabled him to put some of his theory into practice and some of the practice into theory. Many of his colleagues have been mystified by his departure from the clinical field of research, in which he had previously made his name, and they have mistakenly assumed that this was a passing interest stimulated by his school-aged children, but there was much more to it than that. Blom had come to the conclusion that education furnished one of the largest and most significant inputs for the developing child and that to understand the clinical situation fully, it was imperative to assess the nature of this ongoing assimilation. Through his work the image of the child psychiatrist had been expanded to include a vital educational component that could prove of great value to educators over and above the clinical assessments of learning disabilities and disruptive classroom behavior. The child psychiatrists who worry that Blom is "clinical" and the child analysts that he is less "deep" are to a large extent embedded in their traditional roles and quite unable or unwilling to cross the interesting interface that lies between disciplines and refurbish their ideas. This they should recognize as a limitation in themselves and not in Blom. He is concerned with the "whole" child, emotionally and educationally, and in crossing over he is not confusing his identity but adding to it. Having said this, I should add that it remains unclear how and why he came to follow this particular line of development. It is also difficult to gauge how far he can go while retaining his connection with psychiatry. It makes me wonder whether any of that hard, indefatigable work of content analysis will eventually bear fruit in the clinic.

STUDIES OF BEHAVIOR
IN CHILDREN WITH
DOWN'S SYNDROME

Leon Cytryn

My interest in mental retardation goes back to the years of my pediatric training. My chief at the time was Harry Gordon, one of the country's outstanding pediatric teachers, who later became the director of the Rose Kennedy Research Institute at the Einstein Medical School. Gordon inculcated in all of us a basic respect for the mentally retarded and their families both as patients and as subjects of scientific investigation. Continuing on my professional journey I came into the orbit of Leo Kanner and Leon Eisenberg at Johns Hopkins. There my interest in mental retardation deepened and I first began to be concerned with the personality development of the mentally retarded, their emotional vulnerability, and the link between mental retardation and mental illness, particularly the childhood psychoses. Kanner introduced me to his pioneering thoughts on early infantile autism and pseudofeeblemindedness, as well as to his historical perspective of mental retardation. Eisenberg added to this his profound interest in the social forces that shape human behavior and the basic defects in our social and value system responsible in large measure for the existing psychopathology in our society. From there, I went to Children's Hospital in Washington, D.C., to complete my training under Reginald S. Lourie. Lourie's interest in the mentally retarded and dedication to their rehabilitation was a source of inspiration to me. He contended that the mentally retarded are capable of attaining optimal personality development under favorable circumstances. He backed up his contention with a departmental policy under which mentally retarded children were treated on a par with normal children if in need of psychotherapy. I was

LEON CYTRYN, Research Associate, Children's Hospital, Washington; Clinical Professor of Psychiatry and Behavioral Sciences, Clinical Professor of Child Health and Development, George Washington University School of Medicine, Washington; Clinical Associate, Adult Psychiatry Branch, National Institute of Mental Health, Bethesda, Maryland.

271

also strongly influenced by Lois Murphy in the same setting. Her concepts of constitutional vulnerability as predisposing to psychopathology fitted well into my own developing ideas about the emotional vulnerability of the mentally retarded. Her method of studying single children in depth, in rich detail, rather than studying large numbers in a rigid design suited my personality and predominantly clinical orientation.

My decision to enter the field of child psychiatry after the completion of pediatric training resulted for a while in a vague sense of "identity diffusion," of being neither fish nor fowl. The resulting discomfort was probably one of the most potent motivating forces to search for a central focus of relevance to both these disciplines. My search was rewarded with the finding of not one but many such nodal points, where psychiatry and pediatrics interdigitate. Child development presented one focus of vital importance to many disciplines, and the study of the antecedents of human personality development from the point of view of a psychologist, neurologist, pediatrician, and social worker provided me with a firm foundation for my subsequent work. While struggling to delineate the role of the child psychiatrist in the study and treatment of normal and deviant personality development, I was trying to define my own professional identity. As my thinking evolved, I began to see the child psychiatrist as a synthesizer who can transcend the boundaries of the many disciplines involved in the study of the child and blend them into a unitary framework.

Mental retardation provided another focus of major importance. The many facets of the problem clearly call for an interdisciplinary effort. The equal weight accorded both the physical and the psychological aspects permitted me to feel comfortable both as a pediatrician and as a psychiatrist. At first my efforts in the area of mental retardation were not focused. I began to study mentally retarded children and their families in a variety of settings, such as a pediatric hospital, an outpatient department, a diagnostic public health clinic, and schools and institutions for retarded children. This rich experience was followed by a growing realization of the enormity of the problem and of the many uncharted areas yet to be explored (Cytryn *et al.*, 1967).

Of all the aspects of mental retardation, personality development seemed the most neglected, despite the fact that emotional and social adjustment are often decisive in the life course of a mentally retarded person. Admissions to state institutions may serve as a case in point. Many patients, especially during adolescence, are admitted mainly because of their disturbed behavior and social maladjustment rather than because of intellectual impairment. Considering that we have around 6 million retarded people in the United States, of whom the great majority will have to fend for themselves in the community outside of institutions, the personality development of this group becomes a matter of great practical importance. In addition better understanding of the personality development of the mentally retarded may shed some light on the normal personality development, especially on the interaction of cognitive, emotional, constitutional, and social forces.

The extreme heterogeneity of the mentally retarded group is probably responsible for the often conflicting and confusing views about the personality development of its members. There has also been a paucity of well-conducted studies and surveys that use standardized methods of investigation. Assumptions in this field are often based on studies using residents in state institutions or patients in psychiatric clinics and hospitals. I became convinced early in my career that only detailed studies of well-defined, uniform subgroups of mentally retarded who live at home would provide more valid answers in the future, to replace the current speculative confusion.

As fate would often have it, I arrived at a choice of a subgroup through serendipity. Richmond Paine in our department of neurology got interested in the biochemical makeup of children with Down's syndrome with trisomy-21. He found high levels of several enzymes in the leukocytes of these patients, as well as very low levels of platelet serotonin (5-hydroxy-tryptamine), often one-third to one-half of normal values (Rosner et al., 1965). Because of the recent interest in this neurotransmitter and its relation to mood and behavior, it was decided to attempt to raise the levels of serotonin by feeding these children a serotonin precursor (5-hydroxy-tryptophan). A multidisciplinary effort (which included neurologists, pediatricians, and a psychologist) was launched under the direction of Mary Coleman. I served in the capacity of a psychiatric consultant. The ambitious program called for the inclusion of over a hundred patients with Down's syndrome, who were to be followed at close intervals from the first week of life for several years. I became aware that this presented a fine opportunity to study one of the most uniform subgroups in mental retardation.

This decision was aided by my gradually emerging interest in the emotional and social aspects of Down's syndrome. I was fascinated, in particular, by the long-standing controversy concerning the behavior of children with Down's. Most investigators stress placidity, good social adjustment, cheerfulness and the relative absence of psychopathology in this group (Domino, 1964; Kanner, 1957; Penrose, 1963; Silverstein, 1964). On the other hand, there are some who claim that children with Down's syndrome are probably no more homogeneous in terms of emotional and social adjustment than any other unselected group of normal or mentally retarded individuals (Menolascino, 1965, 1967; Rollin, 1946). The many methodological difficulties often found in behavioral research concerning this problem were recently pointed out by Belmont (1971). Many studies of children with Down's syndrome describe institutionalized children, often coming from socioculturally deprived segments of our population. Thus, in addition to their innate retardation, they are often subject to considerable environmental deprivation, which makes the interpretation of the findings extremely difficult.

As a first step in my overall strategy, I wished to ascertain the validity of the concept of lesser emotional vulnerability of children with Down's syndrome. In order to avoid some of the methodological pitfalls mentioned above, I decided to study children (1) who were from middle-class families; (2) who had been exposed to a good educational program; (3) who lived at home; and (4) who had not been referred to any agency because of behavioral difficulties.

Behavioral Disturbances in Children with Down's Syndrome

Method

MCARC nursery is a private nursery-school system for retarded children ages three to five in suburban Washington. The parents are predominantly middle class and all families were intact at the time of the study. We studied the entire population of this school system, consisting of 46 children, whom we divided into two groups. There were 21 children with Down's syndrome, of whom 1 had the mosaic form, 2 had the translocation form, and the rest had trisomy-21. There were 25 children with other forms of mental retardation, of whom 1 had PKU, 1 had Lawrence-Moon-Beadle syndrome, 2 had seizures of unknown origin, and the rest had no medical diagnosis.

The mental age of 15 children in each of these two groups was established by use of the Stanford-Binet and Bayley tests. All parents were seen in a $1\frac{1}{2}$-hour-long psychiatric interview, on the basis of which they were assigned to one of four categories of family disturbance ranging from 1 (no disturbance) to 4 (very disturbed). The interviews were all tape-recorded. An independent psychologist rated 7 parents in each group on the basis of these tape recordings. There was an 89 percent perfect interrater agreement.

All the children were rated by three members of the teaching staff on a 4-point scale on seven types of behavioral disturbances commonly seen in MR children: hyperactivity, aggression, lack of cooperation, withdrawal, lack of relatedness, irritability, and impulsivity. Each child was rated independently by the principal, the teacher, and the teacher's assistant. Care was taken to

TYPE OF RETARDATION	N	SEX M F	CHRON. AGE (MEAN)	MENTAL AGE (MEAN)	FAMILY DISTURBANCE (MEAN) 1-4 SCALE
DOWN'S	21	10 11	45 MONTHS	30 MONTHS	2.1
NON-DOWN'S	25	14 11	48 MONTHS	31 MONTHS	1.8

FIG. 1. Sex, chronological age, mental age, and degree of family disturbances in both experimental groups.

	PRINCIPAL	ASSISTANT	TEACHER	COMPOSITE
HYPERACTIVITY	NS	NS	NS	NS
AGGRESSION	NS	NS	NS	NS
LACK OF COOPERATION	NS	NS	NS	NS
WITHDRAWAL	.OI	.05	.05	.OI
LACK OF RELATEDNESS	.05	.05	.05	.05
IRRITABILITY	.OI	.05	.OI	.OI
IMPULSIVITY	.05	NS	.OI	.05

FIG. 2. Summary of significant differences in behavioral disturbance ratings (Down's versus non-Down's children).

preserve the independence of the ratings. The following agreement among the three raters was obtained: perfect agreement, 50 percent; agreement within 1 point difference, 95 percent. The children with ratings of 1 or 2 were combined into a low-disturbance group and those with ratings of 3 or 4 were combined into a high-disturbance group.

Results

As indicated in Figure 1, there were no significant differences between the two groups on such indices as sex, age, chronological age, mental age, and degree of family disturbance. There was no significant correlation between the presence of behavioral disturbances and any of those factors

The children with other forms of MR showed significantly more disturbance than those with Down's syndrome on four of the seven behavioral variables: withdrawal, lack of relatedness, impulsivity, and irritability. The two groups did not differ significantly on the other factors: hyperactivity, aggression, and lack of cooperation (see Figure 2).

These results lend at least partial support to the behavioral stereotype of better social adjustment in the child with Down's syndrome. However, the findings of a lack of difference between the groups on the variables of hyperactivity, aggression, and lack of cooperation make it unlikely that the children with Down's syndrome differ as completely from children with other forms of mental retardation as has often been supposed.

Personality Development in Patients with Down's Syndrome Receiving 5-Hydroxytryptophan or Placebo

Next I considered the possibility that the behavior of children with Down's syndrome might be mediated by biochemical factors. Much of recent animal research attempted to link various aspects of behavior to the levels of various neurotransmitters in the brain, although the data were inconsistent and did not present a predictable pattern. In this context the previously mentioned low level of 5-hydroxy-tryptamine (serotonin) in blood platelets became of great interest. Although there is at present no method available to measure directly the serotonin content in the brain, there are indications that the blood platelet may present a model of the serotoninergic neuron (Coleman *et al.,* 1973). A double-blind study was carried out in which two groups of infants with Down's syndrome were given 5-hydroxy-tryptophan (a serotonin precursor) or a placebo. The personality and the neurological and intellectual development of all these children were studied extensively over a three-year period. The neurological and psychological testing was carried out by appropriate disciplines, while I was entrusted with the study of personality development in both groups.

Method

A personality inventory for infants and toddlers was constructed, based on the concepts of coping developed by Murphy (1956, 1952), and of constitutional vulnerability developed by Heider (1966, 1971). The inventory consisted of 45 five-point scales arranged in four groups, namely, motor development and sturdiness, social relatedness, coping and mastery, and emotional integration. In addition, a parent-rating instrument was devised consisting of 4 five-point scales, namely, acceptance of child, maternal responsiveness, maternal initiative, and maternal encouragement of independence. Both the children's and the parents' rating scales were unidirectional. A rating of 5 was given for optimal behavior and a rating of 1 was given for least desirable behavior. Each child was visited twice at home, with a one-week interval between visits, by a team of two observers who observed and rated the child independently, following which they adjusted their findings after an exhaustive discussion. In addition during each visit one of the observers wrote a running description of the child's and the mother's behavior, as well as that of other members of the family. These extensive reports permitted us to preserve the richness of relevant behaviors and interaction to an extent impossible with only the use of rating scales. Throughout all rating sessions the raters were unaware of the child's blood 5-hydroxyindole level.

I tested the inventory on six 20-month-old toddlers with Down's syndrome known to have received 5-HTP (not in the double-blind study) as well as on three normal 20-month-old toddlers. These preliminary results indicated a full interrater agreement on 84 percent of the scales and a 99 percent agreement within a 1-point difference. The test–retest, after a one-week interval, indicated a full agreement of 56 percent, with a 97 percent agreement within a 1-point difference. The inventory also distinguished well between normal infants and those with Down's syndrome and pinpointed specific areas of personality strengths and weaknesses. For instance, it is accepted that the social development in Down's syndrome is usually good; in the area of social relatedness the differences between the normal toddlers and those with Down's syndrome were much smaller than in other areas.

Since my observations and ratings were based on repeated home visits, I was forced to eliminate 3 of the 19 children in the project, who lived outside of a 50-mile radius from Washington. Thus we were left with 16 children. I rated each child at 20 months and again at 32–34 months (see Figures 3 and 4).

Results

The children who were given 5-hydroxytryptophan had normal serotonin blood levels. Neurologically there was a transient early improvement in muscle tone in those children who were given 5-hydroxytryptophan; this improvement did not persist. In the same group, however, there were several children who developed hypsarrhythmia. The intellectual level was not significantly different in the experimental and the placebo groups.

I added up all the scores of our 16 patients on the personality inventory,

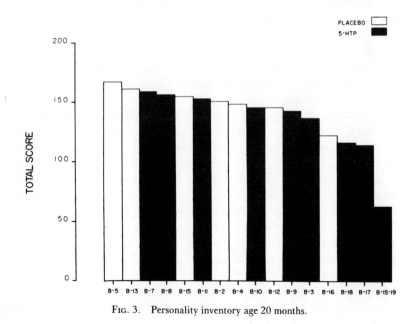

FIG. 3.   Personality inventory age 20 months.

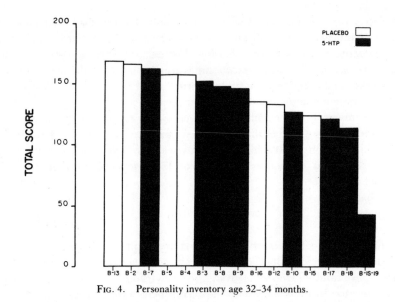

FIG. 4.   Personality inventory age 32–34 months.

rank-ordered them, and divided them into a high group (the first 8) and a low group (the last 8). There were more untreated children in the higher group on the total personality score and several of the subscales, but the differences did not reach statistical significance.

I planned to rank-order the mothers as well, but this proved impossible since they all clustered between 16 and 18 points on a 20-point scale.

Thus there were no significant differences in personality development between the two experimental groups. When I examined the various subscales of the personality inventory, and especially the detailed reports of the home visits, several general factors emerged that distinguished between the children in the high and low groups, regardless of whether they were given medication or a placebo.

First, the children in the high group were more *cheerful* and *lively*, corresponding to the stereotype of *joie de vivre* that many investigators feel characterizes the majority of children with Down's syndrome (Belmont, 1971). In contrast, the children in the low group were either more apathetic and lethargic, with a very low energy expenditure, or extremely irritable and restless. This supports the position taken by Engler (1949) and Wallin (1949) about the existence of three major types of behavior in children with Down's syndrome: (1) the majority are alert, placid, and friendly; (2) a minority are dull and listless; and (3) some are negativistic, restless, irritable, and very hard to handle.

Second, the children in the higher group showed more *awareness* of and more *responsiveness* to their environment, which included people as well as inanimate objects. For instance, although their responses to the examiners varied greatly, their general behavior was definitely affected by the presence of the examiners. In contrast, most children in the low group seemed hardly to notice the presence of two strangers in their house.

The importance of maternal influence on the personality development of the child is generally accepted, and we looked for the possibility that superior personality development correlated with high ratings of maternal behavior. As stated before, we were unable to rank-order the mothers since they all clustered within the 16–18-point range on a 20-point scale. This makes it likely that all the mothers in our sample performed near the optimal level of maternal behavior. The finding corresponds to our general impression of these mothers and is probably related to the enthusiasm and hope generated by their participation in the research project, as well as the mutual support within this maternal group. Thus the differences in personality development of the children in our study seemed related not to the differences in maternal handling but rather to differences in innate endowment.

My experience in this project taught me at least two important lessons. First, it is probably naïve to expect a single one-to-one relationship to exist between behavioral and biochemical factors. Second, the frequency of hypsarrhythmia in our treated group indicates the need for great caution in any attempt to correct an inborn biochemical imbalance.

Attachment Behavior in Infants with Down's Syndrome

My experience with the previous two studies indicated that despite the appearance of social normality children with Down's syndrome are often much less aware of their parents and strangers than normal children. This observation led me to a longitudinal study of the timetable of emerging attachment behavior of this group.

Methods

I studied 76 infants and toddlers with Down's syndrome. The overwhelming majority of these children had trisomy-21, 3 had translocation, and 2 had the mosaic form of Down's syndrome. All the children were seen in a research project in the department of neurology. The object of the research was to raise their blood serotonin level, either by the administration of 5-hydroxy-tryptophan (a serotonin precursor) or vitamin B_6, which acts as a cofactor in tryptophan metabolism.

The children were seen in different settings:

1. Each child was seen by the research neurologist at approximately 2-week intervals during the first 3 months of life, at one-month intervals for the remainder of the first year, and at 3-month intervals during their second and third years of life. The visits were in the neurologist's office and included a standard neurological examination.
2. Each child was admitted for several days to the hospital research ward at the end of the first, second, and third years of life for intensive psychological, neurological, and encephalographic study.
3. Twenty children were also seen in their homes during extended visits at 10, 20, and 32 months of life.

The behaviors observed included: (a) focused scanning;   (b) cooing;   (c) babbling; (d) smiling (nonsocial); (e) smiling (social); (f) recognition of mother; (g) separation anxiety; and (h) fear of strangers.

I was concerned (1) with the earliest observed occurrence of each behavior, and (2) with the degree of intensity of each behavior. A 3-point scoring system was used, ranging from absence of behavior through mild, moderate, and strong intensity. For instance, in the category "recognition of mother" the child's merely staring at his mother would be scored as 1, while his obvious joy upon seeing her, accompanied by squealing, kicking, and a bright smile, would be scored as 3.

During my visits at home and on the research ward I merely observed and recorded the child's interaction with his environment, without actively intervening in the process. During the visits to the neurologist the mother was encouraged to interact with the child by talking to him, smiling at him, and picking him up. When the child passed 6 months of age, she was also asked to leave the room for several minutes, leaving the child with the examiner and the neurologist. The examiner approached the child in a prearranged sequence.

1. Facing the child with an impassive face.
2. Smiling at the child.
3. Talking and smiling.
4. Picking the child up.

My ongoing relationship with the parents over a period of three years gave me ample opportunity to collect much detailed information on the child's family, such as the general emotional climate, the presence and nature of emotional strains, the marital relationship, and attitudes toward the child with Down's syndrome.

Average onset of attachment behaviors in infants with Down's syndrome

Behaviors occurring in the first 6 months of life		
Focused scanning	2–3 months	(range 1–4 months)
Cooing	2 months	(range 1–3 months)
Babbling	3–4 months	(range 3–6 months)
Smiling (nonsocial)	6–8 weeks	(range 4–8 weeks)
Smiling (social)	3 months	(range 2–5 months)
Recognition of mother	4 months	(range 3–6 months)
Behaviors occurring between 6 and 12 months of life		
Separation anxiety	22 months	(range 8–30 months)
Fear of strangers	20 months	(range 8–36 months)

FIG. 5.

Results

As seen in Figure 5, the onset of attachment behaviors characteristic of the first six months of life was only slightly delayed as compared with normal infants. The intensity of these behaviors ranged from mild to moderate and seldom reached the highest degree of intensity.

The infants were interested in their surroundings and scanned the room in the first two to three months of life. They focused on presented objects, especially if shiny and bright-colored. Cooing developed about the same time, followed closely by babbling sounds. Smiling was at first indiscriminate for a few weeks but was soon replaced by preferential smiling at human faces. This in turn was followed by reserving smiling exclusively for the face of a parent— a sequence occurring naturally in normal infants. In addition to the preferential smiling the recognition of the mother was indicated by excitement, hyperactivity, squealing, and laughter when she appeared in the child's visual field.

The attachment behaviors characteristic of the second half of the first year, i.e., separation anxiety and fear of strangers, did not begin until close to the end of the second year in about 85 percent of the sample (65 children). The majority of the children also did not progress beyond mild intensity in these behaviors. All children (except 1 with very severe brain damage) showed at least mild fear of strangers by the end of the study, at the age of three years. However 20 percent (15 children) did not show any separation anxiety even at this age. This latter behavior was best observed during the child's hospitalizations, when the mother left the child in the evening. At the end of the first year very few infants showed any reaction to the mother's departure. The majority were unconcerned and reacted freely to the nursing staff. At the end of the second year most of the infants showed some discomfort and concern after the mother's departure in the form of whimpering, whiny behavior, and occasional crying. In most cases this negative reaction to the mother's departure did not last long, and the children were easily consoled by nurses, who had often had no previous contact with the child. This behavior is, of course, a striking contrast to the behavior of normal two-year-old children in the same circumstance.

As mentioned above, 85 percent of the children presented this delay in attachment behavior which occurred in the second half of the first year of life. However 15 percent (11 children) had the onset of separation anxiety and fear of strangers at the usual time, i.e., in the second half of the first year. The intensity of these behaviors was also stronger in these children than in the rest of the sample.

My first guess was that these children happened to be the most intelligent in the group. However, this didn't prove to be the case, since the developmental quotient (DQ) in both subgroups at three years of age hovered around 50 with no significant difference.

On examination of my descriptive notes I found a plausible solution to this puzzling finding. I realized that in all the children with normal attachment behavior there was an unusually close, almost symbiotic relationship between mother and child because of unusual life circumstances. Seven of the 11 children had congenital heart disease and often were in mortal danger during the study period because of heart failure and heart surgery. The anxiety over the child's life led to an overprotective, hovering attitude on the part of the mother and an unusual degree of closeness. Two mothers had serious marital difficulties and 2 were foreigners without relatives or friends. Because of these difficulties the women sought solace in a very intensive involvement with their children with Down's syndrome.

Along with many other investigators (Dameron, 1963; Koch et al., 1963; Share et al., 1969), I found the development of children with Down's syndrome to progress normally up to six months of age. IQ scores gradually decreased from near normal at six months to 30–40 at older ages. This decline in intelligence can be real or apparent. It could be that infant tests do not reveal the full extent of the defect, which becomes manifest only when more sophisticated tests are used in early childhood.

Our findings support the generally growing recognition of a correlation between the general level of intelligence and the evolution of object relations and human attachment patterns (Guin-Decarie, 1965). It seems that a certain minimum level of intellectual activity and comprehension is necessary to the development of meaningful human ties. The infant's recognition of his mother as an entity, separate from himself and clearly distinguishable from others, is an intellectual process that precedes or parallels its affective counterpart. This process of self-differentiation, in turn, depends on intact sensory and perceptual mechanisms, memory, and the ability to organize bits and pieces of information into a meaningful whole.

In my study I noted that in the first 6 months of life the normality of intellectual level was paralleled by the relatively normal development of attachment patterns appropriate for this age. Between 6 and 12 months the significant decline in intellectual functioning was paralleled by a delay in the development of attachment patterns characteristic of this age.

The other important finding indicates that the inherent risk of an insufficient or delayed attachment behavior in the mentally retarded can be at least partially overcome by an overcompensating, intense involvement on the part of people in the child's environment.

The development of early attachment patterns may be crucial to all future social interactions of an individual. Thus the possibility exists that infants with Down's syndrome acquire in the first six months of life a capacity to relate that positively influences their socialization process despite a subsequent delay in the passing of attachment milestones.

Furthermore, one must consider the well-known fact that the ambivalent feelings of parents of retarded children are a significant factor contributing to the emotional disturbance of their offspring. Most mentally retarded children without Down's syndrome are not diagnosed until the age of two to three years. Prior to a definitive diagnosis of mental retardation the parents often go through a period of puzzlement, confusion, uncertainty, and dashed hopes that may adversely affect their rapport with the child. In contrast, the overwhelming majority of the children with Down's syndrome are diagnosed in the first week of life, causing all parents to go through a period of grief over the loss of the ideal child they expected, lasting in most of them two to three months. Following this grief reaction most parents are able to adjust to the child's handicap and develop coping devices permitting them to deal with the situation in a realistic manner. The obviousness of the disability prevents the parents from using excessive denial, which interferes with the adjustment to any chronic handicap.

Thus it appears plausible that the lesser emotional vulnerability of most children with Down's syndrome is due to their good social adjustment, which is helped by their normal development of early attachment patterns and a realistic acceptance by their parents, favored by early diagnosis.

Conclusion

My research strategy has been strongly influenced by the ethological research model. According to Lewin (1951), ethological research proceeds through several levels of "successive approximation." Ainsworth (1969) elaborated on this strategy, in which one begins with a global observation of behavior while the subject is in his own habitat. Following the collection and evaluation of these global behavioral data, which include the interaction between the subject and his habitat, one proceeds to more refined methods. One can enter the habitat, focus on a smaller sample of subjects, and observe a few very specific behaviors, their frequency, and their timetable, or one may bring the subjects to a laboratory and subject them to a specific experimental routine. My own path in the field of mental retardation has followed both patterns to some degree. I started with an intensive study of the mentally retarded in a variety of settings. This was followed by a delineation of the area of personality development as worthy of study. Finally, the decision emerged to concentrate on one subgroup of the mentally retarded, namely, the children with Down's syndrome.

The first and second studies were conducted in the child's natural surroundings, namely, the school and the home. The third study was conducted in a laboratory situation, namely, a hospital office. The methods used included naturalistic observation and ratings of behavior, as well as the introduction of experimental procedures geared to evoke specific behaviors.

There are several lessons that can be learned from these research efforts. To begin with, behavioral research, because of its complexity, seldom yields clear-cut, "elegant" results. There may be ambiguity and partial rather than total confirmation or rejection of hypotheses. This ambiguity, in turn, invites speculation, which, of course, is intellectually very stimulating but carries the danger of distortion in the direction of the investigator's bias. Second, because of the many facets of behavior, research in this area should preferably be interdisciplinary, to enable one to attack the problem from a variety of vantage points. Third, in addition to standardized research instruments that measure and evaluate behavior, one should carefully collect and record clinical observations in very rich detail. It is the clinical material that often offers the most meaningful findings.

I wish to elaborate a bit on several principles that guide me in my work. As a rule, I stay away from abstract ideas that do not seem related to everyday clinical experience. I do not deny the value of basic research whose significance is not immediately apparent, but my own orientation makes me more comfortable with issues that bear an obvious relationship to clinical reality. When I survey the entire field of research in child psychiatry, I note that a strong clinical orientation characterizes most workers in this field.

Thus my interest in mental retardation and my realization of the importance of the emotional and social adjustment of the mentally retarded preceded my research activity in this field by many years. Work with emotionally disturbed retarded children and adolescents made me aware of the many hazards they face in the process of growing up and the paramount importance of prevention, which must be based on the thorough knowledge of personality development. It would give me profound pleasure if my work were to make a contribution, however small, to the welfare of these "forgotten" people.

References

AINSWORTH, M. D. S. Object relations, dependency, and attachment. *Child Development*, 1969, **40**.

BELMONT, J. H. Medical-behavioral research in retardation. In N. R. Ellis (Ed.), *International Review of Research in Mental Retardation*. New York: Academic Press, 1971, Vol. 5.

COLEMAN, M., BARNETT, A., LODGE, A., & CYTRYN, L. *Serotonin in Down's syndrome*. Amsterdam: North Holland Publishing Co., 1973.

CYTRYN, L., & LOURIE, R. S. Mental retardation. In A. M. Friedman and H. I. Kaplan (Eds.), *Comprehensive textbook of psychiatry*. Baltimore: William and Wikins, 1967.

DAMERON, L. E. Development of intelligence of infants with mongolism. *Child Development*, 1963, **34**, 733.

DOMINO, G., GOLDSCHMID, M., & KAPLAN, M. Personality traits of institutionalized mongoloid girls. *American Journal of Mental Deficiency*, 1964, **68**, 498–502.

ENGLER, M. *Mongolism*. Baltimore: Williams and Wilkins, 1949.

GUIN-DECARIE, T. *Intelligence and affectivity in early childhood*. New York: International Universities Press, 1965.

HEIDER, G. M. Vulnerability in infants and young children: A pilot study. *Genetic Psychology Monographs*, 1966, **73**, 1.

HEIDER, G. M. Factors in vulnerability from infancy to later age levels. In J. Hellmuth (Ed.), *Exceptional Infant*. New York: Brunner-Mazel, 1971.

KANNER, L. *Child psychiatry* (3rd ed.). Springfield, Ill.: Charles C Thomas, 1957.

KOCH, R., *et al.* Gesell development scales in mongoloids. *Journal of Pediatrics*, 1963, **62**, 93.

LEWIN, K. *Field theory in social science: Selected theoretical papers*, D. Cartwright (Ed.). New York: Harper, 1951.

MENOLASCINO, F. Psychiatric aspects of mongolism. *American Journal of Mental Deficiency*, 1965, **69**, 653–660.

MENOLASCINO, F. Psychiatric findings in a sample of institutionalized mongoloids. *Journal of Mental Subnormality*, 1967, **13**, 67–74.

MURPHY, L. B. *Personality in young children*. New York: Basic Books, 1956, Vols. 1 and 2.

MURPHY, L. B. *The widening world of childhood: Paths toward mastery*. New York: Basic Books, 1962.

PENROSE, L. *The biology of mental defect* (2nd ed.). New York: Grune and Stratton, 1963.

ROLLIN, H. Personality in mongolism with special references to the incidence of catatonic psychosis. *American Journal of Mental Deficiency*, 1946, **51**, 219–237.

ROSNER, F., PAINE, R., COLEMAN, M., & MAHANAND, D. Biochemical differentiation of trisomic Down's syndrome (mongolism) from that due to translocation. *New England Journal of Medicine*, 1965, **273**, 1356.

SHARE, T., *et al.* Longitudinal development of infants and young children with Down's syndrome. *American Journal of Mental Deficiency*, 1969, **68**, 685.

SILVERSTEIN, A. An empirical test of the mongoloid personality. *American Journal of Mental Deficiency*, 1964, **68**, 493–397.

WALLIN, J. *Children with mental and physical handicaps*. New York: Prentice-Hall, 1949.

STUDIES OF FAMILY ADAPTATIONAL RESPONSES TO A SPECIFIC THREAT

EDWARD H. FUTTERMAN

Observing, describing, and defining the complex interaction of adaptational processes over time has characterized our work with the families of dying children. In this paper I will be scrutinizing the process of the research itself and its evolution over time, recounting how we confronted the tasks, dilemmas, and challenges involved in studying the families of fatally ill children. The poignancy in the plight of these families motivated us, stimulated us, and engaged us in a more intensive examination of their coping than we might have made if the stakes were not so high. Our shared response to the ultimate fate of the child influenced our research strategies, including the fluctuations in our approaches and avoidances.

Dealing with Death

Several earlier workers (Glaser and Strauss, 1964; Gorer, 1965) have explained their entry into the field of death and dying by describing personal experiences that moved them in this direction. Perhaps motivation must be particularly compelling when one is dealing with issues ordinarily considered taboo. Death was not a stranger to me. Several uncles and all of my grandparents died before I was out of my teens. When I was in college my father succumbed to a terminal cancer. At the advice of his physician, we did not talk about the possibility of his dying. I continue to regret the lost opportunity for meaningful communication. This regret is reflected in my

EDWARD H. FUTTERMAN, Director, Clifford W. Beers Guidance Clinic, New Haven; Associate Clinical Professor, Yale University Child Study Center and Department of Psychiatry, New Haven.

persistent efforts as a psychiatrist to confront the taboos surrounding death. Another event, the near fatality of my second child from hyaline membrane disease, immediately preceded the beginning of my studies of leukemic children and their families.

Survival and Adaptation

I began my professional career working in community psychiatry in a black ghetto neighborhood in Chicago. Survival was a key issue in Woodlawn. There it was important to learn how people coped, particularly considering the variety of conditions and situations to which they had to adapt. It was a community in which there were many institutions and systems to which the residents had to relate but that were not necessarily geared toward their value systems and needs. Therefore we were deeply enmeshed in the dilemmas involved in trying to define adaptation, maladaptation, normality, and psychopathology in a social setting.

The Initial Question

Like many investigations this one began with a question that I was unable to answer. Vernick and Karon had just published their paper entitled "Who's Afraid of Death on a Leukemia Ward?" (1965). They challenged the prevalent practice among pediatric oncologists of concealing information about the disease and its prognosis from the child. Since I was serving as consultant to pediatrics, Joseph Simone, who was then a fellow in hematology, asked me to consider with the pediatric-oncology group whether their approach to the psychological management of the disease was more harmful than helpful. Having no ready answers, I invited Henry Coppolillo, a child psychiatric colleague, to join us in a conference to discuss the management of families with leukemic children. From this conference we came to the realization that we had no data about children's level of awareness of their illness nor how changes in their awareness might affect them and their families.

With my increased sensitivity to the fact that the death of a child was not something that might merely affect some distant strangers but might be at my own doorstop, as well as being confronted continually with issues involving the emotional care of very sick and dying children in the hospital, I found myself groping for answers that were not readily available. I reviewed the excellent early investigations that described many of the important issues facing families dealing with a leukemic child (Bozeman et al., 1965; Chodoff et al., 1964; Hamovitch, 1964; Natterson and Knudson, 1960; Richmond and Waisman,

1955). Still unsatisfied, Simone and I decided that we could master these issues only by learning from families who had coped with such a crisis. In the fall of 1965 we decided to interview some families and we approached Melvin Sabshin for consultation and advice.

Redefining the Questions

From the beginning we vacillated between concern with the moving, human aspects of the problem and conceptual, methodological issues. In addition to the challenge in the original questions posed by the pediatricians, here was an opportunity for an empirical investigation concordant with Sabshin's other work on normality (Offer and Sabshin, 1966). We recognized that we were confronted with a disease that, at that time, had a uniformly fatal outcome. We were interested in adaptation rather than psychopathology, and we felt that families of children with leukemia would be ideal subjects for such studies. We defined some of the parameters as follows: "The threat to family integrity is severe while falling short of family disruption (such as the loss of a parent). The crisis is acute with an inevitable outcome calling for new adaptations over time. The course of the illness, characterized by remissions and exacerbations, allows for a comparison of adaptive processes under varying conditions [Futterman, 1965]."

So began a search for conceptual tools. We were interested in family systems and we went to the literature to understand how we could study families as a whole. We looked at family interaction scales; we explored the material available on social group interactions; we investigated the literature on value orientations, role assignments, communication patterns, and family coping styles. We were hoping to discover or develop instruments that would provide us with a typology of coping from which we could predict outcomes.

Engaging the Issues

With some trepidation we plunged into the task of becoming more familiar with the issues facing these threatened families. As a pediatrician–psychiatrist team we began interviewing families in the hospital and in their homes. Our own hesitation to confront death and dying was evidenced in our initial, gingerly approach to the interviewing. The first subjects were parents whose child had already died, since we were reluctant to deal with families in which a child was still alive but dying. We interviewed the mother and father together, each of them separately, and each of the siblings. This particular family was quite eloquent and very willing to share on an emotional level what they had experienced and what they were now experiencing in response to the death of the child. In her bereavement, the mother could articulate her feelings as follows:

"The baby came three months before Harold died. . . . I wish I had spent more time with him alone and not have had the distraction of the baby. But, on the other hand, when he was ill at home I used to go into the bedroom and sit with him and her and talk to them both. I used to feed her sitting there next to him so I could be with him and talk to him and then I told him about his own birth. I remember telling him about the ride to the hospital, which I thought was particularly beautiful. Sentimental, perhaps, but it made me happy to tell him and I think he was happy to hear about it. And I told him how much we wanted him and how proud daddy was that he had sons. . . . I felt I had to cram in a lot of things in a short time. Many times children don't know these little things. You just never get around to telling them. But this is a time when I planned: 'What do I want this child to know about us, about himself, about our family, about our philosophy, about our relationship? And even if nothing else matters, even if all our philosophy and religion or anything is rather irrelevant, at least I felt we did the best job I knew we could do at that time. I don't mean to say there were no failures. There were times that I felt that, perhaps, I should have done differently. But I feel satisfied before God and man and for myself. And I don't say this proudly. I just say it as a fact."

This family saw the interviews as opportunities to integrate their experiences and to open up communications in which they had been reluctant to engage. We were encouraged when other families also responded positively, appreciating the chance to talk, to teach, and, potentially, to give to others. Our initial fears about being intrusive, and even destructive, were converted into hopes that our interventions might have some therapeutic consequences. Most of the feedback was positive:

"It helps to talk to someone like you because you're not involved emotionally . . . like all our friends down there, they're always, we get to talking about it and they say, 'Well, how do you do it, how can you stand to be away from all the other kids so long, how do you make ends meet?' and they get me upset."

We began to interview more families, turning to those whose children were still alive. Not all of the responses were enthusiastic. For instance, one father included the interviewers in his feelings of isolation:

"You people don't mean nothing to me. You are strangers. And our case here is just another number to you. You have no personal connection to us . . . you people here couldn't care less of the ups and downs of us other than just another patient. You're just too detached."

Fortunately, the negative responses came after we had become convinced that we were doing more good than harm. Other pediatric oncologists joined in the project, and as a group, along with other pediatricians, psychiatrists, and social workers, we provided each other with mutual support and listened to the tape recordings with Sabshin to see what we could learn.

Early Speculations

As we continued to become more deeply involved in the clinical material, interviewing more families, meeting informally with the pediatricians, and making more contacts in the tumor clinic, we also formulated observations and further questions. After intensively interviewing eight families, we made a first attempt at quantification of results by developing a semantic differential scale with poles such as empathy versus aloofness, isolation versus communication, trust versus mistrust, and coping versus overwhelmed. We failed to reach agreement in our ratings since the scale was not sufficiently precise nor the variables sufficiently defined. However, we did discover that there was close accord among the psychiatrists and pediatricians when we rank-ordered families on the basis of coping ability. On a qualitative level, we were able to observe variations in affect, coping strategies, defensive maneuvers, restitutive efforts, anxiety levels, grief, and adaptation over time in the families whom we had seen.

We wondered why we had not observed serious psychopathological outcomes in our sample. We questioned whether this was because the illness was not so severe a stress as we had originally anticipated or because such a stress taps family resources in a way that mitigates against pathological resolutions. We could only speculate on the possibility that our own interventions and the supportive approach of the pediatricians might account for the differences in outcome in our population as compared with those studied by Binger and his colleagues (1969), in which there was no continuity in the primary physician relationship with the families. We also recognized that we might be operating with a bias against identifying pathology since our interest was in coping and normality.

Seeking Models

While continuing to search for conceptual models and to seek appropriate tools for analyzing and obtaining data, we were reluctant to discard the interview, which captured the richness and complexity of the families' experiences. Nevertheless we felt the need for ancillary techniques, observations, and methods for reporting. We investigated many conceptual approaches to describing families. We were looking for a model that could characterize the family as a system rather than as a group of separate individuals, that would not be biased by a pathology–nonpathology orientation, and that might have the capacity to predict coping success or failure with some specificity. We felt that most communication and interaction models tended to retain a pathology bias to the extent that communication and interaction were considered good and isolation was considered bad. We were also trying to deal with the complications involved in rating communication, either on a global basis or by analysis of samples.

In the fall of 1967, when Irwin Hoffman joined the research team, we took stock. We knew that we had obtained some remarkably rich data. Consultants who listened to our interview material were greatly impressed by the wealth of genuine information and feelings that emerged from these interviews. Yet we felt the need for hard research methodology to countermand the softness of our vague, clinical impressions. However, none of the molecular approaches to data analysis seemed to capture the essence of our clinical material. When David Bakan visited with us, he encouraged a break from our attempt to dissect the interviews systematically since he felt we would be doing injustice to the data and be retreating from anxiety-provoking material by attempting hard statistical analyses. He suggested that we adopt the kind of empiricism that entails immersion in the data in order to allow theoretical possibilities to emerge directly from intimate familiarity with the material. Later Rudolph Eckstein reminded me that this was also the advice that Jean Martin Charcot gave to Sigmund Freud: "To look at the phenomena so long until they seem to tell the story by themselves [Ekstein, unpublished]." When we met with Jules Riskin, who had devised detailed family interaction scales, he recalled that the late Don Jackson faced problems similar to ours in trying to organize his material on families with ulcerative colitis, that is, being overwhelmed with rich data that were difficult to handle in a quantitative approach. Riskin (1964) conjectured that while there might be some advantage to using his own family interaction scales, they might not provide the kind of richness we were seeking.

Simultaneously, Hoffmann (1967) introduced us to the work of Glaser and Strauss on "grounded theory." They made the distinction between generating theory and verifying theory, with theory generated from data being considered grounded. They also made the distinction between substantive and formal theory. Substantive theory remains close to an empirical base, staying specific and concrete. Thus theoretical formulations about families adapting to leukemia in a child would be primarily substantive and grounded. Glaser and Strauss emphasized the necessity to maintain a maximum flexibility of research design, with the collecting, coding, and analyzing of data undertaken simultaneously to feed into one another. They also recommended the continual classification of observations, using direct raw data rather than generalizations.

With Hoffman and his colleagues recommending this kind of empiricism, we were faced with the irony that I, the child psychiatrist, aware that my approach to research was soft and lacking in methodological rigor, was desperately searching for hardware and quantification, whereas the psychologist, who subsequently became co-investigator, was encouraging more exploratory approaches and immersion in the data. Obtaining sanction to follow our original inclinations and to capitalize on our clinical skills relieved our anxiety and ultimately contributed to the richness of the findings and conceptualizations. Thereafter we continued to meet regularly as a clinical research team to listen to tape-recorded interviews, to share observations, to commiserate, to theorize, and to categorize bits of information from all sources.

Early Findings

In reviewing minutes of the meetings and progress notes from that period of time, we can discern many partial conceptualizations that subsequently were more formally articulated. In our struggle to avoid the psychopathological bias implicit in a language of defenses, reactions, conflicts, and symptom formation, we were developing a vocabulary of adaptation. We were beginning to describe some of the psychological tasks required in parental adaptation, e.g., the need for parents to maintain a high level of concern and involvement with a child who would no longer be a family member, the task of withdrawing emotional investment in the child as a person with a future, and the task of attending to the needs of other family members. We noted fluctuations in cathexis between parents and children in relation to stages of the illness. We recognized a trend toward idealization of the sick child, and we began to speculate about the relation between this phenomenon and anticipatory mourning. The overriding importance of the process of mourning in anticipation of the death of the child was becoming clear.

Some of the early perspectives were not extensively developed. For example, based on data obtained from two families early in the study, we speculated on a "Rashomon" effect. The term comes from a Japanese story that tells several contradictory versions of a murder biased from the vantage point of the particular witness-participant. We theorized that each family member experiences the crisis from his own vantage point, and to the degree that there is congruence in their perceptions, mutual supports for adaptation might develop. Any member of the family whose perception or method of adaptation was incongruent would be considered at risk. While this line of thinking was not fully pursued, its reverberations can be recognized in our later observations on the issue of awareness, in which we became convinced that children universally have greater awareness about their illness and its implications than their parents or physicians realize (Futterman and Hoffman, 1970a).

Hoffman's interest in the development of self-concepts helped us to appreciate the extent to which the crisis of leukemia stimulates an increase in issues involving self in terms of worth, mastery, and capacity for trust. These issues became included as aspects of the task of *maintenance of confidence* in the self, in others, and in the nature of the surround.

Refocusing Information-Gathering

While we had attempted to randomize the selection of families for intensive interviewing and to interview periodically during the course of the disease and after the child's death, in the fall of 1968 we adopted a more formal interview schedule. We identified important phases during the course of the illness and interviewed randomly selected families during each of these phases (diagnosis, remission, relapse, terminal phase, early bereavement, and late bereavement) whenever possible. We also decided to enlarge the data base by keeping records of informal contacts with families on the wards and in the clinic and by recording our contacts with physicians, nurses, and other medical-care workers.

In cooperation with occupational therapists, nurses, and medical social workers, we organized a waiting-room play program that subsequently evolved into separate parent and child groups (Hoffman and Futterman, 1971). The project began a shift from the primacy of research to the primacy of clinical service. Our intervention as researchers sparked clinical interest in the problems of families coping with dying children and became a source of mutual support among personnel working with severely ill children and their families. It also became a valuable and valued clinical experience for students of all disciplines. In turn, those who were clinically involved with the children and their families fed back data obtained informally on the wards, in the halls, and through all their contacts. In addition children in the waiting room were interviewed, as were the physicians treating the families.

An example of our efforts to obtain data from as many sources as possible was one-time experiment of leaving a tape recorder with a family in their home to pick up spontaneous interactions around the dinner table. While we used these records to supplement our understanding of the family interaction surrounding a child who developed transient school phobia (Futterman and Hoffman, 1970b), we subsequently abandoned this technique. We decided that it was exploitative and that it was an inefficient shortcut to placing an observer in the home over time. Later, when Myra Bluebond, an anthropologist, joined the team, she mingled with the children in the waiting room and became highly involved with the families, visiting their homes and joining them at times of distress, even at funerals. Her work reemphasized the advantages of intensive, personal participation with families.

Identifying Processes of Adaptation

As we assembled, sorted, and assimilated the data, we began to identify a series of dilemmas confronting families in their adaptation to the fatal illness of a child. They were faced with the problem of balancing apparently polar adaptive tasks, e.g., acknowledging the ultimate loss of the child and maintaining hope; attending to immediate needs and planning for the future; cherishing the child and allowing him to separate; maintaining day-to-day functioning and expressing disturbing feelings; active personal care of the child and delegation of care to medical personnel; trusting the physician and recognizing his limitations; and caring for the child and preparing for his death. Among these adaptive tasks and dilemmas the weight of empirical data thrust certain issues into prominence by virtue of their compelling and persistent presence. Almost unwittingly we continually returned to issues centering around separation, loss, mourning, mastery, confidence, and awareness.

Separation anxiety in families with a leukemic child is intense. We began by focusing on a single family, in which this issue was highlighted by the observation that the child developed transient school phobic episodes at times of hematological relapse. Many of the insights from attempts to understand this family were useful in our later approach to the general course of adaptation. This case study illustrated the necessity of considering the importance of time in understanding psychopathology and adaptation. By observing fluctuations in the degree of separation anxiety in the family related to changes in the child's clinical state, we could identify linkages between psychosomatic symptom-formation and the increase in threat to the child's life, with remission in the school phobic symptomatology as the danger subsided. Insights derived from this case study helped to guide our approach to the course of adaptation and to the relationship between psychopathology and adaptation (Futterman and Hoffman, 1970b).

We also tried to identify processes associated with adaptational tasks related to the phases of the illness. For instance, we outlined the sequence of adaptive operations that seemed to help families maintain a sense of mastery during the course of the child's illness and after his death. Accordingly we described families prior to the diagnosis engaged in what we called *search* operations, which involved active questioning to discover what was wrong with the child. Immediately after the diagnosis families seemed to undertake *rescue* operations, which entailed attempts to locate the best possible care as well as frantic efforts to unearth miracles. During remissions we identified *preservation* operations in early remission and *reversal* operations after long remissions. By *preservation* we meant attempts to do everything necessary for care, and by *reversal* we meant the process whereby, after a long first remission, parents began to doubt the diagnosis and made some efforts to disprove that the child had leukemia. Such schemata were developed for the entire course of the illness along several adaptive lines. As we proceeded in this way, however, we found that not all of the descriptions rang true and that this framework tended to introduce arbitrariness. These particular lines also were not sufficiently general to encompass the complexity of adaptational processes. So we found ourselves going back and forth from data to conceptualizations to discover the best way to characterize the processes over time in the manner in which they were being experienced.

Again, the most fruitful approach proved to involve starting with a particular. We were impressed by a process that we later called *enshrinement*, whereby the child was conceived of as possessing otherworldly characteristics, being viewed as saintly, with wisdom, character, sufferance, and goodness far beyond what is usually ascribed to children. For instance, a mother described the following interaction with her son a few days before his death:

> "Marshall asked me how Jesus made people. And I started to explain like you would normally to a four year old. And he said, 'No mommy. I know now!' And that helped more than anyone could have said or done. I think he was shown a way through God to answer the question I could not answer."

We did not see this in all families, but we wondered about its meaning and relationship to the general course of adaptation. As we studied it, we realized that this phenomenon was an aspect of the process of *memorialization*, whereby parents developed a relatively fixed mental representation of the dying child which tended to endure beyond his death. This, in turn, was related to the process of *detachment*, whereby parents gradually withdrew emotional investment from the child as a growing being with a real future. Subsequently we recognized that we were dealing with several interrelated processes, which all contributed to adaptation, encompassed under the task of *parental anticipatory mourning*. In relation to this task we could identify five major processes that seemed to peak in sequence in the course of the illness. The first is *acknowledgment*, which involves the continual struggle between hope and despair, with progressive deepening of parental awareness and narrowing of hope. *Grieving*, the vicissitudes of emotional expression and experience of the impact of the anticipated loss, is contingent on the degree of *acknowledgement*. Next comes *reconciliation*, whereby the expectation of the death of the child becomes integrated into the family's values and their sense of themselves. These, along with *memorialization* and *detachment*, were identified as part processes in the course of adaptation preparing for postbereavement mourning (Futterman *et al.*, 1972).

We were subsequently similarly able to combine a cluster of adaptational processes that seemed to fall together in the general realm of *maintenance of confidence*, which included the mastery and worth issues mentioned previously (Futterman *et al.*, 1973).

What started in a groping, experimental fashion became an implicit working model for the team, which did not emerge so clearly as a pattern until this particular writing. It seems that, in every instance, when we analyzed the material we had collected we began with bits of information, pieces of insight, and tentative hypotheses. From these we developed generalizations and formulations around which to organize the data. We did not summarize the material. We tended to group observations and statements and to view these as a whole, later seeking some unifying concept. For instance, a medical student working with us became interested in the relationship between families and medical care-givers. She extracted all statements from the interview material that had anything to do with physicians, hospitals, medical care, and related issues. The concepts that emerged as most relevant after scrutiny of the data were anxiety, ambiguity, and trust. Ambiguities and uncertainties about diagnosis, prognosis, and treatment plans over the course of the child's illness were clearly related to parental anxiety and influenced the development of trust in the doctor–family relationship (Kirkpatrick *et al.*, 1974).

Similarly Hoffman, in preparing his doctoral dissertation on parental adaptation (1972), initially categorized all of the material from content

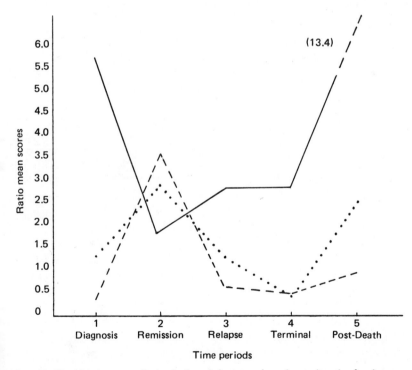

Fig. 1. Profiles of ratio means: Ratio of acknowledgment to hope (———), ratio of maintenance to grief (– – – –), ratio of confidence to doubt (· · · · ·).

analysis of the interviews into about 60 categories that had evolved from the process of immersion with the data. These included categories such as "awareness-shielding," defined as "protecting others from knowledge about child's illness or simply keeping relevant information from others," and categories of "clinging," "blaming," and others. With further content analysis these were condensed to 48 categories and grouped under major headings. Hoffman then identified a few major adaptive tasks and employing the concept of an adaptive balance as a parental response to an apparent dilemma, he evolved three ratios under which he could group the results of his content analysis. These were the balances between acknowledgment and hope, between maintenance and grief, and between confidence and doubt (see Figure 1). From these ratios he was able to describe a modal course of adaptation for the parents in our study and, by combining the content analysis with illustrations from the actual data, conveyed the meaning with considerable richness. He was able to describe parents' development of a sense of growth from having coped with the crisis of having a fatally ill child, as reflected in the following statement by a father:

> "This is one thing that changed—my outlook on life. I used to plan a lot for the future. This is why I was working sixteen hours a day, seven days a week. You know—to get ahead so I could give them a good education, but not anymore. Tomorrow will take care of itself. I worry about today. You appreciate what you've got now, instead of worrying about what you want to have. Be thankful you've got what you have and be contented, and do the best you can with it."

Offshoots

As we became immersed in the data, we learned that we had created a new milieu that persisted beyond our own personal investment. It was a milieu in which research continued to be done. An anthropologist studying symbolic communications worked with children and their families in the tumor clinic in the hospital, in their homes, and in their other living areas (Bluebond, unpublished). A nursing dissertation focused on the differences between families who participated in the parent group and those who did not.

It remained a therapeutic milieu in which a psychiatric social worker and a psychologist continued to work with the parents in a group, which became more and more central to the clinic's functioning, in which nurses and physicians participated, and to which parents came in increasing numbers while the child was ill and even after the child had died (Borstein and Klein, unpublished). An occupational therapist assumed responsibility for the play group in the waiting room. A nurse from the inpatient unit began to participate in the waiting-room program to bridge the gap between the outpatient and inpatient experiences.

It was also an educational milieu. The program has been viewed as a model of preventive intervention with opportunities to observe the potential for humanizing an institution as large and impersonal as a university hospital. Medical students, pediatric and psychiatry residents, psychology residents, social work students, occupational therapy students, and nurses in training have all participated in various aspects of the program.

Conclusions

This particular approach to research is a costly, painful, long, stumbling, plodding foray through many blind alleys and circuitous routes. It lacks the crispness of a well-designed experiment and the rigor of quantification. In addition, by establishing an environment in which communication was encouraged, we contaminated our findings since we undoubtedly affected the quality of medical care, the relationship between the family and the hospital, and even the course of their own adaptation. In fact, we knew from the beginning that we influenced what we studied and we were encouraged when we perceived that it was in a positive direction. We had to cope with the dilemma of being healers and researchers. We chose to plunge in, counter to our fears, and to use our most effective clinical tool, namely, clinical interviewing, to attempt to get to the core of what people were experiencing and feeling and how they were coping. Our research approach, in retrospect, followed our clinical model of intermittently and simultaneously becoming deeply enmeshed and observing from a more detached vantage point.

In the course of our investigations we were confronted with adaptational issues of our own related to the task of studying families with a fatally ill child. On the one hand, we were grappling with concerns regarding loss, transience, and death aroused by our empathic relationships with families. At the same time, we were also trying to resolve a series of dilemmas in our approach to the research tasks, e.g., maintaining scientific rigor while retaining the richness of the available data, avoiding a psychopathological bias while also avoiding a bias toward normality, and maintaining objectivity while identifying with family concerns.

Implications and Prospects

In recent years several investigators have written about families of dying children (Bozeman et al., 1955; Chodoff et al., 1964; Hamovitch, 1964; Natterson and Knudson, 1960; Richmond and Waisman, 1955; Binger et al., 1969). While we wish to contribute to this literature, we are particularly interested in the ways in which studies of family adaptation to this specific threat might broaden general understanding of maladaptation, normality, and psychopathology. We believe that we have been successful in developing a language that is not pschopathologically oriented and that can begin to describe the process of adaptation. We are coming to a greater understanding of the subtle vagaries in the distinction between adaptation and psychopathology. Observing processes over time seems to be essential to understanding adaptation in relation to psychopathology and to comprehending the interactions of adaptive mechanisms with each other as well as with defensive and reactive mechanisms.

We are beginning to realize that the processes that we have described may be applicable to adaptation to other external threats. Similar processes can be identified in families coping with other problems, such as those encountered with chronically handicapped children, retarded children, and children with severe illnesses. For instance, the mastery operations that we have identified as *search* and *participation in care* are described elsewhere in families of children with cystic fibrosis: "They both began searching immediately to find the cause of this disturbance . . . they began to deal with some of their guilt, depression and anxiety by 'doing' for the baby [Leiken and Hassakis, 1973]." The same authors state, "the most frequently used helpful coping mechanism was the 'doing defense.'" Similarly the issue of *acknowledgment* is described in the same study:

> All of the families in our study have made it clear to us that they must think of the death of their child only very rarely. If the thought of the ultimate prognosis was always with them each day, it would bring dreadful pain and suffering. They must indeed suppress or even deny, at times, that the future is filled with uncertainty.

This finding resonates with our own comment regarding the families of leukemic children, that "hopeful statements are often tinged with resignation while pessimistic remarks are laden with hope [Futterman *et al.*, 1972]." We differ with these authors and others in vocabulary, trying to avoid the language of defense and reaction when dealing with coping and adaptation, but the phenomena are familiar. It may be that the adaptive responses of families to a wide variety of threats follow similar lines. Having wondered about this, I find that it becomes time for immersion again.

References

BINGER, C. M., ALBIN, A. R., FEUERSTEIN, R. C., KUSHNER, J. H., ZOGER, S., & MIKKELSEN, C. Childhood leukemia: Emotional impact on patient and family. *New England Journal of Medicine,* 1969, **280,** 414–418.
BLUEBOND, M. H. I know, do you? A survey of awareness, communication and coping in terminally ill children. Unpublished paper.

BORSTEIN, I. J., and KLEIN, A. Parents of fatally ill children in a parents' group. Unpublished paper.

BOZEMAN, M. D., ORBACH, C. E., & SUTHERLAND, A. M. Psychological impact of cancer and its treatment: adaptation of mothers to threatened loss of their children through leukemia I. *Cancer,* 1955, **8,** 1–19.

CHODOFF, P., FRIEDMAN, S. B., & HAMBURG, D. A. Stress, defenses and coping behavior: Observations in parents of children with malignant disease. *American Journal of Psychiatry,* 1964, **120,** 743–749.

EKSTEIN, R. From the language of play to play with language. Unpublished paper.

FUTTERMAN, E. H. Family adaptation to fatal illness of a child. Research proposal, 1965.

FUTTERMAN, E. H., & HOFFMAN, I. Shielding from awareness: An aspect of family adaptation to fatal illness in children. *Archives of Thanatology,* 1970, **2,** 23–24.(a)

FUTTERMAN, E. H., & HOFFMAN, I. Transient school phobia in a fatally ill child. *Journal of the American Academy of Child Psychiatry,* 1970, **9,** 477–494.(b)

FUTTERMAN, E. H., & HOFFMAN, I. Crisis and adaptation in the families of fatally ill children. In E. J. Anthony and C. Koupernik (Eds.), *The child in his family: The impact of disease and death.* New York: Wiley, 1973.

FUTTERMAN, E. H., HOFFMAN, I., & SABSHIN, M. Parental anticipatory mourning. In B. Schoenberg, *et al.* (Eds.), *Psychosocial aspects of terminal care,* New York: Columbia University Press, 1972.

GLASER, B., & STRAUSS, A. L. *Awareness of dying: A study of social interaction.* Chicago: Aldine, 1964.

GLASER, B., & STRAUSS, A. L. *The Discovery of Grounded Theory,* Chicago: Aldine, 1967.

GORER, G. *Death, grief and mourning.* Garden City, N.Y.: Doubleday, 1965.

HAMOVITCH, M. B. *The parent and the fatally ill child.* Los Angeles: Delmar, 1964.

HOFFMAN, I. *Parental adaptation to fatal illness in a child,* doctoral dissertation, Department of Psychology, University of Chicago, 1972.

HOFFMAN, I., & FUTTERMAN, E. H. Coping with waiting: Psychiatric intervention and study in the waiting room of a pediatric-oncology clinic. *Comprehensive Psychiatry,* 1971, **12,** 67–81.

KIRKPATRICK, J., HOFFMAN, I., & FUTTERMAN, E. H. Dilemma of trust: Relation between medical caregivers and families of fatally ill children, *Pediatrics,* 1974, **54,** 169–175.

LEIKEN, S. J., & HASSAKIS, P. Psychological study of parents of children with cystic fibrosis. In E. J. Anthony and C. Koupernik (Eds.), *The child in his family: The impact of disease and death.* New York: Wiley, 1973.

NATTERSON, J. M., & KNUDSON, A. G. Observations concerning fear of death in fatally ill children and their mothers. *Psychosomatic Medicine,* 1960, **22,** 456–465.

OFFER, D., & SABSHIN, M. *Normality.* New York: Basic Books, 1966.

RICHMOND, J. B., & WAISMAN, H. A. Psychological aspects of management of children with malignant diseases. *American Journal of Diseases of Children,* 1955, **89,** 42–47.

RISKIN, J. Family interaction scales. *Archives of General Psychiatry,* 1964, **11,** 484–494.

VERNICK, J., & KARON, M. Who's afraid of death on a leukemia ward? *American Journal of Diseases of Children,* 1965, **109,** 393–397.

LANGUAGE AND EGO FUNCTION OF YOUNG PSYCHOTIC CHILDREN

THEODORE SHAPIRO

The task of describing the origin and roots of one's research activities demands a change of observational stance, which disrupts the usual distance of the investigator from his work. The disruption may stimulate anxiety similar to that evoked within psychoanalysis when the observing ego takes the self as its object. All the intellectual comfort in working at a distance on a presumably external object becomes under the new scrutiny at once self-conscious and awkward. The new circumstance holds a presentiment of arousing even more archaic fantasies, which are themselves the likely precursors to scientific investigation. While this is troublesome, it may also have its purpose and reward, for it is an opportunity to see anew the narcissistic contribution to one's scientific work and to renew a dim surmise that our research conforms to a pattern closely related to the ground substance of our mental organization and conflicts. The patterns of our archaic fantasies are the "root stuff" of our sublimated activities, which our egos classify as contributing, creative, and in the image of our ego ideals and actual teachers.

The background of my research literally mimics a duality in my interests that I can trace at least to my college years. My intent to become a physician was long, and training in biological sciences was necessary, but my interest in philosophy, history, and the humanities was closer to my temperament. The conflict frequently threatened the straight and narrow path to medicine. Only after I began my clinical work did the seduction of "pure ideas" cease. Practical work with patients and application of the knowledge learned in medical school and internship commanded my interest. After exposure to many clinical disciplines I soon learned that in psychiatry I could make a happy marriage of the two strains of interest in philosophy (especially directed toward ways of knowing) and my physicianship.

THEODORE SHAPIRO, Professor and Director of Child Psychiatry, New York University School of Medicine, New York.

Having put the conflict to rest temporarily, I pursued my studies and chose psychoanalysis as a further reconciliation of my interests. At the same time I became a child fellow doing clinical research under Dr. Barbara Fish and was quickly involved in studying the effect of drugs on schizophrenic children. Just as I had mastered an old conflict between the physical and the mental, the happy reconciliation was threatened by the old dualism between body and mind. Though I participated in drug studies, my earliest collaborative papers in which my contribution was greatest concerned new diagnostic typologies and descriptive clarifications for research application. I was more involved in the impact of psychic organization on behavior than in the physiological impact of drugs.

At this point serendipity participated in what was to become the most recent reconciliation of a conflict that was turning out to be more adaptive than disruptive.

The most significant parameter of the behavioral repertoire of the small psychotic youngsters we studied was their limited language behavior. At that time I had no tools to study this significant developmental line. Coincidental with this realization, a new course in ego psychology stressing linguistic development was offered by Dr. Victor Rosen at the New York Psychoanalytic Institute. A new literature of linguistics was opened up to me at a time of ferment stimulated by Chomsky's contributions. I read avidly, all the time curious as to whether a complementary model to Bender's and Mahler's views of childhood psychoses could be generated that used language behavior as a means of characterizing the development of psychotic children and quantifying their progress. I was looking for a way to count and measure something that would illuminate ego organization, where previously the only data were anecdotal, clinical description and theoretical inference. Moreover, I saw another opportunity to be involved in an abstract science that complemented psychoanalysis and that could be applied, for investigative purposes, to the children I was so interested in studying clinically. This second opportunity to do hard science, and epistemology as cognitive psychology, compelled my attention. The crossover seemed natural, and at that time it was a possibility that I could not leave without trying. I can be retrospectively pleased that I was not so learned as to be paralyzed by the doubt of experts who either feel "it's all been done before" or whose close knowledge of argument and counterargument within a specialized field discourages application to more remote systems. To some degree I rushed in where more sophisticated students feared to tread. The subsequent results can only be recounted. The fact that I must now accept is that I probably could not have done otherwise than I did. The fit to my needs, my curiosities, and my tendency toward complementarity as a scientific viewpoint were the givens of my prior psychic structure.

My efforts produced a number of false starts. These were largely in the area of an overly inclusive vantage point. I had read a number of linguists whose discussions of the function of language fascinated me and promised to be fruitful if applied. For example, K. Buehler (1934) suggested that language begins as an *expressive* function and then takes on an *appeal* function in evoking a response by the auditor and emerges as a *propositional* faculty by which an individual symbolically states this or that about a referent (thing) in a suitable vehicle (speech utterance or graphic representation). Not only was Buehler developmental in his vantage point, but he provided a functional scheme that might be harnessed to measure the elusive communicativeness of a subject's maturing speech productions.

The latter idea caught my imagination, because the existing literature on language development presented a strange dichotomy: the normative sequences of language learning and performance were well documented and included in many developmental tests ranging from Gesell's Developmental Scale (Gesell and Amatruda, 1941) through the standard IQ batteries. Investigators too numerous to mention (e.g., Irwin, 1947, 1948; McCarthy, 1930, Sampson, 1945) had established the sound sequences of speech development, ranging from prespeech babbling to phonemic patterns that represent the minimal differences in sound form that native speakers recognize and in turn are the phonetic bases of each specific language. On the other hand, the functional aspects of communicativeness had received less attention, except for Piaget's (1963) early distinction between egocentric and socialized speech, which was not easily verified by workers in the United States (McCarthy, 1930) and was criticized by the Soviet psychologist Vigotsky (1962), whose early death robbed psychology of a major creative thinker.

In my search for a method I did not wish simply to place the children we studied on a normative scale leading to propositions such as, "This eight-year-old schizophrenic child speaks at a two-year-old level." Too many of our psychotic children were not "simply retarded" (besides which I do not believe any child is simply characterized by his diagnosis). They had a characteristic deficit and/or deviance that could be described clinically as poor communicativeness, and had been further characterized only in anecdotal terms as echoing, making metaphoric substitution, etc. (Kanner, 1946). If one could but combine existing standards of retardation with an assessment of functional communicativeness, a two-dimensional description of any child's linguistic skills could be made at any point in development. Moreover, if one could categorize one could count and compare, and then the general aim of objectifying data in a Baconian sense would be achieved. Buehler's scheme offered some hope, but it was difficult to assign behavioral categories using his outline. Moreover, we knew more about the speech of these children than his scheme provided for.

At this point a check-sheet questionnaire was formulated that we have faithfully filled in since we began our work but have never used for later correlations. Included are phonemic, comprehension, and Piagetian estimates of a

Addressor ◄—————————————————————————————► *Addressee*
(Expression)   *Channel*   (Appeal)
                                     (Phatic)
                                     Message
                                     (Poetic)
                                     Code
                                     (Lexical)
                                     Context
                                     (Designative)
                                     Metalinguistic
                                     (Descriptive of language)

FIG. 1.   Jakobson's scheme.

child's ability to locate objects in representational space. Perhaps some day I
will be pleased I have this data. Then the work of R. Jakobson (1955, 1960)
caught my eye. He augmented Buehler's functional description of linguistic
performance. His scheme is reproduced (see Fig. 1).

Jakobson breaks the communicative scheme into an *addressor*, whose
function is expressive, and an *addressee*, whose function is to register the appeal implied by the addressor, evoking some sort of action or its equivalent.
The *channel* that they use is said to provide a phatic function. It may comprise
of a two-way, open, vocal–auditory channel as in human beings, or, in the
instance of a one-way radio, only one expressor or addressor at a time may use
the channel. The message may carry a *poetic* denotation, that is, be rich or
poor in meaning, which in turn is related to a *code* made up of a lexicon or a
series of words that have reference and designative correspondence to things,
persons, actions, and ideas—at the least. This is all carried out in a *context*
that aids the addressee in his task of pinning down the words expressed to a
particular meaning as intended or evoked.[1]

This seemed a very comprehensive approach to the functional aspects of
language. However, my collaborators and I were dealing with very small, very
retarded, and very deviant children, and we had to fit our data into a scheme
that would maximize the possibility of generalizing the fewest regularities that
would dictate their unique language performance in all its complexities. The
linguistic scheme offered an exciting prospect for breaking down the categories
to which we had to attend, *but* it remained cold and removed from the human
matrix of development. What of Mahler's descriptions of the separation-individuation process's going awry at different substages in the psychotic process of
children? We argued that one of the vehicles that aid children in their

[1] The metalinguistic function has been omitted here, but Jakobson includes it. This function refers
to language about language, which was not relevant to the severely impaired children with whom
we were working.

separation-individuation process is the capacity for communicative language. Adequate language abilities at an appropriate maturational stage permit a child to delay his immediate needs and put them into word forms, which serve as maps of the territory to be traversed and as vehicles to communicate needs, while modulating drive derivatives that emerge with separation. Culturally determined phonemes transmitted by mothers provide a double satisfaction: mothers take pleasure in the child's performance and also enjoy gratifying the child's wishes as his vocalizations elicit satisfying actions by the mothers. We were thus aware that speech is learned and used in a human matrix, but we were not at all certain to what degree the maternal supporting systems or the particular stimulus circumstances would effect the child's capacity to encode his wishes in speech.

Recent linguistic research in the area of grammar (Chomsky, 1965) and the biological aspects of language development (Lenneburg, 1967) had led us to the tentative conclusion that there were maturational structures and timetables included in the child's average biological equipment that must emerge in explicit functional forms in an "average expectable environment" (Hartmann, 1958). Thus we believed that grammatical relationships would emerge as an autonomous function of the maturing ego. The recent data temporarily permitted us to proceed in our studies of the children with the hope of later developing tools to study mother–child interaction. Mahler's (1968) idea that these children are unable to utilize the "mothering principle" was interpreted as referring to an ego deficit that effected both language and personal social behavior. This interpretation permitted us to focus on the productive language of our children in context, so that data could be limited, categorized, and counted.

We risked leaving out essentials, *but* every researcher must first narrow his field from the broad clinical holism that stimulates his work. Moreover, as new ideas are generated from data, new projects can be contemplated. A never-ending cycle of investigative joy is possible! We knew that our first task was to record and categorize speech events in such a way that we took into account not only the developmental sequence of intelligible phonemic units but also coded them in terms of their communicative value. We also knew some of the relevant clinical categories from our anecdotal data. Thus our scheme devolved from a melding of clinical experience and theoretical modeling. Even in the scheme outlined we were going beyond linguistic and grammatical studies, which tend to ignore context, and away from simple behaviorism, because we inferred psychic and cognitive structure.

We settled on a working scheme that was revised a number of times before it was usable but whose basic structure remained unchanged (Table 1). A *morphological* table was outlined with a *prespeech* area of items ranging from gestures without vocalization through jargon, which has none of the

TABLE 1

MORPHOLOGY

Prespeech
Vowels and vowel–consonant combinations
Babble and jargon
Speech
Conventional sequences
Single words
Two–five-word combinations
Disjunctive syntax

FUNCTION

Noncommunicative
Isolated expressive speech
Context disturbance (complete)
Imitative speech
Context disturbance (partial)
Communicative
Appeal speech (wish-oriented)
Signal/symbol speech (propositional)

phonetic discreetness of speech but does have the speech melody. The *speech* category ranges from conventional sequences, such as counting or songs, and from single-word designations for things and people, through complex phrases and sentence fragments, up to sentences of five words or more, with a special category for disjunctive syntax. The *functional* scale was a compromise application of both Buehler's and Jakobson's schemes. There is a large noncommunicative sector, which includes isolated expressive, imitative, and context-disturbed speech. Isolated expressive utterances are those in which a child seems to be talking to no one, vocalizing either with gross motion or with music or play or perseverating in a way that has no essential communicative value. Context-disturbed speech includes utterances that show a poor or tangential relationship between what the child has to say and the immediate surroundings or that confuse the examiner by the essential irrelevancy of the remarks. Even if he could pick out a referent it would be very difficult to pinpoint how the particular sequence of events in the play led to the child's calling up this referent. Imitative speech includes immediate or delayed echoing within the examination period.

The *communicative sector*, on the other hand, includes appeal and signal–symbol speech. Within the appeal sector any phatic remark that is a reciprocal opening of the channel of communication is considered as having the property of forwarding a communicative contact. The remainder of the items in this area are protests, wishes with or without gestures, or exclamations and commands—all of which have a wish-oriented focus. We initially thought that these would have developmental priority over later designative items. The fact is that they do not. This fact brought us to the realization that frequently an attempt to apply a theoretical model leads to concretizations of concepts. If, as Freud notes, our first thoughts are wishes, why not our first words too! Image of a researcher as naïve child!

The last and most-developed category describes what we call signal–symbol speech or propositional items. This is a rather large category, ranging from referential naming to question answering and asking. At a higher level items are present that include the sharing of information (in the present or the past or future), role playing, or even metaphors.

Perusal of this scheme suggests the rather narrow limits in which we expected our children to perform. At the point at which a normal child of three spoke functionally good language, he would rather quickly be catapulted off our scale. As I describe the progress of our work, it will become apparent why we had to add other linguistic techniques to complement this scale as we wished to pursue other aspects of language development in psychotic children. We were open to doing this and we recognized that the attempts at scaling these more immature children's performances was a first step in the direction of charting their course of linguistic performance as a measure of ego integrity.

While we included an area of syntactic disturbance in our primary scales, we did not find that this was a significant area of disorder for our children if taken simply at face value, i.e., only as disarrayed word-to-word relationships. In some ways we had hoped that this would be the characteristic feature of childhood schizophrenia, as it would have brought the disturbance into simple relationship with Chomsky's propositions about normal syntax as an innate human category. How easy it would have been to report that schizophrenic children do not share that "humanness" with other children. At a later point I will show how some of our work does indeed suggest aspects of Chomsky's hypothesis, but more in the relative ease with which grammatical transformations from simple sentences are made and used.

A slight digression is warranted now because our work was influenced by the new work in psycholinguistics that was pressing around us. The general thrust of Chomsky's contribution to linguistics rests on the notion that analysis of sentences in the traditional grammatical forms, such as subject, verb, object, etc., leads to a multiplicity of cumbersome formal categories of words in sentences, so that the surface structure of a sentence is all-important and does not permit a reduction of data into usable units. He was looking, rather, for the smallest set of general laws or propositions that could be used to describe the "infinite" number of possible sentences that a native speaker of the language might generate. Thus he challenged metaphorically the Ptolemaic universe of complex epicycles, and like Copernicus he was looking for a

Lexicon   Deep Structure (DS)
(Words Categorized by Features)   (Simplest Kernel Sentence Forms)

Transformation rules

↓

Surface Structure (SS)
(Sentences: imperative; passive voice, interrogative; compound, etc.)

	Example
John hit the ball.	SS declarative, past tense.
Hit the ball, John!	SS Imperative transformation.
The ball hit John.	Meaning change by word rearrangement and not a transformation.
The hit ball John.	Meaninglessness on basis of position in sentence that is not permitted by features of words used.

FIG. 2.   Generative grammar model.

simpler system to describe the data of the language universe. Concisely (Figure 2) what he suggested was that there are a number of *deep structural* forms of sentences that undergo a set of *transformations* to yield a particular manifest or *surface structure* of sentences. These deep forms and transformations are limited in number and may be analyzed according to a fixed set of phrase rules. Thus passive-voice sentences and active-voice sentences and interrogative sentences, among others may be looked at as being made up of a *lexicon* of words that are available to an individual. This individual will use them in particular formal arrangements that are subject to transformational rules, which in turn guarantee grammaticality. These ideas, originally based on the analysis of contextless model sentences, have been expanded and extended by others, so that innate psychological structures corresponding to these linguistic analytical structures have been sought. Lenneburg (1967) is one of those who has studied the development of language from a biological standpoint and seem to be in accord with such a proposition.

Recently Roger Brown (1973), who initially studied children's language development outside the Chomskian frame of reference, has also come to a view that the linguistic abilities of children are most likely a species-specific behavior with a strongly maturational basis. This digression was introduced only to suggest that while Chomsky did not influence our scales directly, the climate of thinking during the course of our work was having its effect on our formulations. All our clinical models derivable from Bender, Kanner, and Mahler had emphasized the biological unfolding of specific maturational sequences. Now the linguists and psycholinguists all emphasized the substrate potentials of children. While some of the clinical investigators focused on core biological disturbances as influencing and distorting ego structures, linguists were discovering language behavior as a maturing function to be studied as an integrated system. In my inquiries I was still looking for a means of using language as a simple indicator of more global disturbance attributable to deficient ego structures, which at other levels may parallel central nervous system deficits or deviant maturational plans. Language behavior now seemed to be such a natural, measurable parameter.

While it was not our specific aim, we were also seeking a clinical description of these children in linguistic terms to see how they differed from normal children. We hoped in this way to illuminate the deficiencies or variants in language of these children compared to those structures inferred for normal development. At the back of our intent was the age-old model of working from pathology to normality and using pathology to illuminate normal development.

The Studies

Initial studies (Shapiro and Fish, 1969) utilizing our method over a six-month period showed that our scale could differentiate between a child who had a severely fixed psychotic picture from one with a developmental language lag. The psychotic child's speech was characterized by a heavy complement of poor syntactic utterances, which included echoing and context disturbance. An incidental finding in this study soon became an object of further interest. The child who went on to develop normally functioning speech had a burst of echoing during his more general explosion in linguistic development. This echoing soon disappeared, but it made us curious about the role of imitation in the early development of normal and pathological language.

Behaviorists suggest that language learning, like all other learning, arises through imitative strategies and generalizations, while the Chomskians offer the proposition that inborn grammatical potential comes to fruition as an autonomous biological structure. Thus from the beginning children ought to be creative in their usage of grammatical forms. The intramural battle between these new empiricists and the rational idealists continues to rage as though Locke and Descartes and Kant lived still.

We determined to make further study of imitation in our children as compared to normally developing youngsters (Shapiro et al., 1970). We knew that normal three-year-olds are quite productive in a wide range of linguistic forms. Since our population suffered a handicap, we selected a sample of psychotic children close to their fourth birthday. We had records of eight such children and three with nonpsychotic diagnoses, and we compared them with four-year-old peers as well as to three-year-olds and two-year-olds, using samples of their naturally occurring imitative and echoing responses. Because the method we had developed did not discriminate among the varied forms of imitative response, we devised a new scale that described a spectrum of imitative behaviors ranging from exactly congruent echoing to verbalizations made up of newly created sentences. The latter would require linguistic integrations and selections of words originally heard adapted to flexible use in new combinations.

We discovered that while schizophrenic children use predominantly congruent imitations, normal four-year-olds use predominantly creative, newly formed utterances. Moreover, and somewhat to our surprise, normal three-year-olds and two-year-olds also have a very healthy complement of newly creative utterances and many fewer congruent echoes. The psychotic children, in turn, have almost no newly created imitative forms. The small group of nonpsychotic children (three) who were also hospitalized showed a spectrum of imitations that approximated our normal two-year-olds, i.e., they were more retarded in their format than deviant.

In order to understand these data, one might construct the range of possible functional substrates from which such variants in behavior might derive. What functional elements are necessary to do the required task of echoing and/or reshuffling, and what strategies are preferred for social exchange? Children who can repeat in the same form what they heard moments before require at the least a receiver-recorder-repeater mechanism. If the same words in same sequence are to be uttered at a more distant time, storage capacity would be necessary. However, if new sentences are to be formed from words heard in other sequences, a reshuffling and integrating apparatus would be needed. In human terms a child's mimicking her mother exactly is quite different from her playing mommy at a distant time with a doll that represents a baby. This difference represents the crucial distinction between introjection and identification.

Our curiosity about which strategies are preferentially selected and used by psychotic children as the developmental course proceeds led us to consider the longitudinal course of a single child. We shifted our focus from a cross-sectional approach to a single case study and followed a child from ages two to six over 18 examinations (Shapiro et al., 1972). Beginning with minimal productive capacity this child increased in intelligible speech (phonemic approximation) and also in general communicativeness. However, he remained both retarded and deviant, never achieving the 30-month-old level of intelligibility according to age standards for each sample and never going above the 50 percent mark in his communicativeness. On close analysis of both the noncommunicative and the communicative aspect of his sample we could draw a model curve that described this particular child's developmental course and that we found could be generalized for understanding the processes that underlay the linguistic performances of our psychotic children (see Figure 3).

Initially the noncommunicative sector of this child's speech was characterized largely by echoing. There was a period during which his echoing became equivalent with his context-disturbed speech, and then the context-disturbed speech became more prominent than the echoing. By way of contrast, normal children begin to use their new phonemic forms in newly structured sentences from age two onward. On the other hand, this psychotic child echoed what he heard, then acquired a storage of phonemic and phrase forms, and then used them later in a rigid, formalistic manner and often without reference to external context. The reshuffling, word-integrating element in our mechanical scheme seemed to be inoperative (or an alternative mechanism akin to introjection, taking stimuli in whole, was at work), and no assimulative breakdown for future syntactic use could be demonstrated.

As a complement to our findings in the noncommunicative sector, we studied the communicative sector of this child's performance. Here the predominant group of utterances were sentence fragments and sentences cast in the present indicative tense, usually designations. He never used the future tense, the passive voice, or negative sentences; he asked but one question; he used only two telegraphic forms; and in general he revealed little evidence that he was able to make grammatical transformations of any variety. Thus even in his communicative speech he did not display a quality of linguistic ease. These difficulties afforded his productions a stilted style with simple reference to the here and now. He seemed to be caught in a world of immediate signals rather than symbols.

These data encouraged us to look further at our entire group to see if the echo–context relationship had further application (Shapiro *et al.*, 1974). We turned our attention to a longitudinal study of all 30 children whom we had

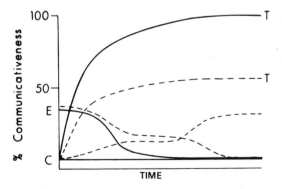

Fig. 3. Communicativeness—two idealized curves. T—total % communicativeness, C—% context disturbance, E—% echoing, ——Child who develops language skills, - - - Child with poor language skills.

studied using an initial examination, a short-term follow-up in the hospital two
to three months later, and a final examination. The length of our study ranged
from less than one year in 10 children to more than one year in 20 (24 were seen
past the poor-prognosis-index age of five). Eleven of the children were under
three years and six months at first examination and an additional 13 were under
five. I haven't the space here to give the details of this study of our youngest sub-
sector, which will soon be in print (Shapiro, in press), but a number of conclusions were drawn:

1.   The percentage of communicative utterances at the second language
examination retrospectively segregated those who would make a good
adaptation to school from those who required special schools for psychotic
children.

2.   Our data suggested that we could push our prognostication back from
age five to 42 months on the basis of linguistic data.

3.   More important to our current discussion, the context–echoing relationship noted in the single case study was also evident in the group and had
prognostic value.

Our studies of severely disturbed children stress and elaborate on the deviance in their language development. However, all of us who have followed
young psychotic children are aware that some "develop out" of their initial rigidities and begin to communicate rather well. These children retain the mark
of their disorder in bizarre fantasies, fragmented isolated adaptations to their
environment, and an uncanny, inappropriate compulsivity. Their speech and
language may even attain excellent abstract and grammatical structure.
Though I too have observed this development, I have not seen it studied in detail. Existent studies of children with severe psychotic disorders who are taught
by operant conditioning methods show an increase in vocabulary but do not attain less rigid formal speech characteristics. Moreover, we all recognize that
many schizophrenic children grow into adult schizophrenics who present a variety of disorders of language that are variously referred to under the general
shibboleth of "thought disorder." This has been cataloged in the literature as
concrete attitudes, paleo-logic etc. However, except for some recent studies of
adult schizophrenics' language behavior, we have not been able to trace any longitudinal studies from childhood onward to document systematically and quantitatively how children with psychoses change in their language performance
and if they "grow out" of the severe difficulties that we have been studying at an
early stage.

We have reported one such longitudinal study in progress (Shapiro,
Huebner, and Campbell, 1974) on a child whose speech developed sufficiently to
require that his productions be dealt with by other methods. He blew the top off
our scale. We therefore turned to content analysis along with other linguistic

techniques. At his best level of hierarchic integration, content analysis revealed massive anxiety regarding body fragmentation and castration anxiety, as well as poor integration of fantasy life. His language still retained a greater frequency of fragmented and simple sentences than of complex constructions. Moreover, the longitudinal view showed that he moved through an intermediary stage of disrupted syntax. From our vantage point we viewed these changing forms of manifest behavior as reflecting a constant core of deviant integrative difficulties. This view, of course, does not answer the clinical questions of which children can be helped by what kinds of intervention. However, our linguistic analysis done at crucial points in development does correlate with prognosis within the current therapeutic scene.

This overview of our work in progress suggests a number of propositions regarding not only the ego structures of those who are diagnosed as childhood schizophrenics but also the course and type of research that I have chosen—the latter first:

1.   Clinical training seems to permit a flexibility in the application of techniques that might not fulfill all the demands of some highly trained researchers. In many ways clinicians are more easily apologized for when they do research, because they "know not what they do." We tend to work seminaturalistically with small samples and to apply our statistical methods less systematically. While our results may be less conclusive than those obtained with more rigorous research methods, I do believe we have clinical practicality in mind and are question-centered at all times. You will notice that persistence in the use of method has been demanded for this work, but flexibility was also required when new questions arose. We opted for shifts in technique as we changed from longitudinal to cross-sectional to individual studies and as new questions were to be approached. Each technique developed p. r. n. to generate new data because of questions arising from a prior investigation. Moreover, the single case study again takes on new importance in the hands of a "clinician as researcher." This is, I believe, a very favorable trend.

2.   The following is an attempt to summarize what a study of the language abilities of schizophrenic children[2] reveals about the structure of the disorder.

---

[2] It should be clear that we recognized the clinical differences between the designations *autistic* and *schizophrenic*, but we made no segregation in the sampling for the studies described. While there is some evidence to recommend a primary distinction (Rimland, 1964; Rutter, 1968), we chose to maintain a position that childhood schizophrenia currently is sufficiently designative to include childhood autism, symbiotic psychoses, and other mixed forms that appear in the course of development. Following Bender, we would tentatively suggest that autism is a variant of childhood schizophrenia. Moreover, the clinical value of discriminating among these subgroups may be important only when the parameters of natural history and ultimately etiology have become more certain. Indeed, if we slighted the differences among groups, it was also because we anticipated that language profiles might offer another taxonomy of differential forms.

If we return at this point to Jakobson's scheme (Figure 1), his categories provide a rational breakdown of the areas of disturbance in language seen in childhood schizophrenia. The major disturbances may be categorized in terms of the *appeal* function of language. While these children maintain an expressive mode, at times verbal and at other times nonverbal, the evocative appeal function of the language is, more often than not, elusive. The unclarity in form and message leads, in W. Goldfarb's words, to "perplexity." But reasons for this perplexity may be further pinpointed within the poetic function of the message and the designative ambiguity, which are secondary to not sharing a common context with the listener. These children are very simply pointing with designative words to concrete here-and-now objects, but the message lacks specificity when more complex descriptions are required. They cannot make propositions that state more than a simple relationship in their phrases. They also do not enrich their messages with nuances and variants in reference as in normally developing speech. That is, they use the conventional code available to them—the words and phrases available to them within the language with which they were taught to mimic and point—but they do not employ the code for the many flexible possibilities of pointing in the past and future or describing action in progress. Moreover, the context referred to is clearly at variance with the context that can be understood by the auditor. Frequent extraneous words are spoken that refer to a personal world, or they are spoken after a long delay so that the eliciting context has long since eluded the companion in conversation.

The availability of a channel for interchange is something that has to be taught specifically. Until they are taught to do so, these children do not self-consciously and naturally recognize that the auditory vocal channel is available for evocation of wish fulfillment or for stating relationships perceived. The autistic aloneness that has been so well described is clinically reinforced by this apparent ignorance. Moreover, the vital relationship between learning the code and using it appropriately involves a third factor, which we ignore in normal development because it occurs naturally, so that only when pathology seems to disrupt an expected process do we see what is missing. In the most disturbed forms of childhood schizophrenia the children are able early on to learn phonemic forms, which are presented to them very largely via echoing. Then, once the storage is completed, echoing falls off only to be replaced by rigid productions out of context, as though the children are trying to fit their ideas into words, which they have some dim awareness are used for communicative purposes. However, they do not seem able to fit the rigidly stored phonemic forms appropriately to the text of their ideas. They have a lexicon of acceptable phonemic sound patterns or words stored for use, but they have difficulty in coding their ideas. Nowhere else do we see the distinction between thinking and language as a vehicle for thought so radically separated. This breakdown of functional systems in childhood schizophrenia permits us to view anew which componants are necessary for a normal child to perform in coherent and relevant language forms. Vigotsky's (1962) distinction between prelinguistic thought and preintellectual speech is put to a crucial test in the difficulties schizophrenic children have in linking words and syntax to ideas. Figure 2 suggests that any surface structure of a sentence that expresses a syntactic relationship referable to a logical or referential occurrence demands that there be a deep-structural, potential form from which any surface structure may be derived. A lexicon must also be available that is made up of words categorized according to their features and ready for use. For example, the feature arrangement requires that verb forms be cataloged as action words, and then a further feature of some verb forms is that they demand use for animate objects only. Word usage then must comply with the structure of the lexicon as well as the individual's need to code relations that include time (past, present, and future) or the inflections of the language (that is the suffix endings in English that are applied for person and place). The two- and three-word phrase structures of normally developing children already reveal the ability to carry out some of these transformations. Incorrectly inflected endings emerge in the surface structure in sentences such as "He *standed* on my back," suggesting the overgeneralization of rules quite early in development. Such errors are relatively absent from the speech work of schizophrenic children, who are severely disturbed. Thus, while our data document that the lexicon of designated forms can be rich, the number of transformations appears to be many fewer. These children seem to live in a here-and-now, designative world and code only the simplest relationships. From time to time they use pat phrases that they have stored as echoed memories and that they call out on new occasions for rigid use. By and large, when they speak they speak in sentence fragments, and even when they speak full sentences they are generally grammatical as heard. Grammatical to be sure, but short and few in number. There seems to be a tendency toward curtailment of length and coding that favors cognitive strategies probably based upon early echoic forms.

These disturbed children, then, seem to fall into a category of disordered language in which any of the flexibilities that are postulated for normal development, requiring integrative mechanisms such as transformation and general rule application, are seriously impaired, stilted, and foreshortened. It is not, then, in the periphery (that is, on the receptive level) that the disturbance exists but in the integrative aspects of cognitive organization. These children are not able to structure their world with the aid of language.

The inability to use the "mothering principle" as described by Mahler may be looked at as a parallel difficulty in world structuring. These children are impaired at the level of ego-integrative mechanisms in such a manner that they cannot pull their experiences with objects and the world together into the unified amalgamation that we ultimately call an identification. The structures within seem to remain discrete, as though introjected. Clinically we see other evidences of this mode in the little people within our patients who tell them what to do in rigid echoes. Their objects are "swallowed whole." Development never reaches the stage of full accommodation in which the external person is internalized.

Similarly the individual words and individual phrases seem locked into rigid recording devices or ego systems that do not permit reshuffling for use in varied contexts. This rigidity leads to a nonadaptive psychological core of object representations, which shows externally not only in the rigidity of their clinical behavior but specifically and objectively as language behavior that may be studied by the methods I have described.

What about those children who go on to develop adequate language? Our one longitudinal study of the course of an individual who had a more favorable developmental outcome shows that there were stages in his development during which the struggle for syntactic fluency and adequate phrase structure were temporarily disrupted. Having matured past such a stage, he spoke fairly good syntactic but curtailed speech. We had to look at other parameters that revealed the postulated core disturbance at a different hierarchic level. Such data suggest that we cannot look at childhood schizophrenia as a static disease with a fixed language deficit but as a process that, as Bender says, affects all functions subsumed under the central nervous system at each and every level of development. I believe that it is particularly salutary to be able to observe language behavior, which itself has a definable developmental course, a structure, and a pattern against which retardation and deviation can be measured. From the observation of language behavior we can make a taxonomy whose reference is an ego-integrative core of great complexity that unifies identifications, object relations, and biosocial capacities for adaptation.

Epilogue

I have described a path of investigation and its discoveries that have commanded the past eight years of my professional work. The personal roots of the enterprise are dimly outlined and the work is described in more detail, but the hours of collaboration with others and personal rethinking can only be surmised. Lest this presentation give too romanticized a view of research, I would like to comment that the work is frequently dull and arduous and the results meager, but on the other hand, it is difficult to measure the pleasure gained— nevertheless it is generated and experienced as the puzzle unfolds.

References

BROWN, R. *A first language: The early stages.* Cambridge, Mass.: Harvard University Press, 1973.

BUEHLER, K. *Sprachtheorie.* Jena: Fischer, 1934.

CHOMSKY, N. *Aspects of the theory of syntax.* Cambridge, Mass.: MIT Press, 1965.

GESELL, A., & AMATRUDA, C. S. *Developmental diagnosis.* New York: Hoeber, 1941.

HARTMANN, H. *Ego psychology and the problem of adaptation.* New York: International Universities Press, 1958 (originally published 1938).

IRWIN, O. C. Development of speech during infancy: Curve of phonemic frequencies. *Journal of Experimental Psychology,* 1947, **37,** 187-193.

IRWIN, O. C. Infant speech: Development of vowel sounds. *Journal of Speech and Hearing Disorders,* 1948, **13,** 31-34.

JAKOBSON, R. Aphasia as a linguistic problem. In H. Werner (Ed.), *On expressive language.* Worcester, Mass.: Clark University Press, 1955.

JAKOBSON, R. Linguistics and poetics. In T. A. Sebeok (Ed.), *Style in language.* Cambridge, Mass.: MIT Press, 1960.

KANNER, L. Irrelevant and metaphorical language in early infantile autism. *American Journal of Psychiatry,* 1946, **103,** 242-246.

LENNEBURG, E. H. *Biological foundations of language.* New York: Wiley, 1967.

MAHLER, M. *On human symbiosis and the vicissitudes of individuation.* New York: International Universities Press, 1968.

McCARTHY, D. A. *The language development of the preschool child.* Minneapolis: University of Minnesota Press, 1960.

PIAGET, J. *The language and thought of the child.* Cleveland: World, 1963. (Originally published in 1923.)

RIMLAND, B. *Infantile autism: The syndrome and its implications for a neural theory of behavior.* New York. Appleton-Century-Crofts, 1964.

RUTTER, M. Concepts of autism: A review. *Journal of Child Psychology and Psychiatry,* 1968, **9,** 1-25.

SAMPSON, O. C. A study of speech development in children of 18-30 months. *British Journal of Educational Psychology,* 1945, **20,** 144-201.

SHAPIRO, T. *(Infant psychiatry.)* L. Sander and T. Shapiro (Eds.). New Haven: Yale University Press. In press.

SHAPIRO, T., & FISH, B. A method to study language deviation as an aspect of ego organization in young schizophrenic children. *Journal of the American Academy of Child Psychiatry,* 1969, **8,**

SHAPIRO, T., FISH, B., & GINSBERG, G. L. The speech of a schizophrenic child from two to six. *American Journal of Psychiatry,* 1972, **128,** 11.

SHAPIRO, T., HUEBNER, H., & CAMPBELL, M. Language development and hierarchic integration. *Journal of Autism and Childhood Schizophrenia,* 1974, **4,** 71-90.

SHAPIRO, T., ROBERTS, A., & FISH, B. *Imitation and echoing in young schizophrenic children,* 1970, Vol. 9. No. 3.

SHAPIRO, T., CHIARANDINI, I., & FISH, B. Thirty psychotic children: evaluation of their language development for classification and propensity. *Archives of General Psychiatry,* 1974, **30,** 819-825.

VIGOTSKY, L. S. *Thought and language.* Cambridge, Mass.: MIT Press, 1962 (originally published in 1934).

RESEARCH IN THE NEW FIELD OF PSYCHOEDUCATION

A CASE STUDY OF A RESEARCH PROJECT ON THE CONTENT OF FIRST-GRADE READING TEXTBOOKS

GASTON E. BLOM

Psychoeducation is a relatively new concept in the child mental health field, even though it has had much longer usage in the field of special education. However what it means conceptually and operationally varies considerably and may indeed represent more of a slogan or a lip-service term than practices and principles that represent a true integration of two broad streams of professional thought: (1) the education and training professions, and (2) the clinical mental health professions. In many clinical and educational settings these professional groups are separate; in other settings they coexist or merely add to each other. What I am referring to as psychoeducation represents an integration in which the result is different from the sum of two parts.

In 1962 an opportunity occurred to develop a psychoeducational program for elementary-school-age children with academic and behavior problems in the Child Psychiatry Division of the Department of Psychiatry at the University of Colorado Medical Center in Denver, Colorado. More traditional professionals might view this program as a psychiatric day hospital for children with educational input if they were medically oriented or as a therapeutic school if they were educationally based. We need not argue with those who wish to place our program in more traditional molds, though we have explained what psychoeducation means to us in a number of publications (Blom, 1968; Blom *et al.*, 1966, 1972).

GASTON E. BLOM, Professor of Psychiatry and Education, University of Colorado Medical Center, Denver.

Our program was conceptualized and initiated by a psychiatrist, a psychologist, a social worker, and an educator, hopefully as equal partners, all of whom were not satisfied with their traditional operations. To be sure the original director of this enterprise was myself, a child psychiatrist and psychoanalyst, and undoubtedly influential in determining the course of our development. Yet over the course of time I have been both criticized and praised for my opinions and accents and in my opinion honored on a number of occasions by being misidentified as a reading specialist, an educator, a psychologist, a laboratory researcher, etc. I was at one time listed on the School of Education faculty as having a M.Ed. degree, a revision made by a secretary from *M.D.!*

From the onset, in addition to viewing our functions as including services to children and families; the training of various professional students including teachers, nurses, occupational therapists, and lay therapists, as well as the more usual ones; and consultation with public schools, we also saw research as a very central activity. The Day Care Center, as we have been called, was viewed as a laboratory in psychoeducation with a focus on school-related issues. Since 1962 the staff has published 72 papers, which include in their range clinical reports, conceptual contributions, evaluation studies, educational issues, and experimental studies. They have been based on our own population of children as well as those in public elementary schools. The subjects of these publications have included teacher management issues, the concept of perceptually handicapped children, behavior modification, instructional programs, classroom social engineering, and others. We have also focused on the nature and effectiveness of curriculum materials, a particular one being first-grade reading textbooks—the subject of this case study research report. We have been fortunate to have relationships with many public schools in the Denver metropolitan area. We have made certain contributions to them, while they have returned more contributions to us in facilitating our work in service, training, consultation, and research. Without such relationships we could not have been as productive in our work. In addition to basic funding from the university and from patients' fees, funds have been obtained for special purposes from private donors, private foundations, and government agencies. These funding sources have also made a most significant contribution to our work.

The psychoeducational setting of the Day Care Center created the climate for the research study that I will report—a collaborative research project on the content analysis of reading textbooks from the United States and other countries and the influence of content on reading and other behaviors of children. I will present a case study of this research that covers 11 years, from 1962 to 1973. There have been 26 published studies of our findings, most of which have been collected and rewritten in a recent book edited by Sara G.

Zimet (1972). I will not condense these many findings, which the reader can obtain through the references at the end of this chapter. Rather, I will focus on the process of this research study. In this way perhaps I can convey some of the excitement and despair, the tedious disciplined activities, the poor leads, the unreplicated results, and the overall satisfactions that came from this endeavor. This is also a good time to write about this research experience, since two of us who remained with the project over most of this time felt that 11 years was long enough to study primers! Last summer the current group of us decided to go in a new direction—to study the relationships between aggression and learning.

The case study begins at a PTA meeting in 1962 at the suburban elementary school that all four of our children attended. I was a parent at that meeting, but as it was concluding, one of the first-grade teachers and I began to discuss the much higher incidence of boys than girls with reading problems. We went through the usual possibilities of identification problems of boys with women teachers, the schools' expectations relative to girls' behaviors, and the lip service given to sexual differences in behaviors and other biological, psychological, and social factors. Then one of us brought up the question of reading textbooks and whether they were written primarily by women for girl readers. We also thought further about content in relation to some of the jibes, criticisms, and subjective statements that were appearing in the press and books at that time, sometimes called the "Sputnik era." We wondered whether it was possible to analyze the content of primers systematically so as to make generalizations about them that were meaningful and that related them to the problem of reading disability. The following day I spoke to a psychologist colleague on the Day Care Center staff about our discussion, and he recalled the agonies he experienced as a child reading "that stuff" and as a parent going over primer reading with his children. We thought it might be interesting to see if the three of us could develop some impressions from reading various primers.

So the three of us began to meet on Saturday mornings in a regular way. The teacher brought the books, which were published before 1962—an important detail, since it explained some research findings that were generated one and a half years later. We read them together, looking at the pictures and characters, and began developing impressions, which we wrote down as our minutes: young age interests, few older children, family settings, middle-class environments, no aggressive words or themes, boys' activities unsuccessful, Anglo-Saxon people and names, suburban settings, cleanliness, etc. Then we read books separately, noted our impressions independently, and compared them. Our impressions began to coalesce around three central ideas: (1) that the content presented more girl activity themes than boy activity; (2) that when boys' activity was presented, it ended more often in failure then did girls' activity; and (3) that the activities were those of interest to children of a younger age than first grade. At this point we developed a questionnaire that contained primer stories and requested the respondent to rate them according to these three dimensions. We first asked first-year psychiatric residents to reply, and their responses agreed with the assessments of the three investigators. The same procedure was repeated with freshman English classes at two local universities, arranged by the teacher on our research team. She was at that time doing graduate work in librarianship and began a systematic review of the educational and psychological literature on our topic for a master's thesis, which served our research purposes very well. Our original impressions of the story content were supported by psychiatric residents and freshman English students, but when we were ready to write up our findings, the 150 questionnaires were missing! We recovered by devising a semantic differential scoring system for stories, which was soon discarded in favor of more direct measures.

At this time we had not found any published systematic studies on the content of primers, although McClelland's (1961) work on third-grade texts and Child's studies (Child, Porter, and Levine, 1946) were known to us. Both reports indicated that the stories from grades lower then third were too simple for content analysis studies. We did not agree with that impression. However, I was never sure that someone had not already done work similar to our own in spite of searching the literature. That concern still remains slightly after repeated and continuous searches, though it has abated from those early years, and I am almost inclined to believe that our work represented original contributions. During the second year of the study the group obtained a small research grant from the National Institute of Mental Health, and another member joined our research group. She had an unusual background of graduate education training, teaching experience, and psychological interests. She was later able to do a doctoral dissertation in education on sex roles as depicted in American primers from the colonial period to the present. This represented a contribution to the research and a personal gain to her—a kind of having-your-cake-and-eating-it-too phenomenon and a repeat performance from the previous year, at that!

We had in a sense demonstrated in a systematic impressionistic way that other adults' views of primer content were similar to those of the research group. Then the question was considered: Would first-grade children see content in a similar way to adults? At first we interviewed first-grade children individually, showing them various books, reading stories with them, and then doing an inquiry into their reactions and impressions. The tape-recorded results were not very satisfactory for scoring purposes, so we designed a focused study that made use of pictorial rating scales on the dimensions of the sex of the activity of the story, the age of the activity, and the outcome of the activity. A number of stories were read to children individually in two first-grade classes, and they were asked to rate them on the pictorial scales one by one. The results were clear, particularly for age and sex of activity, and agreed with adult ratings of the same stories. The results on the outcome scale were ambiguous, and we recognized that it was an affect scale of happy to sad and that the stories frequently had laughter and smiling associated with a failure outcome and no evidence of sadness in any of the characters. The children were responding to this confusion in what was being communicated.

The four members of the research group decided we had demonstrated that both adults and children tended to view primer content in a similar way, but we needed to develop a precise way of determining that content. Therefore we started to construct a content-analysis coding manual in 1963 that contained scaled dimensions, such as predominant theme, character distribution, age of activity, sex of activity, and outcome of activity. This manual went through a number of revisions, so that the final 1969 version contained 14 dimensions with defined categories within them. One of our major problems was developing scales for the age and sex of activity. These did not exist in the literature, though behaviors associated with age and sex were present in diverse sources. We worked on this problem into the following year, eventually defining criteria and guidelines for these ratings. It so happened several years later that we were accused of male chauvinism by some feminists for developing a stereotypical sex-behavior rating scale! As this was going on, we formulated our initial impressions of the content as three hypotheses and applied for NIMH funds to continue our work. As if this was not enough to do, one member of our group made inquiries of publishers regarding their selection of authors and decisions about the content of stories. The responses from publishers were indignant, defensive, and often rationalized. Many claimed they were written by authors knowledgeable about child development and were reviewed by "experts" in this field!

With grant funds we were able to proceed into the third year. Three medical students became interested in our project during the year (1964–1965) and assisted us in the collection of data, hopefully learning something about research in the process. The following year (1965–1966) two psychiatric residents joined our research group, as well as one medical student. Our original first-grade teacher could not continue, since the project had become much more than a Saturday morning and evening affair.

During the third year we refined our coding manual on motivational content dimensions, so that it could be applied to American reading textbook stories by trained raters working independently. These raters were consistently able to achieve 93 percent agreement on independent ratings, but it took time to train them and refine the rating process. There was some struggle in defining and obtaining the sample of stories to be rated so that it would be representative of American primers. We came across an unpublished study of a national survey of commonly used first-grade readers and finally tracked down the author in Normal, Alabama, by telephone. He graciously made his data available to us (Hollins, 1955). As a result our sample consisted of 1307 stories from 12 of the most commonly used reading textbook series in the United States. This was identified as the National Sample and the findings were published as our first paper. The three hypotheses were tested out and only one of them achieved statistical significance. This was a disappointment, since we had a degree of conviction about the validity of our impressions. Then one Saturday morning one member of our group was going over the textbooks from which we had derived our impressions and happened to look at a page with the publishing date. He got a hunch that perhaps there was a difference in content in relation to date of publication. So the data on the 12 series were split between those books published before 1962 and after. The analysis of the data treated in this way showed that all three hypotheses were confirmed by statistical significance on the stories published before 1962 and only one hypothesis had significance for those published after that data! This was a mixed blessing: a confirmation that we were correct but that the hypotheses came from books of an earlier publication date and did not generalize to the entire sample. So there was no Nobel Prize in that effort, yet it was interesting. Still many schools in our country were using reading textbooks from this early period and probably still are. Furthermore there was considerable evidence that the content of primers remains inappropriate in relation to sex roles, cultural differences, developmental interests, and the depiction of real life. The idea of change over historical time did not escape us, since sometime later a study was made of the content of primers from the colonial period to the present, covering six historical periods of cultural change.

During the summer of that third year (1964–1965) two medical students worked with the research group and used our pictorial scale study with a group of migrant children in an area of Colorado north of Denver. The findings from this group did not agree with those obtained from middle-class first-grade children on the dimensions of age, sex, and outcome. Inquiry led to the impression that the activities in the stories were in general alien to them, and they frequently rated them as older age activities because maybe they would occur later in their lives.

It goes without saying that we could not have dealt with such quantities of data without computer methods. Using a computer necessitated collecting data in a form that could be handled by such methods and having technicians and consultants who could advise us. While all of us learned how to do chi-squares by hand, I would hardly recommend it as a steady diet, nor is it realistically necessary or feasible to do so. The computer also made it possible to factor-analyze our content-analysis data on 1307 stories. The results, while intellectually interesting, were of no particular benefit in reducing the dimensions to fewer factors. Actually there were seven factors, which accounted for 40 percent of the variance, and it was difficult to conceptualize them any better than what we had from our original dimensions. This was an illustration of how elegant statistical treatment, including loadings on factors, was not fruitful or beneficial to what we wanted to discover and communicate. Descriptive and probability statistics were sufficient for our purposes. I suppose as a side benefit I was learning more about statistical methods and developing a respect for their meaning, value, and limitations.

This third year (1964–1965) was really a turning point in our research. We were invited to join a consortium called Project Literacy, which was located at Cornell University in New York. This group was organizing reading research efforts in the country through government funding, with the goal of developing a more sound basis for reading instruction approaches. Periodically researchers in this consortium met to discuss their research ideas and results and to obtain reactions, responses, and suggestions. These meetings provided us with an interesting forum not only to present our research but also to learn from a wider group of professionals: linguists, educators, and psychologists in various fields of endeavor. Through Project Literacy's good offices we were assisted in obtaining a more fully funded research grant from the Office of Education for three years (1965–1968). While Project Literacy did not accomplish its ambitious aims, it fostered research of high quality and eventually compiled a number of interesting studies in a publication (Levin and Williams, 1970).

The next three years of our research (1965–1968) were highly productive. We became interested in the newly appearing "multiethnic urban" series, many of which turned out to be not very ethnic nor particularly urban. Some of our published findings "burned" a few publishers, but it was hard for them to argue about percentages and chi-squares. We had developed at that time two further content dimensions: environmental setting and ethnic composition of characters based on skin color. Then we became interested in the attitudes and values that were communicated in some of the multiethnic stories. One of our group did a type of TAT analysis of black and white families in one series that pointed to prejudicial stereotypes in spite of the publisher's conscious efforts to avoid stereotypes (Zimet, 1972). An increased interest in attitudinal content developed, and new attitude scales for content analysis were constructed. This construction was again a very tedious effort, but eventually it paid off in the development of 40 attitude scales grouped according to cultural posture, other-directed posture, and inner-directed posture. On these scales we were able to obtain consistent reliabilities of above 75 percent agreement between trained independent raters. This lower reliability of 75 percent as compared to 93 percent for the motivational scales was expected in view of the greater difficulty of the rating task. However, we decided to use consensus ratings on all our attitude findings.

Prior to the construction of the attitude scales we had started to collect a few primers from some other countries: French Quebec, Russia, Argentina, and Japan. We did this through professional friends, and we were quite excited about the differences in content among them from visual inspection. Since our attitude scales were paying off, we wondered how we might get representative samples of primers from a number of foreign countries. At that time one of the psychiatric residents in our research group was planning to attend a conference in Washington, D.C., and we suggested he might go up and down Embassy Row requesting primers. It happened that this was not the strategy that paid off, nor did going to various offices in the Office of Education. Rather, through a Colorado Senator's office, contact was made with a director in the United States Information Agency who was also a Coloradan. He agreed to contact agents in a number of countries to send us representative first-grade reading textbooks. A delightful description of this episode was presented in a memo to our group, entitled "Consultation with Washington Regarding the Attainment of Foreign Primers (Childe Roland to the Dark Tower Cometh)." Through the cooperation of the USIA we obtained primers from 18 countries. Since the agent in South Korea thought an English translation of the stories was part of the instructions, we included South Korea in one of our earliest studies. With these additions to our collection and some that subsequently came from other sources, we have primers from 20 countries: England, Norway, Sweden, Denmark, Finland, Russia, West Germany, France, Italy, Greece, Turkey, Israel, India, Japan, South Korea, Australia, Argentina, Mexico, French and English Canada, and the United States. Translations of primers from 11 countries were done by graduate students, and a stratified random sampling of 60 stories from 13 countries was used on which we obtained attitude-content ratings. We slowly developed this data bank, publishing findings along the way. Through statistical consultation a partitioned chi-square was used as a way to compare findings among countries in terms of differences and similarities (Castellan, 1965). We also compared our findings from the content analysis of primers with other cross-national studies (Hess and Torney, 1967; Holmes, 1960; McClelland, 1961). So we saw primers not only as serving instrumental functions (i.e., of teaching and learning to read) but also as having contents with motivational elements and socializing functions. Furthermore, the success of primers in facilitating reading acquisition might be dependent on motivational and attitudinal content, regardless of the method of reading instruction emphasized.

We thought that content might have a particular influence on nonwhite children. So one of our research staff trained a Chicano and a black college student to interview first-grade children of Chicano and black ethnic origins (respectively) regarding stories that they would like to read in school. These interviews were tape-recorded, but we did not have sufficient staff time to analyze their responses systematically (10 interviews of 30 minutes each). We did think of using the general inquiry method of computer analysis for this purpose but felt that we already had enough irons in the fire to manage. In listening to these tapes we got the impression that they contained far more fantasy, aggressive actions, and strong affects than any primer stories displayed. So what children wished to read and what they were offered were in striking contrast. This issue was studied in a number of other ways. Another member of our research group interviewed black and white first-grade children in a number of school settings, comparing their reactions and choices to a series of questions about an all-white primer and a multiethnic primer. Other research staff did two library-selection studies of first-grade children, one in a suburban school and the other in a urban school. The content that children selected to read and did not select was compared to the content findings in our national sample. These findings confirmed our impressions about the differences between what children want to read and what they have to read. A consultation visit with Daniel Fader further confirmed that but with the added input of his stimulating, interesting, and enthusiastic comments (Fader and McNeil, 1968).

Following this three-year period (1965–1968) we obtained a five-year grant from NICHD to study further the impact of content on the behavior of children. As indicated previously, we had the psychoeducational laboratory of the Day Care Center in which to do clinical naturalistic studies of individual children. The teaching staff was sensitive to content issues in facilitating or impeding learning, and specifically in reading. Our findings pointed to the need to individualize choices of stories, since in one instance we were shocked to discover that one child preferred Dick and Jane stories because they were more orderly and predictable than her real-life situation! Another child could even eroticize *Dick* and *but* in these stories! So with this in mind we published a book that indexed the contents of 116 primers from 16 publishers containing 2443 stories (Zimet, Blom, and Waite, 1968). We hoped that first-grade teachers, reading teachers, and school librarians might find this index useful in selecting stories for individual children. It was no best seller and provided no royalties, because the minimum number of copies were not sold!

Then we did a rather neat little study in which the computer was asked to select stories whose content varied on only one variable and kept nine others constant. We used a paired-comparison design in which first-grade children were asked to indicate a preference between two stories contrasted on one variable, such as older age activity versus younger age activity. Our results made sense in terms of what children preferred.

For a considerable period of time we became involved in writing high-

and low-impact stories and rating words (mostly monosyllabic verbs) according to emotional impact. One of our studies demonstrated that late kindergarten children recalled high-aggressive verbs more frequently than low-aggressive verbs (Camp and Zimet, 1973). When frequency of usage was taken into account, both high-aggressive and low-aggressive words of middle frequency were remembered best. It seemed that when frequency of usage goes up, emotional impact goes down. However, the study did not establish that better recall is accompanied by better retention over time. If this could be demonstrated, then mid-frequency words, in general, and high-aggressive mid-frequency words, in particular, should receive greater emphasis in primer vocabularies. The vocabularies of reading textbooks used in most schools today are characterized by a plethora of low-aggressive–high-frequency words.

Because of limitations in funds and time we decided not to continue to write stories with high-impact content. However, we developed greater empathy for authors of textbooks during that process. There were the strictures imposed by vocabulary and syntactic control to be considered. We recognized that a total emphasis on high impact might turn many children off or overly excite them. So there should be variety. We also experienced conflict between presenting situations as they are versus how they ought to be and between resolving difficult realistic dilemmas in stories versus leaving them unfinished. So there were problems in presenting realism or idealism, including language usage: should our stories be written about slums, ethnic bias, divorce, and handicap, or about successful, happy ethnic integration, family life, and recovery from illness? Our answer was to include both what is and what should be, a mixture of realism and idealism—a task that was difficult indeed, especially for a group of researchers with social activist attitudes. For a short time we also wrote stories with low-impact content, which created even greater difficulties for us!

We gave up writing stories when two recently published first-grade reading series were discovered that had strikingly different content. So primers with contrasting content were available for testing their differing effects on reading achievement and other behaviors of children. Considerable pilot work was done, as well as some short-term studies on various measures that we considered using in a first-grade study: aggressive behaviors, systematic daily observations and ratings of children on deviant and on-task behavior, attitude toward reading, and teachers' management styles. After we decided which test measures and ratings to use, 54 children in two first-grade classes in a racially integrated, lower-middle-class, urban elementary school were selected as the object of study for the entire school year. The purpose of this study was to assess the relationship between the content of stories in two reading series and four variables (deviant and on-task behavior, attitude toward reading, and reading achievement). The results showed no significant differences on the mean scores of reading achievement between the two classes. Unlike other studies, no sexual differences were found on any of the achievement measures within or between classes. Both experimental classes reached significantly higher achievement in reading than the previous year's classes of the same two experienced teachers. The Hawthorne effect was probably responsible for this finding. There were also no differences in attitude toward reading scores between the two classes. The difficulty of singling out content as a significant influential variable for study in a dynamic classroom setting was very apparent. There were obviously many variables operating in this field and interacting in a complex way. Similar problems were found by other researchers when attempting to evaluate the effectiveness of different instructional methods in first-grade reading (Chall, 1967). We were also not very satisfied with the attitude toward reading measures. In retrospect one might say we should have known better than to have done the global experiment, even though it was a pilot in nature. However, it had not been done before, and the lack of results did not in our mind lead to the conclusion that content was unimportant. Other approaches of assessing its influence had to be used that had better control over the variables involved.

In addition to these national studies our interest in cross-national studies continued during 1968–1973. A comparison of attitude content in reading primers from 13 countries was completed. Both motivational and attitude content in textbooks from 6 countries were examined, representing our most complete comparative data. In this study attitudes associated with male and female characterization were determined, i.e., how sex-role attributes were displayed. A particularly interesting finding was that antisocial attitudes were displayed almost exclusively by animal characters in the United States primers. Similar but less strong trends were present in England, while the 4 other countries (Russia, South Korea, Italy, and West Germany) displayed them by humans (children and adults). A possible interpretation of this finding is that the United States displaces and projects aggression rather than directly socializing it in its culture—a provocative, disputable viewpoint worthy of further examination. National gestalts were formulated for each of the 6 countries based on the content-analysis data. Another study examined attitude ratings of stories from Israel in the light of stated educational goals by the Israeli Ministry of Education and compared the content of secular school textbooks and religious school textbooks. Our results indicated that findings were not entirely consistent with educational goals and philosophy. Such discrepancies can be brought to the attention of educational authorities for appropriate modifications in textbook content.

A further cross-national study developed during 1972–1973 as a result of my taking a seven-month sabbatical leave in Copenhagen, Denmark. During that time I visited 32 reading specialists in 14 countries to obtain information

and impressions on a large number of factors related to reading achievement
and reading disability. Some of our research findings were shared with these
professionals. During a visit to the School of Education at the University of
Oulu in Finland, I conducted a class over several days whose students applied
our content-analysis procedures to Finnish textbooks! On another occasion I
presented impressions on factors related to reading to the Danish Reading
Association. I revised a previous position paper on sexual differences in
reading achievement and reading disability (Blom, 1971), which has yet to be
published. Based on the professional visits indicated above, I developed an
opinion questionnaire on factors related to reading achievement and reading
disability in collaboration with Mogens Jansen, Director of the Danish Institute for Educational Research. This is a questionnaire containing ratings
and judgments on a large number of structured questions. There are 162
scorable items. It was printed and sent to three reading professionals known to
Jansen and/or me in each of 14 countries (Iceland, Denmark, Norway,
Sweden, Finland, France, West Germany, Russia, England, Ireland, Scotland,
Italy, Greece, and the United States). As of this date we have received 27
replies from 12 countries and expect to analyze these opinion data so as to
make statements about the reading situation in each country and about comparisons among countries.

During the last five years of the research project a number of us have
been invited to join various national efforts regarding reading. I was a member
of one of these groups, the National Advisory Committee on Dyslexia and Related Reading Disorders (HEW) from 1968 to 1969; this committee published
a report of its findings and recommendations (Reading Disorders in the United
States, 1969) and a compilation of a number of position papers (Reading
Forum, 1971). While the committee's impact on government action and planning was limited, attention was called to reading disability as a national
concern and problem. My perspective on reading was greatly enhanced as a
result of this national activity. Currently another member of our research
group has collaborated with the National Education Association in the
publication of a reading kit for teachers to develop critical reading in children.
The goal of this program is to help children to be aware of biases, unrealities,
and misinformation in the content of what they read. These two examples
represent attempts to deal with the social implications of our research.

To provide one index of the quantity of work done over these 11 years in
content analyses, we developed 467 variables for the American historical
primers, 103 motivational variables, and 94 attitude variables. This makes a
total of 664 variables rated on various story samples. There were 360 stories in
the historical study, 2503 stories in various national studies, and 720 stories in
primers from 12 other countries. This does not include the great number of

other variables from tests, ratings, and observations of and by children, teachers, researchers, and other adults. Again, it is clear that the processing and analyzing of so many variables could not have been done without computer methods. So while the ideas were designed by humans and the interpretations made by humans, the processings between were done by machine. So in addition to the acknowledgements made at the beginning of this presentation to the Day Care Center, to public schools, and to funding agencies, a final one should be made to the computer!

Conclusions

To some extent our first-grade study represented the culmination of our efforts in this content-analysis research. The fact that in a complex field content was not a strong enough variable by itself to show significant results was of course a disappointment. There were many adventitious findings, such as the influence of substitute teachers on pupils' behaviors and the discovery that certain teacher and pupil behaviors could be systematically measured. At some later time we may go back to some of these findings and will indeed use the experiences and training that came from our endeavors.

However, we are now tired of studying primers, even though we have collected a unique library of them from the United States and 19 foreign countries. We have published our findings and presented them to many professional and lay groups in this country and abroad. Both praise and criticism have come our way in both written and verbal forms. Many of the unpublished studies would be especially appropriate for the *Journal of Irreproducible Results*. We have also collected jibes, cartoons, and comic strips that refer to first-grade reading textbooks. We have tried to influence textbook publishers, book selection committees, and superintendents to be sensitive to appropriate content for both instructional and socialization purposes. We have an interesting library of professional books related to our studies and an indexed compilation of reprints and studies in our files. We have had many stimulating thoughts and helpful suggestions from consultants.

So while we had wished for more definitive proof, our work has not been without substantive results. However, one of the most important satisfactions that came from this long endeavor was the dialogues in our research team and the problem-solving tasks that we did together. It was hard work that contained moments of discovery, disappointment, humor, and diligence. While these are satisfactions in their own right, they also have influenced my behavior as a clinician and a teacher—to think more clearly, systematically, and knowledgeably and to do that with a perspective of humor and modesty.

References

Blom, G. E. The psychoeducational approach to emotionally disturbed children. *Medical Record and Annals*, 1968, **61**, 348–351.

Blom, G. E. Sex differences in reading disability. In NINDS Monograph #1, *Reading Forum*, 31–46. Washington, D.C.: Government Printing Office, 1971.

Blom, G. E., Ekanger, C. A., Parsons, P., Prodoehl, M., & Rudnick, M. A psychoeducational approach to day care treatment. *Journal of American Academy of Child Psychiatry*, 1972, **11**, 492–510.

Blom, G. E., Rudnick, M., & Searles, J. Some principles and practices in the psychoeducational treatment of emotionally disturbed children. *Psychology in the schools*, 1966, **3**, 30–38.

Camp, B., & Zimet, S. G. Recall of aggressive words by kindergarten children. *Psychological Reports*, 1973, **33**, 575–578.

Castellan, N. J. On the partitioning of contingency tables. *Psychological Bulletin*, 1965, **64**, 330–338.

Chall, J. *Learning to Read: The Great Debate*. New York: McGraw-Hill, 1967.

Child, I. L., Porter, E. H., & Levine, E. M. Children's textbooks and personality development. *Psychological Monographs*, 1946, **60**, 1–54.

Fader, D., & McNeil, E. *Hooked on books: Program and proof*. New York: Berkley Publishing Corporation, 1968.

Hess, R. D., & Torney, J. V. *The development of political attitudes in children*. Chicago: Aldine, 1967.

Hollins, W. H. A national survey of commonly used first-grade readers. Unpublished data, Alabama A and M College, 1955.

Holmes, M. B. A cross cultural study of the relationship between values and modal conscience. In W. Muensterberger and S. Axelrod (Eds.), *The psychoanalytic study of society*. New York: International Universities Press, 1960, Vol. 1.

The Journal of Irreproducible Results—Official Organ of the Society for Basic Irreproducible Research. Chicago Heights, Ill. 60411.

Levin, H., & Williams, J. (Eds.), *Basic studies on reading*. New York: Basic Books, 1970.

McClelland, D. C. *The achieving society*. Princeton, N.J.: Van Nostrand, 1961.

Reading Disorders in the United States. Report of the Secretary's (HEW) National Advisory Committee on Dyslexia and Related Reading Disorders. August, 1969. U.S. Department of Health, Education and Welfare.

Zimet, S. (Ed.), *What children read in school: Critical analysis of primary reading textbooks*. New York: Grune & Stratton, 1972.

Zimet, S. G., Blom, G. E., & Waite, R. R. *A teacher's guide for selecting stories of interest to children*. Detroit: Wayne State University Press, 1968.

NATURALISTIC
RESEARCH

INTRODUCTION

Naturalistic studies, as described in this chapter, are closely modeled on the approach taken by anthropologists entering a target culture. The observer attempts to obtain a dual perspective on the culture: he looks at it through the eyes of individuals belonging to the culture and also through his own eyes. This dual perspective provides him with a bifocal experience from the inside as well as from the outside, and the contrasts between the two furnish yet a third set of data.

There is a second bifocal experience that is equally illuminating: the differences that emerge from individual and group contacts. The individual is more inclined to describe his own special predicament within the group and the existential concerns that go with it; the group brings its own dynamics to bear on the problem being considered, and its interactional account adds a further dimension to the individual viewpoint.

The families being studied are those with an adult psychotic member, a parent, which immediately marks them as "different"—the notion of *difference* having a negative connotation. Considered in anthropological terms, the attributes characterizing these families lie over and beyond those distinguishing the modal families of the culture. They take the following forms:

1. *Emotional inbreeding* is the common tendency of the family members to concentrate all their emotional energies on one another with the exclusion of anyone else, putting, as it were, all their emotional eggs in one basket. The process is therefore highly centripetal. The families remain isolated from other families and mostly self-contained. Contacts outside the group are relatively infrequent, and the longer the isolation persists, the more the ability to form affiliations is attenuated.

2. The isolation of the family and its emotional overinvestment in itself is further accentuated by an "egocentrism" that leads it to believe that its own ways of behaving are the only ways of behaving. As a result, its tolerance for its own eccentricities may be considerably raised since no external standards are available for comparison.

3. The conditions of life within the family are bewilderingly "ambiguous," so that family members are unclear in their own minds what is taking place between them in any given place, at any given time. Misperceptions and misconceptions are therefore fairly common but unobserved within the group.

The stranger in the group, however, has quite a different perspective on the situation. She is immediately aware of its exclusiveness, its self-absorption, and its nebulous frames of exchange as she enters the alien world. As described

337

in this chapter, she becomes a barometer that sensitively registers the cultural gap between herself and the new milieu.

Living with patients has been done for many centuries within institutions. In order to tolerate the proximity of psychotic individuals, the staff of such institutions normally develop defensive "distancing" mechanisms that help to keep the patients within certain bounds. In recent years this distancing process has been examined and held responsible for some of the "chronic" behavior seen and described in institutionalized individuals.

The living-in undertaken in this research is different in that the observer has had no time to develop immunities to psychotic life, and consequently the observer invariably (and perhaps inevitably) develops minor disorders. Instead of being treated as contaminants, these are carefully examined for the light they throw on the situation. This is in the tradition of the great psychiatrist, Johann Weyer, who in the sixteenth century occasionally took patients home to live with him so as to understand them better; and in our times Minkowski, the well-known French psychiatrist, elected to live with his patients for as long as two months at a time in order to further his *"inward experience of their illness."* The British psychoanalyst Winnicott took a disturbed boy into his wartime household and subsequently described what happened in a well-known paper the title of which speaks for itself: "Hate and the Countertransference"!

Therefore, not only is our observer very visible but her presence is a provocation to those she is observing as they respond to her and she to them. She knows why she is there but they have to find an explanation for her presence, and this need will further influence their behavior when she is around. Who she is and what she is will also have their effects. Anthropologists are well aware of this, to quote Barnouw (1963):

> Another kind of difficulty which may affect the process of observation concerns the nature of the observer. An observer may project; he may have blind spots to certain aspects of behavior and be unduly attentive or sensitive to others. What he sees may be influenced by his mood or by his attitudes and values. . . . His mood, as he works, may be influenced by any number of things—the nature of his living quarters, the response he has met within the community. He may feel somewhat homesick and ambivalent about fieldwork. He may fall ill. Any of these factors, or others, may bring about distortions in what he observes and records. As some have put it, a culture may be seen as a sort of huge Roschach blot, in which different ethnologists with different personality tendencies, may detect different patterns [p. 191].

We accept this as an inherent feature of participant observation and attempt to turn an apparent weakness into a strength. We use the "inward experience" of illness.

This method of inquiry has its antecedents. The modern psychoanalyst makes use of his countertransference to alert himself to what is going on in his patient; here we are making use of the disturbance engendered in our observer for the purpose of learning what is taking place in the family. This kind of sampling of experience is different from the usual type of sampling, in which the validity of the sample depends on the number of cases; here, to quote Mead and Metraux, validity is a function of "the proper specification of the informant, so that she can be accurately placed [p. 41]." Knowing her, we can know through her.

The presentation demonstrates how much we stand to gain from our colleagues in the behavioral sciences. Of these, the anthropologist is perhaps closest to us in outlook and approach, and we can anticipate the time when he will become an indispensable member of the psychiatric research team.

References

BARNOUW, V., *Culture and personality*. Homewood, Ill.: Dorsey Press, 1963.

MEAD, M., & METRAUX, R. *The study of culture at a distance*. Chicago: University of Chicago Press, 1953.

NATURALISTIC STUDIES OF DISTURBED FAMILIES[1]

E. James Anthony

Preamble

I sat on the side of a wall and watched him, and the longer I sat the more mystified I became. I wanted to ask questions but I knew it would be unwise to do so. He was a 10-year-old boy, very much inside himself, and from previous interviews I had come to realize that the more I questioned him the further he withdrew. He belonged to one of the earliest families with a psychotic parent that I studied when I was still groping for some glimmer of understanding of the lives of these people. I had come out of the house, which was little better than a hovel, in search of fresh air and had found the boy by the roadside drain making and floating little paper boats that traveled some distance and then disappeared suddenly down a manhole. As he launched them on the water he put bits of gravel on board and appeared to be whispering something to himself. What struck me most was his lack of concern at losing his fleet of paper boats. He seemed to watch them go almost with satisfaction. Eventually my curiosity got the better of me and I asked him very gently what he was sending away. For a while he did not answer and then said, very brusquely, "Dirt"! After a further pause, he added, "I'm sending the bad things away from our house and they'll never come back." I wondered aloud what sort of bad things these were and this time he took longer to respond. Then he said very slowly; "All sorts of bad things like my mom being sick and all." After this disclosure he fell back into his usual impenetrable seclusiveness and our interview was over for the day.

[1] This work was supported by Public Health Service Grants MH-12043 and MH-14052 from the National Institute of Mental Health. It was the basis of the Saul Albert Memorial Lecture, McGill University, 1969.

E. JAMES ANTHONY, The Harry Edison Child Development Research Center, Washington University School of Medicine, St. Louis.

341

An Extended Frame of Reference

I thought that I understood the boy's reaction in my usual psychodynamic context, but a few days later I discussed my notes with my co-worker, the anthropologist Jules Henry, who talked of primitive beliefs in the transference of evil and referred me to a passage in Frazer (1949) in which villagers from the island of Ceram, when beset with illness, fill a small ship with food contributed by all the people and send it sailing away. When the disease-laden bark is lost to sight, the people come running out of their houses joyously beating on gongs and on tinkling instruments to celebrate the departure of the sickness.

I mention this little episode as an example of the type of feedback provided by neighboring disciplines in the behavioral sciences. My collaboration with the anthropologist has extended my frame of reference and offered me fresh perspectives, invigorating assumptions, and different approaches to the task of investigation. This was my experience with Jules Henry, who died in St. Louis on September 21, 1969. Without his supervision this part of our work could not have been undertaken. I was profoundly influenced by his belief that "the best way to new discoveries in the field was through study of the disease-bearing vector, the family, in its natural habitat, pursuing its usual life routines—eating, loving, fighting, talking, seeking pleasure, treating sickness, etc.—in other words, following the usual course of its life [1965]." This brought home to me the importance of studying pathology against the background of normality, of becoming increasingly aware of what he referred to as "the uncountable and unremembered series of events" that make up day-to-day living, and of savoring all this at firsthand rather than on the basis of reports.

Since the time of Malinowski anthropologists have lived in with cultural groups, and when Henry turned to the study of the family, he regarded it as a particular subculture that also required penetration and direct experiencing. He carried out his first studies in this new field of the abnormal family in conjunction with Bettelheim, and the collaboration proved remarkably fruitful. When he came to work with me, he was soon able to realize that the dynamic configuration of the family altered significantly when the parent and not the child was psychotic. We had to start afresh and be guided by experience. As Henry pointed out, no one had as yet entered this type of family and it was essential to clarify our concepts of normality and abnormality.

The view of the family as a particular subculture set in the ambience of the general culture allowed us to compare the attitudes and behavior of the smaller with the larger system. There were, in fact, a series of concentric systems—the individual within the family, the family within the class, and the class within the race—so that the preponderant influences shaping family life could derive from individual pathology, family tensions, class pressures, racial discriminations, or a mixture of several of these. We wondered whether our living-in experiences would tell us whether the unusual behavior of a particular family stemmed from the presence of a schizophrenic parent, from the poverty-strickened environment with chronic unemployment, or from racial dissatisfactions, but even if none of these proved to be the cause, we still hoped to learn much more about the separate factors and their interrelationships. With experience we came to realize that what was almost at once clarified was the association between normality and abnormality. Even most abnormal families in our sample did not behave abnormally, in the gross sense, except for certain periods.

> Our crucial experiences in living-in taught us that between the rational and the irrational there lay a complete series of transitional behaviors along a continuum and that watertight compartments of rationality and reality were not compatible with the actuality of human life.
>
> A similar continuum prevailed with regard to reality and unreality along which we also slide in both directions during the course of everyday life. At many moments in the day, under conditions of average stress, we make like compromises with reality refusing to acknowledge its existence at times when it fails to serve our more urgent needs [Anthony, 1972].

It likewise became clear that the abnormal family, like the normal family, ran the whole gamut of custom and tradition and that, apart from episodic deviances, they were as custom-dominated as so-called "normal" families. This was very much in keeping with Dewey's view that the part played by custom in shaping the behavior of individuals far outweighs the effects of their idiosyncrasies. In addition the abnormalities that appeared were often not observable in the tangible sense but were *experienced* by the observer *within himself* as something out of the usual. This meant that the observer had to be studied as much as his observations, since it was his inner apprehension of discrepancy that often threw most light on the phenomena under study. Moreover, if psychosis were in large part a product of family functioning, one might anticipate that the disturbing influence could generate disturbances in the observer, whereas if psychosis were largely an autochthonous production, one would be less likely to expect a profound effect on the observer. (This somewhat simplistic hypothesis was quickly demonstrated to be nonsupportable and, in fact, nontestable, since it was found that the problem of causality remained as complex and ineluctable inside as outside the family milieu.)

The response of the observer to the irrational and unrealistic was summarized thus in Anthony (1972):

> As investigators intermittently in contact with psychosis, we are becoming increasingly aware that our response to the irrational and the unrealistic is not quite the same as that of individuals living at home with a close psychotic relative.

We seem to lack, or to possess in short measure, certain adaptive capacities that
develop only with exposure to the vicissitudes of everyday psychotic functioning.
However, when we intensify our contact over time by entering the family circle, a
curious enculturation gradually takes place and early discomfort, stemming from
mystification, gives way to a surprising acceptance of eccentric phenomena. The
more participant and the less objectively observational that we are, the more
striking is the change in this attitude to acceptance. Nevertheless, we never achieve,
and never hope to achieve, full familial status within the disturbed milieu, and one
of the main factors impeding total assimilation is the exaggerated rationality with
which we tend defensively to counteract exposure to the irrational. Families within
the subculture of psychosis do not, in general, take kindly to strangers, especially
when they unconsciously flaunt their sanity like a professional badge of office. It is
only after we begin to appreciate the elements of irrationality within ourselves, provoked into fuller awareness by the living-in experience, that the degree of acceptance by our ever-suspicious hosts is enhanced.

In naturalistic studies of the family we have, therefore, paid special attention to the reactions and interactions of the participant-observers or par-
ticipant-interviewers with regard to both objective and subjective ideas and
feelings. They have fulfilled a variety of intermediate roles between
observation and participation: at times they are cameras accurately recording
the scene from the outside; at times they are an integral part of the family
interaction; and finally, there are times they become internal reactors to family
pressures directed at them. Thus they can be weather vanes pointing in the direction of prevailing abnormal currents or, when the family is walled off
against them, Trojan horses that gain admission into the very center of the
psychotic citadel.

The Strategies of Penetration

Several naturalistic strategies of penetration have evolved in relation to
family studies; two of these have been developed, not surprisingly, by anthropologists and applied to clinical or quasi-clinical settings. The two techniques
may be described in the following way (see also Figure 1):
1.   *Henry's technique,* in which the observer-participant enters into a
week's living arrangement with the family without preconceptions or expectations. From time to time he dictates his observations into a tape recorder, and
these tapes are later typed without paragraphs, with each page line separately
numbered. The account includes both what he sees and hears and what he
thinks and feels about what he sees and hears, the latter representing, as far as
possible, his immediate, spontaneous reactions. At the end of the week the observer is interrogated closely about his comforts and discomforts in the situation
and any dreams or daydreams occasioned by the experience. (Anthony, 1971)

2. *Lewis's technique,* in which the observer-interviewer meets separately, preferably in their own setting, with the different members of the family, each of whom focuses on the impact, positive or negative, that the sick parent has had on him or her during a remembered lifetime. I have referred to this method, which I have used extensively in my investigation, as "focal interviewing" (Anthony, 1970) and compared it to a type of film making in which a target figure is reconstructed in depth through the different accounts given by members of the family. The observer-interviewer filters these several accounts through himself into the final protocol, adding his own reactions to the total experience.

With Henry's technique the agent either lives in the house or stays with the family from breakfast until bedtime. During the day she hangs about helping with the household chores, the supervision of the children, the shopping, etc., all the while attempting to chat, as naturally as possible, about the everyday things that are of concern to the family, the husband, the wife, or the children. She joins the family on visits to relatives and friends, and if they attend churches and clubs, she goes with them. She is introduced as a visiting friend or relative. She strives at all times to remain passive and compliant unless some emergency or family crisis arises.

Female observer-participants are used, since we have found from experience that they are more smoothly and rapidly assimilated into households and are better able to interchange with the mothers on such topics as infant and child care, household management, the purchase and preparation of food, and the perennial tasks of cleaning and tidying. The woman-to-woman communications reach a level of easy intimacy more quickly and erupt into emotional exchanges without embarrassment.

The observers undergo various degrees of "cultural shock" on the initial encounter but over a week's time are inclined to settle down in the psychotic milieu and assume some of its characteristics. The unstated message from the family is: "If you want to live with us, be like us and act like us." The observer's dilemma is that she must balance the family's need to absorb and control her and her own need for independent thought and action. Anthropologists in new cultures are frequently exposed to a similar conflict. They have reported frustrations, anxieties, paranoid perceptions, inner complaints, and depression. One of them, Golde (1970), has this to say about it:

> The learning of a [new] culture is not an intellectually dispassionate process, nor is it ever necessarily mediated by words; it is direct intuitive learning that seeps through all the senses as it did when we were children being socialized to our own world. Field work can be a replication, condensed in time, of childhood learning with its attendant anxieties, mystification, impotence, and occasional and gradual mastery. We might label this "initiation anxiety" expecting to find perplexity, feelings of powerlessness, unsureness and strain accompanying the process of being inducted into any ongoing, structured situation that is new.

This approach demands a total immersion and a giving over of oneself to a differently organized reality. There is no doubt that this experience of dislocation has a pervasive and compelling consequence. However, it is one of the few ways open to us of realizing an alien (or alienated) point of view, a vision of the world that is another's and not merely a reconstruction within the framework of our own.

Three questions inevitably suggest themselves: How does the observer gain access? To what extent does she distort the family life she is observing? And how does she stand the pressures involved?

The family is told that the living-in arrangement serves the purpose of validating the clinical and experimental findings of the research center. It is pointed out that this is an invaluable method for discerning strain, since the child is observed in his own setting under normal conditions. It has been our experience so far that a fairly strong bond is rapidly created between the observer and the family. Her multiple roles ensure multiple contacts at many different levels. At one end she is a baby-sitter and at the other an omniscient observer with the capacity for powerful psychological insights. She tries to be what the family makes of her. In practice she never "psychologizes" and never intervenes in a therapeutic role. For this reason she should not be a clinician, since it is neither ethical nor usually possible for someone with therapeutic training to refrain from giving help where it is needed. The observer-participants are relatively unsophisticated, undergraduate students who are selected on the basis of their unobtrusiveness, their calmness under stress, their objectivity, and their manifest interest in the human situation. We expect that the family will react to them and that they, in turn, will react to the families, and we expect, therefore, to obtain two sets of data from the two sets of reactions.

During the training period, the observer-participant is exposed to a number of "critical incidents" artifically manufactured and graded in complexity. The incidents are timed to occur when she is unoccupied or participating, when she is near the incident or some distance from it, and when she is visually or aurally oriented toward it. (The last exercise is effected by the simple procedure of blindfolding or "deafening" the observer with ear plugs.) From observing a situation from behind a one-way screen to observing a situation directly while engaged in it is a large step in the process of becoming a proficient reporter, since the distractions during participation can be manifold. The observer-participants must learn to "focus" on the critical incident to the exclusion of all other stimulations. This means that they must develop a hierarchy of significant occurrences and to recognize what is psychologically salient among numerous concomitant incidents.

Both observer-participants and interviewer-participants are expected to become sensitive not only to what they see and hear in others but also to what they perceive in themselves and to realize the value of their own responses to the understanding of any particular situation.

Anthropologists, ethnologists, and psychiatrists have become aware that there is no substitute for observations made in the natural habitat, in unhampered living conditions, and at close range. Schaller (1964), in his firsthand observations of the behavior of gorillas in free-living jungle conditions, has offered some important advice to would-be observers. They should enter the new situation, he says, with the dual expectation that they will learn something not only about the target subjects but also about themselves and that the two learning experiences should go hand in hand. He also thought it essential for them to shed their arrogance and feelings of superiority, to enter the field not expecting hostility and aggression, and to try to maintain under all conditions a "completely consistent observational framework." It is necessary to be as relaxed as possible since the unusual person or stranger can generate a high degree of tension in the group under scrutiny. The response to the observer in the jungle vacillated between the tendencies to run away fearfully and to approach more closely out of curiosity or hostility. If these two incompatible tendencies were well balanced, as was frequently the case, the animal either stayed in one place or exhibited "displacement activity" to reduce the tension. He might feed or scratch himself intensively.

There is something bizarre (as seen from the outside) in the act of living in with animals, and the same is true of living in with psychotics. Schaller (1964) remarks:

> I am sure that the Africans thought me slightly crazy. Why would I leave the cabin day after day, in fog and in rain, to sit and watch gorillas. . . . But to be thought of as peculiar has its advantages, for people tend to accept one's unpredictable behavior and sometimes they show sympathy.

There is, he says, a world of difference between studying apes in captivity and apes in the jungle, just as we have found an equal discrepancy between observing families at home and in the clinic. To carry out home observations is, however, easier said than done. It is not easy to enter the home of a psychotic family, especially when a paranoid parent is guarding the door. Obtaining admission can be a cumbersome business, fraught with anxieties on both sides, and success may depend on the method of approach and on the nature of the family.

Obtaining Admission of the Family Home

To understand the resistance to living in of the family with a psychotic parent, one must first become congnizant of the nature of this type of family. It can be schematized in various ways: in terms of its ambience, its network system, and its degree of openness.

A prominent feature of the ambience is the kinship and friendship system of the nuclear family group. It has generally been found that their "social orbit" has a higher incidence of mental disorder than the orbits surrounding normal families. This, however, is true only of families that have been well established in a neighborhood for at least two generations; it is not true of families that have entered a neighborhood more recently. In the first case the families may be relatively "open" so that various kinship-friendship networks are established, which generally implies that the family is amenable to outside influences and to the processes of change. This openness may, however, alter with any alteration in the psychosis. As the psychotic member deteriorates, affiliations may be severed, and the family may close up and become encapsulated. Other families, especially paranoid ones, may be sealed off from the beginning. The network system may be poorly established, and consequently the family is less susceptible to influence and change.

It is understandably easier for observers to gain admission to open than to closed families. Although admission is not impossible, in certain beleaguered paranoid families the lowering of the drawbridge may be exceedingly slow and accompanied by a good deal of suspicious hesitancy. In the case of one paranoid family that had shifted its habitat several times because of "persecutions," the psychotic father immediately refused to have anything to do with a living-in observer. He suspected that it was a fiendish trick engineered by those plotting against him. After a great deal of talk he reluctantly consented to read a full account of the research. He then called several times to make sure that we did indeed occupy the building from which our letters were addressed. A few weeks later he visited us unexpectedly and to his surprise was

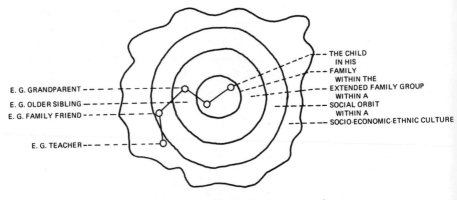

FIG. 1.   An interchangeable functional and network system.

taken on a conducted tour through all the offices and laboratories. He put us to one or two further searching tests and then, quite suddenly, capitulated and very graciously invited the observer "to enjoy the hospitality" of his home.

There is no doubt that once the family becomes "closed," the intrafamilial pathology is intensified, and the levels of reality and rationality steadily decline. The observer in this kind of situation often feels remote from the outside world and cut off from it: "It's like being incarcerated within a setting where the doors and windows no longer let in the familiar world."

The process of closure may take place in well-defined stages: during the "open" phase the psychotic member is treated like any other family member, and the group may deny the sickness by including the patient in all its social activities without mentioning his illness. At a less open phase the family may continue its affiliations and activities within the social orbit, but the patient is kept isolated within the household, often within a single room from which he is not allowed to emerge. This form of segregation is often practiced with a great deal of secrecy, so that even friends of the family may be ignorant of the situation. As full closure is imposed, the family as a whole insulates itself from its ambience and carries out its living requirements with a minimum of external contact or communication (Anthony, 1971).

Access to the home in this intensive way requires the making of a "research alliance" that is resilient enough to withstand the complex emotional demands of investigation. The family may well wonder what they themselves are gaining from the project. They become aware of the scientific curiosity that is driving the investigator and may soon come to realize the extent of his investment in the research. Even for the more exhibitionistic subjects, the process of observation is not in itself sufficient to sustain the alliance over a protracted period of time.

To carry a research family through a longitudinal study, or even a short-term, abbreviated one, requires a considerable degree of involvement on the part of both researcher and subjects and a sense of reciprocity. A one-sided situation inevitably makes the subject feel "used." Both sides must give something to the process if it is to endure. The family as a whole should understand the nature of their contribution and its importance to the project, and the researchers as a group should appreciate the gift of time and effort that is being made to them. Condescension must be avoided at all costs, and the concept of partnership fostered. To this extent the family become co-investigators. Today's subjects are not only more conscious of their human rights but also more aware of their human role, and they require more understanding of what they undertake. In the past Ss were treated like Ss; today they need recognition as people with very specific needs within the context of the research. If the research uncovers a need for treatment, it must be made available; if the research uncovers a diagnostic problem that is relevant to the well-being of the family, it must be disclosed to them. In time therapeutic facilities will be built into all diagnostic clinical research so that therapy and research will go hand in hand. This combination will undoubtedly raise contamination problems for the investigation, but their solution can become an important facet of the research strategy of the future. In our family studies we currently offer not only therapeutic help where it is needed but also diagnostic data when they are pertinent.

In order, therefore, to establish a research alliance, we should carry out clinical research as therapeutically as possible. This attitude implies a therapeutic level of concern and consideration for the subjects and a sensitivity to their experience. The "intake" procedure should be undertaken in the same way as in a general clinic, so that the initial contact is a positive one. If these matters are kept in mind, the alliance can become almost as strong as the therapeutic alliance, and dropouts will be the exception rather than the rule.

Some Methodological Considerations of the Observational Method

The process of observation is currently regarded as far more complex and convoluted than formerly (Anthony, 1968). There is also increasing concern with the reliability and validity of observational data, particularly with respect to the observer and his procedures.

1.   The study of observer bias has indicated that observers are susceptible to observing what they expect to observe. What was long demonstrated in the field of social perception has been rediscovered in observational research. As might be expected in an area highly plagued by motivation, the findings have been conflicting. Under some conditions biases are prominent and under other conditions fairly negligible.

2.   The observer's presence undoubtedly has some effect on family interaction, but the nature and magnitude of this effect have also been much disputed. In one study, for example, in which normal families were sometimes observed by the mothers and sometimes by outside observers, no differences were found except for some reduction in the deviant behavior of the older boys in the family when the observer was present. Some "faking" is certainly possible on the part of the family, but it can rarely be maintained over a period of time, and behavior eventually relapses to the family norm.

3.   It is difficult to assess observer reliability, since it has been found to alter when observers know that they are being tested for reliability. When random assessments are made without the observers' awareness, reliabilities are less impressive. Indoctrination can improve the observer's reliability but raises doubts about validity. For all these reasons, researchers have often become disenchanted with the intricacies and inconsistencies of human

observation and have increasingly turned to mechanical recording procedures. It is our conviction, however, based on considerable experience, that there is no substitute in clinical research for human observation. Rather than doing away with the observer, we have attempted to increase her potential and capitalize on her "humanness." We encourage her to react as "naturally" as possible, and this has led not only to greater acceptance by the family but also to a more rapid habituation to the family milieu. Our policy of using naïve observers unindoctrinated with our viewpoint and expectations has certainly helped in the acculturation.

But to keep observers uninformed is an imperfect solution, since even the most unsophisticated do eventually begin to learn something about the project in which they are engaged, and this knowledge contaminates the data. Instead of struggling to preserve a "clean" field in our study, we have accepted the fact that the observer is to a greater or lesser extent, depending on the circumstance, a distorting mirror and that what she sees must be explored along with what she feels, and is just as revealing. This approach is comparable to the manner in which some therapists make use of their own control responses as indications of what is taking place in the patient. We, therefore, decided to investigate not the influence of the observer on the family but:

1. The influence of the family on the observer.
2. The influence of different types of families on the same observer.

We recognized that to make such an investigation thoroughly, we would have to study the observer in depth, preferably therapeutic depth, and that this was neither possible nor desirable. What seemed feasible to us was a mutual examination of the protocols, with particular attention being paid to events in which the observer was reacting *to* the family, *with* the family, and *on* the family. Since she was asked to behave "as naturally as possible" in the milieu, we anticipated that she would react "naturally" to what she was exposed to.

When we logged these reactions in the context of the events being recorded, the following responses stood out significantly: "cultural shock" resulting from class and ethnic differences; emotional disturbances of anxiety and depression; perplexity resulting from incongruous affects and communications; feelings of alienation on exposure to gross psychotic phenomena (hallucinations and delusions); cognitive dissonance in association with thought disorder (irrationality and illogicality); a dislocation of reality resulting from juxtaposition with unrealistic attitudes and ideas; a sense of confusion stemming from environmental disorganization; urges to fight back against aggressions or to escape from them out of the family; feelings of being trapped and of being picked upon and victimized; a withdrawal into oneself as a defense against the possibility of being overwhelmed; psychosomatic complaints (headaches, abdominal pain, GI disorders, and menstrual disturbances); the fear of becoming crazy (of acting or feeling unrealistically, irrationally, or confusedly); and, finally, disturbing dreams and nightmares.

On second and third assignments the observers became as interested in what they were observing in the family as in what they were observing in themselves. What surprised them most was their realization that many of their reactions were not dissimilar to those of family members. It was a common finding that families appeared less crazy toward the end of the week of living in, which could mean either that the family was adjusting to the observer or that the observer, as one put it, was becoming "a little crazy" herself.

The observer's reactions reflect the milieu as well as her personality. For example, involving families were clearly experienced differently from noninvolving families and closed families from open families. The most difficult assignments were undoubtedly those connected with closed, involving families, which felt "like Hell with No Exit!"

These differential reactions are summarized in Table 1.

The Reduction of One Type of Reality to Another

In one of his most perceptive comments Lévi-Strauss (1967) points out that the understanding of the human situation, whether through

TABLE 1

The Influence of the Psychotic Family on the Observer [a]

Observer's reaction	Involving psychosis	Noninvolving psychosis
"Cultural shock"	+++	+++
Emotional disturbances		
Anxiety	+++	+
Depression	0	+++
Perplexity	+++	+
Alienation	+++	++
Cognitive dissonance	+++	+
Dislocation of reality	+++	+
Confusion	+++	0
Urge to attack	++	0
Urge to escape	+++	+
Paranoidal feelings	++	0
Psychosomatic disorder	++	+
Fear of going crazy	+++	0
"Crazy" dreams and nightmares	+++	+

[a] Ratings by independent assessors from protocols: 0, absent; +, mild; ++, moderate; +++, severe.

psychoanalysis or Marxist analysis, involves the reduction of one type of reality to another. Here he affirms:

> that the true reality is never the most obvious; and that the nature of truth is already indicated by the care it takes to remain elusive. For all cases, the same problem arises, the problem of the relationship between feeling and reason, and the aim is the same: to achieve a kind of *superrationalism*, which will integrate the first with the second, without sacrificing any of its properties.

In our naturalistic work, two levels of rationality are involved: the first is the rationality of the unpsychotic observer, who reduces psychotic reality to her reality, and the second is the *superrationality* of the principal investigators, who attempt to reduce the observer's rationality to a more universal, theoretical rationality. These various rationalities can be envisaged as various geological strata that are interconnected in a meaningful way and subsumed under a unifying structural conception. Each level of rationality has its own special mythology and its own logic, through which the individuals at that level depict, articulate, and master their biological, psychological, and social conditions. The "natural study of man" in this context must take into account the traditions and background of the group under investigation; the way it organizes its time, ruminates over its past, or plans its future; the way it eats or cleans or plays or communicates; and, most of all, the way it deals with the minor crises of everyday life. In penetrating beneath this surface the observer gets in touch with the collective symbolism of the group, as expressed especially in its dreaming and wish-fulfilling activities and its symptomatic unconscious behavior. It is at this level that she becomes aware of her own reverberations in response to the experience.

Like Lévi-Strauss we are in the process of studying what he has termed "entropology," which is the study of man undergoing disintegration and eventual extinction. This study implies an inquiry into limitations and inadequacies that develop as the family, along with its designated sick person, becomes increasingly sick as a group (Anthony, 1969).

At some point in the week, crises of greater or lesser dimensions are not infrequent; the visitor may reject the entire experience and cut short her stay or begin a period of adjustment that necessitates the learning of cues to guide her behavior in this alien setting. It should be pointed out that anthropologists are frequently exposed to a similar dilemma, which results in conflicting patterns of behavior. Many, in contact with a new culture, have reported frustrations, anxieties, paranoid perceptions, psychosomatic and hypochondrical complaints, unpleasant dreams and nightmares, and depression. In this context Golde (1970) has this comment to make:

> The learning of a [new] culture is not an intellectually dispassionate process, nor is it even necessarily mediated by words; it is direct intuitive learning that seeps through all the senses as it did when we were children being socialized to our own world. Field work can be a replication, condensed in time, of childhood learning,

with its attendant anxieties, mystification, impotence, and occasional and gradual mastery. We might label this "initiation anxiety," expecting to find perplexity, feelings of powerlessness, unsureness, and strain accompanying the process of being inducted into any ongoing, structured situation that is new.

This type of experience, therefore, demands a total immersion, a giving over of oneself to a differently organized reality. There is no doubt that this experience of dislocation has a pervasive and compelling consequence. However, it is one of the few ways open to us to realize an alien or alienated point of view, a vision of the world that is another's and not merely a reconstruction within the framework of our own. The modern anthropologist, like the modern ethologist, constantly examines his own response when entering a culture for the purpose of observation, and this is the procedure we have tried to follow.

The emphasis here is on different kinds of rationality rather than on a polarization into two agglutinated sets of values labeled "rational" and "irrational." Hartmann (1964) reminded us that rational and irrational behavior are not always rigidly separated from each other, even under ordinary circumstances, and it took us some time in our research to assimilate this very elementary, self-evident fact. We had naïvely supposed that when we entered the worlds of our psychotic patients we would be walking "through the looking glass" and finding everything turned the other way around. We soon learned differently. We found that between the rational and the irrational there lay a whole series of transitional behaviors along a continuum and that the family members slid backward and forward along it to a greater or lesser extent. We now incline to Hartmann's dictum that a totally rational human being is a caricature and not the highest representation of adaptation accessible to man; however, we would add that a totally irrational human being is a similar caricature, unless one institutionalizes the psychotic in a back ward for life and dehumanizes him.

Similar statements could be made about the sense of reality and the presence of a reality–unreality spectrum, along which shifts occur in either direction during the course of everyday life. We all, at times, make little compromises with reality, and these minor refusals to acknowledge outer reality are not only ubiquitous and harmless but also useful. The parents play an important role in inculcating a flexible and workable sense of reality in the child. He takes in their reality and their rationality as he takes in their food, their language, their attitudes, and their behavior. He takes in their reality as they perceive it and as they want him to perceive it. His testing of reality follows their rules, and the differentiation of ideas and perceptions, of subject from object, of inside from outside, and of thought from thing is part of the basic grammar of dualism that he derives from them. He is thus very easily caught up in any temptation on their part to tamper with reality. There are as many emotional rewards for children who conform to the distorted realities of psychotic parents as for children who meet the reality demands of reality-oriented parents. Any parent can seduce his child into living according to prescribed standards of reality and rationality, provided he starts with the process early enough and links it inextricably with his conditions for loving.

Within every developing individual there is this growing sense of inner and outer rationality and inner and outer reality, all of which are sensitive to wayward influences in the environment. Learning to test outer reality is as important as learning to test inner reality, and learning to apply outer rationality must proceed with learning to use inner rationality. In every individual an internal system of rationalities and realities is maintained that must establish an equilibrium with the externally directed system of rationalities and realities. The coherence of the world depends on the extent to which environmental incongruities interfere with this adjustment, and the parents can be conspicuous disturbers of the process. Before the ego becomes the representative of reality and rationality, the parents undertake this role.

The Living-in Protocol

What is true of the group, as described by Freud (1955), is also true of the family. When the organization of the group is disrupted and its leadership undermined, differentiation is reversed and the group becomes impulse-ridden, emotional, violent, fickle, inconsistent, suggestible, unreasonable, irresponsible, lacking in self-respect, and deficient in sense of reality. This level of rationality and reality is made up of paralogical thinking, pseudomutuality, double-bind communications, mystifications, sudden alternations of feeling, projective identifications, ritualistic obsessiveness, oscillations between withdrawal and closeness, lack of organization and direction, "as-if" tendencies, and unpredictability. When the group is competently led, it can function in certain respects better than the individual and can undertake tasks that seem beyond him.

In a well-parented family the environments are highly "expectable," and recoveries from regressions in reality and rationality can be confidently anticipated. In the poorly parented family the ups and downs are more frequent, the regressions more long-lasting, recovery less confidently anticipated, and stability less assured. In either type of family the picture is never uniform, levels of rationality and reality being actively generated with every new stimulus. It is not surprising that a given family may react or overreact to the observer by presenting her with the various profiles that it has been experimenting with over the years. Its collective mythologies are paraded for her benefit and pseudohistories, which never really happened except in the "psychic reality" of the family, are brought out, along with the family album, to convey the suggestion of stability and continuity.

Each individual member of the family, because of the press of his inner realities and rationalities, actively manipulates the family situation to gratify his own needs. In so doing he has to come to terms with the outer realities and rationalities of the other members and establish an intermediate zone of experience that can be shared. It is to this zone, with its relative degree of homeostasis, that the observer at first gains access, and only later is she admitted to the deeper strata.

The protocols are dictated each evening, and transcriptions are prepared as soon as possible, so that the observer's reactions can be correlated with the text. Each transcribed page is headed with the family name, the date, and the number of the tape. Each line on the page is separately numbered so that particular events can be easily retrieved.

The Steiner Family

The first vignette has to do with four members of the Steiner family: Mr. Steiner, a noninvolving process type of schizophrenic in his mid thirties; his wife, Mrs. Steiner, who treats her husband as a naughty child who simply cannot or will not learn; Debbie, an adopted nine-year-old girl; and Gary, an adopted seven-year-old boy. Mr. Steiner is neither interested in nor capable of a sexual relationship. He has, however, been arrested for voyeurism. The family is middle class and well-to-do.

Vignette 1

This first vignette gives some indication of the introduction of the observer into the household.

1.   We began driving around doing various small errands, which Mrs. Steiner
2.   seemed almost to manufacture as we went along. She was commenting on the
3.   fact that there's really nothing that she needs. She had checked the bread box
4.   twice before we left the house to see whether or not they needed bread. They
5.   did not. As we were driving, we were discussing various things, including her
6.   relative nervousnesss and embarrassment at my presence in the house. I
7.   responded by telling her relatively objectively that I was there to observe. She
8.   continually commented that had I been an ordinary guest she would have kept
9.   many of the things I had seen already completely hidden from me but that in
10.   wanting to cooperate, she let me see them although she found it embarrassing
11.   to realize that someone else knew about this. She continued talking about how
12.   she had all of the material things that she could possibly want—plenty of
13.   clothes, a beautiful home, and everything around the house that you would
14.   want—but that there was something really lacking. This did not become clear

15. at first, but as the trip progressed it became clearer. She seemed to be really
16. empty inside. We went first to the cleaners to drop off Gary's coat, and then
17. following that we went over to the Colony Inn, where she dropped off a watch
18. which needed repair at the jeweler. This is interesting in that the jeweler
19. knows her husband from his having come in, and he was commenting on Mr.
20. Steiner's problems with relating to reality and of dealing with facts and his
21. blundering when it came to doing much of anything that really seemed im-
22. portant.

1. Mrs. Steiner was the only one in the household who knew why I was there;
2. it was considered unwise to tell Mr. Steiner the true reason for my visit be-
3. cause of his record of chronic undifferentiated schizophrenia and his suspi-
4. ciousness with respect to people. Therefore I was introduced to the family as a
5. friend of Mrs. Steiner's from school. This created a very easy situation as well
6. as presenting a few problems, which will be brought up later. Mrs. Steiner
7. brought me right in and introduced me to the rest of the family. She is dressed
8. in a gray jersey suit and is an apparently outgoing, very gregarious person;
9. extremely friendly and she talks a lot, usually about herself. Mr. Steiner is
10. not much taller than she. He is bald and what you might describe as pear-
11. shaped. His shoulders and waist are wide, which gives him a rather odd ap-
12. pearance as well as walk. Having been prepared for his rather strange ap-
13. pearance, I was not repulsed—although this probably would have been a
14. normal reaction. Apparently his weight and shape are among the family prob-
15. lems—being a target for overt expressions of hostility. His conversation is
16. relatively shallow, although later on in the evening he was asking questions
17. about the hospital and things like this, some of which seemed to be trying to
18. allay his suspicions and others reflecting a relative lack of knowledge of what
19. he was really talking about. Periodically throughout the evening he would
20. look at me as if he was suspicious; this I think partly was unfamiliarity. Deb-
21. bie is a cute girl. She is a slender blond with long hair. One of the things she
22. was interested in was my long hair. She seems to really remain aloof from the
23. family. She was extremely shy in the car, but when we arrived home she was
24. completely different. She accepted my presence more or less matter-of-factly,
25. and, although she didn't at any time really communicate, she doesn't seem to
26. be shy of acting naturally in my presence. Gary, the younger of the two
27. children, is extremely fat, and he plays the clown considerably. He is
28. constantly making plays for attention, usually by aggressive play or stubborn-
29. ness. He has a sinus condition, which according to his mother is present all
30. during the winter every year, although it seems to become acute at times when
31. he doesn't want to do something. The family has two dogs, male French
32. poodles, one of which belongs to each of the children. Andy belongs to Gary,
33. Pierre to Debbie. These dogs are all over the furniture and constantly under
34. foot except when they are contained in the utility room, which seems to be
35. considered almost the dogs' room. They are confined there most of the time.
36. Shortly after we arrived, dinner was ready, and just before dinner Debbie
37. refused to come to the table if the color television set in the family room was
38. turned off. Mrs. Steiner insisted that she would come and the television would
39. be turned off. Then Mrs. Steiner stated that if she did not come she would
40. have to go to bed and would not get any supper. Finally, after fussing for
41. about two minutes, Debbie came to the table. She sat at the table and fed the

42. dogs chicken from the table until they were finally run out of the room and
43. put in the utility room. No one in this family seems to wait for anyone else.
44. As you arrive at the table you fill your plate and begin to eat.

The observer feels relatively comfortable because the Steiners are a white, middle-class, suburban family. She is quickly caught up in Mrs. Steiner's everyday world, which involves running the family and the household and keeping Mr. Steiner more or less insulated, like a retarded child. She goes out of her way to say that she is not repulsed by her first contact with Mr. Steiner and she handles his suspiciousness fairly well. She is quick to notice where family routine departs from her own experience. However, like the rest of the family, she soon begins to treat Mr. Steiner as a nonperson and to take him for granted like the furniture.

In the second vignette, still on the first day, she is left alone with the children, as the parents go out, and discovers how affect-hungry they both are.

Vignette 2

1. After they had left, Gary talked about the Batman program. Both the
2. children were lying on the sofa or on the floor at various times and watching
3. TV. Gary got out his arithmetic book and insisted that I should help him do
4. his arithmetic problems. During this time Debbie was playing with my hair.
5. He was doing addition problems, and whenever he would come to a problem
6. he would actually count the numbers on his fingers, which most children are
7. not doing in the third grade. Both of the children continued to watch TV most
8. of the evening. They also seemed to be competing for my attention, Gary
9. openly and Debbie more subtly. Gary was talking about animals; for a while
10. he was pretending that his hand was a tarantula, and it was crawling up my
11. arm and across my back, and then it bit me. In other words, he pinched me
12. on the shoulder and back. However, when I asked him why he wanted to hurt
13. me, he answered that it was not he, "It is the tarantula that bit you." He
14. dissociated himself from responsibility for his aggression. About 9:00, while
15. Debbie was taking her bath, Gary took me downstairs and drew pictures of
16. animals on the blackboard they have in the recreation room downstairs, and
17. had me identify the animals as they were drawn. Later, when we were back
18. upstairs, he was running around the room pretending to be a duck or an
19. ostrich with various types of walk and poses. Sometimes he made attacking
20. approaches but yet with a bit of shyness toward me, as if attacking and
21. retreating at the same time. Throughout the evening he was adding to his
22. bubble gum supply. By the end of the evening he had about five or six pieces
23. of bubble gum in his mouth at once, and he was constantly either playing
24. with it in his hands, in other words having it out of his mouth and pulling
25. and stretching it in all directions, or blowing bubbles and bursting them on
26. his face. During the evening, before this, while Gary was performing his
27. various antics on the floor, Debbie said to me, "Whenever anybody comes to
28. visit he shows off." This comment came while she was lying on the sofa
29. watching television, in a very depreciating tone of voice. The one thing that I
30. noticed about the behavior after the parents left was that prior to this time

31. there was absolutely nothing on the floor. Mr. and Mrs. Steiner had not been
32. gone five minutes before Gary had littered the floor with paper and scraps and
33. things like this. This fits in with what I had been told about Mr. Steiner not
34. allowing anything to be on the floor at any time.

The observer now begins to be exposed to the symptomatic behavior of the psychotic. He cannot leave anything on the floor, constantly walks around the house turning off lights, and maintains an empty type of conversation that is both meaningless and affectless. This particular night she has a dream in which all of her notes are being shredded and thrown all over the floor, provoking a monstrous rage in Mr. Steiner, from whom, in a nightmarish way, she is trying to run away. She is also becoming irritated with Mrs. Steiner's "busyness" and begins to feel the need for "a little ordinary love and affection." She feels that things seem unpredictable and relates this feeling at first to mechanical elements.

Vignette 3

1. Throughout the evening Mrs. Steiner got progressively annoyed at the way
2. Mr. Steiner continually ran around the house cleaning things. She yelled at
3. him to leave things where she wanted them and to leave the lights on. He was
4. relatively nonresponsive and kept making comments like "Well, you want the
5. house clean, don't you?" or "Well, why do you need that light on?" In
6. answer to these questions, Mr. Steiner was given no answers. One wonders
7. what would happen if someone answered a "why" question. He really was
8. not very responsive to anything at all. When Mrs. Steiner and I came out of
9. her room, he was standing just outside the doorway of the house talking about
10. how nice and cool the air was. The temperature in this house is erratic. You
11. don't know when you're going to be too hot or when you're going to be too
12. cold because Mr. Steiner continually turns the heat up, down, or off. At this
13. particular time it was about 70 degrees in the house, except that it was cooler
14. in the vestibule because he was standing in the doorway. About 10:00 Deb-
15. bie got up and came into the family room. She was doing handstands on the
16. rug, and it was about 15 or 20 minutes before she was talked into going back
17. to bed. I can't give any reason for why she got up and why it took that long to
18. get her back to bed. About 10:30 Mr. and Mrs. Steiner and I began a Scrab-
19. ble game. Mrs. Steiner enjoyed it very much. She commented that she liked
20. the game and could play it all night. Mr. Steiner was rather slow with it. His
21. vocabulary is not too good and neither is his spelling. Apparently this is also
22. one of her means of attacking him. Because he is slow at the game, she can,
23. and does, more or less legitimately get angry. Her favorite form of the game is
24. to limit each player's turn to one minute. Mr. Steiner was eating constantly
25. during the game. He ate nuts and chicken, which was left over from last
26. night. Toward the end of the game, when all the letters are out of the box and
27. it is just playing with the few remaining letters, it becomes harder to find
28. words. At this point Mr. Steiner quit the game and said that we could finish
29. it if we wanted, but he was tired of it. The game stopped after one game at
30. 12:00. Mrs. Steiner was commenting that Mr. Steiner's behavior is excep-

31. tionally good since I had been there; that he has shown few signs of his
32. problem.

The observer now finds the attitude of the children toward the father quite disturbing, especially since she is starting to share it.

Vignette 4

1. Debbie calls Mr. Steiner stupid. When he came in for breakfast this
2. morning, he was turning off the light in the family room, and she said,
3. "Hey, stupid, leave the light on; we're going back in there." Later on, at
4. about 9:25, when he honked for the kids to go to school, she yelled out, al-
5. though he couldn't hear it, "OK, stupid." Gary this morning broke the box
6. that his buttons were in. He got very upset, almost in the same way that a
7. four-year-old would get upset, despite the fact that he's seven or eight, as if he
8. had broken a toy, and this was the most valuable toy in the world. The one
9. button that he could not find immediately was a pearl button, which he liked
10. particularly well, which his mother had found for him. He treated this, as
11. well as a couple of the green ones, as if they actually were real pearl buttons
12. or emeralds, which of course they were not. His attachments, like those of the
13. other members of the family, are to things—not people. And he, like his
14. father, does not differentiate the real from the fake. Debbie's attitude toward
15. the the whole family reflects this "you are stupid" idea, but it is most overt
16. toward Mr. Steiner. Mrs. Steiner and I then went to a clothes store. She was
17. talking about these women there and how you could come into that particular
18. shop any day of the week, and practically any time of the day, and find the
19. same women there just looking around, not really buying anything but just
20. killing time and running into each other. She kept deploring this. Her
21. reaction to these people seems to be a reaction to her own circumstance as
22. much as anything else. She also commented on the fact that these women were
23. all very friendly to her during the day but she did not go out with them at
24. night because of Mr. Steiner. I believe from this conversation that she is
25. rather bitter, that she would like to do this.

The observer is now beginning to feel, as she put it, "very empty," and at times "quite depressed." She is pleased when Mrs. Steiner asks her to do the rounds simply to get out of the house, where for the most part she becomes apathetic, bored, restless, and withdrawn. It is often a relief to go to her own room. She begins counting the days toward termination.

Vignette 5

What is surprising about these families is their inability to resolve the minor crises of everyday life and bring about a reasonable reconciliation between the members.

1. This also reminds me of the comment Mrs. Steiner made the day before
2. about how she had three children and two dogs, and that she would really like

3. to have a man around the house but that she didn't. This comment sounds
4. like the keynote of Mrs. Steiner's attitude toward the entire family, especially
5. to Mr. Steiner. Mr. Steiner. then went out of the living room, and Mrs.
6. Steiner and her mother were standing there. They got to talking about the
7. dogs being let in; Mr. Steiner had let the dogs in, and they were running
8. around the living room. I was in the kitchen, and through the door I could
9. hear the argument. Mrs. Steiner came through the door from the living room
10. into the kitchen saying, "and you can drop dead with him" to her mother.
11. This storm blew over in a little while, but it was easy to tell that Mrs. Steiner
12. had lost her temper. About 5:00 Mr. Steiner came into the kitchen, and an
13. argument got started over leaving the outside light on at night. Apparently
14. there had been many robberies in the area, and Mrs. Steiner feels that one
15. way to reduce the chances of having her house robbed is to leave lights on out-
16. side all night long. This spat is over turning off lights—one of Mr. Steiner's
17. compulsions. They also got into an argument over where Mr. Steiner could
18. put papers that she wanted to use so that they wouldn't disappear. This again
19. is a reflection of the way Mr. Steiner goes through the entire house as soon as
20. he's home and practically every minute that he is home picks up anything
21. which is out of place. Nothing is left on the floor or anywhere where it's in
22. the open. Mrs. Steiner became very angry and with violent words and actions
23. pushed and yelled at Mr. Steiner out of the kitchen and told him to just get
24. out and stay out because she couldn't do anything as long as he was there.
25. Mrs. Steiner's temper was very much on edge, and it was affecting the entire
26. family. During this time Gary was racing back and forth through the kitchen
27. with a towel tied around his neck cape-style, and each time he came through
28. the kitchen door, which is a swinging door, he banged the door against the
29. cabinet wall. After doing this five or six times, he came in and stood by the
30. sink, rocking back and forth, saying, "What are we having for supper?" de-
31. manding to know what they were having for supper. He was extremely
32. hyperactive the whole evening. He was constantly up when he was watching
33. television, up and down the stairs, and was running around the house with
34. this towel wrapped around his shoulders most of the evening. It is interesting
35. that this very fat boy, who is totally unconcerned with his weight, identifies
36. with the masculinity and agility of Batman and Superman. Mrs. Steiner's
37. mother was sitting in the living room throughout this, with what might be
38. called professional noninvolvement of a mother, making comments like, "I
39. don't want to interfere, *but*," and then commenting on how the children
40. should be better disciplined and how Mrs. Steiner should be better to Mr.
41. Steiner and many comments to this effect, projecting the typical middle-class
42. image of what wives, mothers, and families should be like.

The extent to which the children can become disturbed takes the observer by surprise.

1. Earlier there had been something about Gary playing with my lighter. I
2. had a cigarette lighter in the house, and he was playing with it, lighting it,
3. leaving it on, and not giving it back which had upset his mother considerably.
4. Then everyone came on upstairs and we adults were going to play Scrabble.
5. Gary demanded that he be given the game. There are apparently three Scrab-
6. ble games in this household, but the other one could not be found, so Gary

7. threw a temper tantrum. He went into his room crying and yelling and
8. screaming. He forced everyone, especially Mr. Steiner, away and out of his
9. room yelling, "Go away," "Leave me alone," alternately shouting and
10. yelling, "Go away" and "Leave me alone." This progressed. It started about
11. 10:35 and got progressively worse from there. He yelled and sobbed convul-
12. sively and shook. He was actually shaking and tore shreds from his foam rub-
13. ber pillows. There was a pile of shreds of pillow, approximately ½″ × ½″ ×
14. ¼″ shreds. Mrs. Steiner said that this was an example of his tantrums, and
15. she commented that at least this time he wasn't violent. Very often he would
16. kick and push away and literally throw things actively at anyone who tried to
17. interrupt the tantrum or come into his room at all. She was talking to me
18. about how she could not leave Gary with a sitter and therefore could not go
19. out. She couldn't trust him with a sitter because she was afraid he might start
20. whenever he's crossed, and they don't know how to handle it or what to do.
21. She was also bragging about the way she could handle this and could get him
22. calmed down when nobody else could. She would say things like "You didn't
23. think I would be able to stop his crying, did you?" Of course, it took 45
24. minutes and his complete exhaustion before she managed to do it. Sam com-
25. mented to me that Gary needs consistent discipline, and he feels that a
26. military school would be good for this boy. Mrs. Steiner would like very much
27. to get Gary into a "controlled environment" and seemingly as quickly as
28. possible. Mrs. Steiner was kind of pouring out on my shoulder that she had
29. tried to get help but . . . She had taken Gary to a psychiatrist, who had been
30. seeing Gary twice a week, and the psychiatrist, because of Mr. Steiner's threat
31. to sue him, had terminated the treatment. About 7:00 Gary was playing with
32. my lighter again. He took a cigarette out of the pack and was going to light it.
33. I completely forgot myself and reacted as if I would if he were my child. I
34. said, "You light that and I will hit you." He lit it and I slapped him. He
35. was very shocked and picked up the lighter and threw it across the house. I
36. got it back. Gary broke into convulsive sobbing. It triggered a temper tantrum
37. as had happened the night before. I explained what had happened to both
38. Mr. and Mrs. Steiner, and both said that it was all right, that things like that
39. happen. At that point I would have given anything in the world to take it
40. back, to go back in time. About 7:15, while Gary was still carrying on, Mrs.
41. Steiner began talking again about Mr. Steiner's compulsive cleaning up and
42. how bad it was to be in this house. She really seems to hate Mr. Steiner. In
43. fact, she admits that she hates him, but she is crazy about the kids. She was
44. talking about everything she does for the kids. But it is more of a doting.

The two children were equally disturbed but in opposite directions: Gary
would periodically become uncontrolled, and Debbie was periodically withdrawn. Her teacher had suggested "lighting a fire under her." There was no
doubt that she was strange around other children and unable to mix with
them.

In this noninvolving psychotic milieu the observer reported minimal
cultural shock and little anxiety but a growing amount of depression.
Perplexity and cognitive dissonance were rarely present. At times, however,
she did feel extremely alienated from the environment but was never out of

touch with its reality or confused by its events. During the latter part of her stay she frequently wanted to get away. Although she had some unpleasant dreams that frightened her, she had no fear of going crazy herself. Psychosomatic complaints were also not prominent, apart from headaches and lack of energy.

The Kramer Family

In the next series of vignettes the family in question has a parent with an involving psychosis. In the Kramer family the mother has had recurrent bouts of severe schizoaffective disorder to which her husband responds with a great deal of disturbance himself. There are three children, Freddy age seven, Charlie age five, and baby Sharon.

Vignette 1

1. I arrived at the Kramers' (small white frame house) at 7:00 in the morning
2. for breakfast. I was met at the door by Freddy James and Charlie Kramer.
3. Freddy asked me if I would be staying for two weeks and if I was from the
4. board of education, and I said no that I would be there for one week and that
5. I was from the Child Guidance Clinic. I asked where Mrs. Kramer was and
6. they said she was in the kitchen, so I went in and saw her cooking breakfast.
7. She was dressed in black shorts and a sleeveless blouse. She had on no shoes
8. and looked generally very sour and unwelcoming. I said good morning to her
9. and asked for a place to put my valise, in which I keep my tape recorder, and
10. she said I could put it in the bedroom by the closet. Freddy and Charlie
11. followed me into the bedroom, and Freddy asked very lightly if I wanted to
12. meet his baby sister, Sharon. So I walked to the crib, where Sharon was lying
13. very quietly. She is a very cute little girl but looked very quiet. We then went
14. into the kitchen, where we all had breakfast. Freddy and Mrs. Kramer and I
15. had fried eggs served on very small plates, just about big enough for the egg
16. itself and nothing else. There were also bacon and milk for the children. Mrs.
17. Kramer and I had coffee. Charlie apparently preferred scrambled eggs, and so
18. he had his eggs scrambled. However, he was very reluctant to eat, and Mrs.
19. Kramer was always harping at him to eat his breakfast. The eggs looked very
20. unappetizing. They were colorless and very sloppy looking, wet and drippy
21. looking. Breakfast was a rather disturbing meal for Charlie, especially.
22. Charlie looked over at me and said, "Would you like to take her home?" and
23. I said I didn't think he really would want me to take her home, and Mrs.
24. Kramer agreed and said that she was sure Charlie didn't mean it. He said
25. very decisively that he did mean it.
26. After she made the beds, Charlie came in and saw the valise with the tape
27. recorder in it. He took out the microphone and asked what it was. I told him
28. it was a microphone, and he wanted to know if he could plug it in, and I said
29. no, that it didn't plug into the wall. He wanted to talk into it, so I let him. He

30. said something like "Grandma, mom, are you there computer?" I was
31. holding it, and I asked him if he meant that I was the computer. Then
32. Charlie said that he wanted to take the microphone outside to play with, and
33. I told him no that it wasn't a toy and that he could use it if he stayed in the
34. room, but he kept insisting that he was going to take it outside. I talked to
35. him for a while. I was holding the other end of the cord and talking to him,
36. and finally we gradually broke off the game after I said that it was time to put
37. the microphone up and would he help me wind it up. At first he protested and
38. said no that he wanted it. He was very demanding about this, but I kept
39. asking him if he wouldn't help me put it away and that we would perhaps
40. play with it later. Finally he consented and I put it away. At this time his lit-
41. tle friend from next door was calling him so he went out to play. I went into
42. the kitchen to talk to Mrs. Kramer. Before he went out, however, Charlie
43. went into his room and laid on the floor and was still talking about the
44. microphone, and he said I was a punk. I asked him what that meant, and he
45. said just that I was a punk. Then he did go outside, and I went into the
46. kitchen to talk to Mrs. Kramer. We talked about several things, one of which
47. was the fact that she was now in her second marriage and that she had pre-
48. viously been married to a man who was concerned mostly about cars and his
49. buddies and that seemed to make him very happy. She said that after Freddy
50. came she worked in a bar for four years, and she seemed to feel that her
51. working in a bar had something to do with her present husband and herself
52. having fights. She said that she didn't think they would ever get married, but
53. they finally had gotten married and that she had, during the time previous, a
54. woman taking care of Freddy, whom she partly blamed for Freddy's prob-
55. lems. She said that she thought the woman had given Freddy paregoric and
56. that on occasion the grandmother, on Freddy's coming home, had remarked
57. that Freddy's bottom was very red. Mrs. Kramer said that she thought it
58. would have been better had she not lived with her mother. She said that she
59. felt her parents tend to be bossy and that it would have been much better had
60. she set up an apartment of her own. She also asked me if I lived by myself
61. and asked me if or how my mother felt about my being on my own.

The observer almost immediately feels ill at ease in this household and
somewhat apprehensive "as if a storm was brewing." She feels that the difficulty with the tape recorder has set her off on the wrong foot.

On the second day the children begin to draw her into their play.

Vignette 2

1. During this meal Charlie got up and brought his big gun in. Freddy started
2. asking him if he were a big hunter. Then he asked me if I didn't think
3. Charlie was a small hunter. They they began playing a game. First of all,
4. Charlie went into the living room and Freddy went after him and came back
5. and said he killed the monster. I said "Who is the monster?" and he said,
6. "Charlie." Then Freddy hid in the living room, and Charlie came back and
7. said he had killed the monster Freddy. Then Freddy said that I should be
8. Charlie's wife, and I asked him why and he said because "Wives are big and

9. husbands are small." Freddy began to pretend he was the lion and Charlie
10. was the hunter. They went into the living room again. They came back and
11. Freddy looked at me and said, "you're supposed to ask Charlie if he killed
12. any lions," and I said why. He said, "Because Charlie is the husband."

The conditions begin to warm up, and the observer finds herself becoming increasingly anxious. It is difficult for her to predict how Mrs. Kramer is going to react to the next incident in the family.

Vignette 3

1. Then Charlie tipped over the carton and most of the cheese and meat fell
2. on the floor. Except for an occasional remark, Mrs. Kramer yelled at him and
3. told him to take it back. He didn't do it and she didn't move. Then he
4. brought in some Jello and started eating with his hands. She looked at him
5. and then she looked away. Finally she realized what he was doing, and she
6. started yelling at him not to make a mess with the Jello. Then she forgot it for
7. a while. He took a handful and rubbed the Jello on the little table in front of
8. the couch. This really sent her into a rage. She jumped up and got a cloth
9. from the kitchen and told Charlie that he was really going to get a beating
10. and that sometimes she could *just kill him*. He got this tearful look on his face
11. and went to the bathroom. He went down to the basement and brought up a
12. book. I remembered that he had done that earlier in the day. He also had
13. with him a little toy with wheels on it.
1. She went out of the room for a moment, and I asked him how school was.
2. He said, "All right." I asked him what he did. Freddy said that his teacher
3. wouldn't give him any more paper. I said, "Why not?" Mrs. Kramer was
4. back in the kitchen again saying, "What?"—what she often does when she
5. thinks I said something and I haven't or I am talking to the other children
6. and she hasn't heard what I have said. I said, "Nothing," and she said, "I
7. thought you were talking, I thought you said something." I said, "I was
8. talking to Freddy." Freddy gave this look to me out of the corner of his eye.
9. Out of the clear blue sky Freddy said, "Isn't it a beautiful world?" Mrs.
10. Kramer said, "What makes you think so?" Freddy said, "Well, it's pretty,"
11. and then Mrs. Kramer told him to hurry up and drink down his soup because
12. he was going to be late. He had *just* sat down. He started eating his soup, and
13. I noticed that he had this sort of, he made sort of funny sounds when he ate; it
14. was almost as though he were, that it was catching in his throat, and then he
15. would swallow. It's hard to describe, but it was a funny noise. Then Freddy
16. took an apple and went off to school. Mrs. Kramer fed Sharon. She jammed
17. Sharon's seat in and Sharon's foot got stuck, and she said something like
18. "Now you've *really* done it." Finally Sharon got in and she fed her very fast.
19. During this time Charlie came in and said that his sandwich had gotten dirty
20. so he had given it to the dog. Mrs. Kramer said, "It's not good enough for
21. you but it's good enough for the dog." After lunch Mrs. Kramer asked me to
22. please dress Sharon, which I did. She prepared to give Sharon a bath, during
23. which time Charlie came in again to ask for more money to go to the store,
24. and she said no. She was standing holding the baby and I was standing by the

25. sink and she said, "Peggy, don't let him take the money." I told her that I
26. would hold the baby while she took care of it, that I couldn't do anything like
27. that, so she went over and *yelled* at him and told him not to take the money
28. and that he was going to catch it anyway for taking the other money, so he
29. went out. She had told me before how much Sharon loved her bath. When I
30. was holding Sharon, I noticed that the water was really rather chilly, even for
31. a summer day, for giving a baby a bath. When Sharon was first put in the
32. water, she didn't look at all happy; in fact, she looked very stiff. Mrs. Kramer
33. immediately took her hand and started splashing her hand around in the
34. water. Sharon did splash a little bit but not very much. Mrs. Kramer had told
35. me how she splashed and splashed. She washed Sharon with her hands,
36. saying that this was better than washing her with a cloth. She soaped her
37. hand and then washed, and then she started talking about her neighbor who
38. used a special soap, but she didn't go along with that. She had been raised in
39. a plain family and so had her husband. Her husband had been raised in a
40. family of nine children and there was nothing wrong with any of them. After
41. the bath she examined Sharon's vagina rather roughly. Then she took these
42. toothpicks—Q-tips—and took some baby oil and cleaned out Sharon's
43. nostrils. She said she was supposed to do this. She did it rather roughly. Then
44. she cleaned her ears the same way, and then she again examined her vagina
45. and then poured gobs of powder on Sharon's chest and then sort of just
46. smoothed it over in a very rough way. The powder was up in Sharon's face.
47. She handled the baby as if it were a piece of meat or a sack of potatoes rather
48. than a child. I had noticed early in the morning when she dressed Sharon that
49. she put her shoes on and just pulled them very tightly; she just wasn't very
50. gentle with her bathing.

The observer is beginning to have strong reactions to the type of mothering that she is observing, and she is feeling herself becoming very resentful of Mrs. Kramer. It seems to her that the mother is attacking the baby, and she finds herself wanting to attack the mother. Her interchanges with Mrs. Kramer are becoming increasingly defensive.

Vignette 4

1. She asked me if I had called my mother and I said no, my mother had
2. called me. She asked me if my mother had asked me what I was doing, and I
3. said yes and that I told her I was working for the Child Guidance Clinic
4. doing home visits. She said, "What does she think of that?" I said she
5. thought it was interesting.

The observer is finding it difficult to control her feelings, and at the same time, she finds herself getting headaches, especially as she watches the mother's behavior with the baby.

Vignette 5

1. It has become quite striking to me how much time the baby spends behind
2. bars. She is in her crib or in her playpen almost all the morning, except for

3. one or two days when Mrs. Kramer took her out on the porch, or in her high
4. chair. The feeding was over in five minutes or less. The food was steaming
5. hot again. I could see the steam. The baby didn't put up much of a fight,
6. however. So maybe the food wasn't as hot as it looked. She fed the baby, and
7. the baby spit out and carried on as she always does. The feeding seems to be a
8. very anxious time for the baby because the mother does feed it very fast. She
9. was put in her playpen, and that's where she was when I was in the living
10. room with Charlie and Laura. Charlie has asked me three times today to put
11. on his shoes, and each time I have encouraged him to do it himself. He can
12. put his shoes on; he doesn't tie them. He even did take time to string them up
13. with some encouragement. Mrs. Kramer came in and talked about the fact
14. that if I took my nap when they did I wouldn't have very much time to rest.
15. At that time I was feeling rather tired, and so I told her that I would like to
16. take a nap and she said fine. She came into the bedroom and changed the
17. baby's pants. Then she left and I started to go to sleep. However, Charlie
18. came in and was getting in the refrigerator, and she said, "No, get out of that
19. refrigerator." She came in a couple of times. I don't know what she did be-
20. cause my head was turned the other way. I think she put something in her
21. purse and something else and then went out. I was awakened about 11:45 by
22. the baby's crying. I could hear a spoon clinking against a dish. The crying
23. was coming from the kitchen, so I assumed the baby was being fed. This time
24. the baby really cried quite hard, and Mrs. Kramer kept telling her—al-
25. ternation between "What's the matter?" and "Stop it, Sharon." Then
26. Charlie came in.

The feeding battles continue with both children, and the observer finds herself desperate to interfere yet afraid to do so.

1. Charlie kept saying that he wasn't going to eat his lunch. Mrs. Kramer sat
2. down next to him and took up the spoon and forced Charlie to eat his soup.
3. Charlie would touch her hand, and the hot soup would fall on his chest, and
4. he would say it was burning him, and she would say no that it wasn't burning
5. him. He kept saying it was hot, and she kept putting spoonful after spoonful
6. in his mouth. He had eaten some ham and wanted some more. She said, "No,
7. not before you eat your soup; you're not going to have any more ham."
8. During this time he had this sort of helpless look on this face. He kept saying
9. things like "Mommy, don't," and she kept screaming at him to stop touching
10. her hand and to eat his food. Finally he said, "Let me do it, let me feed
11. myself," and she said all right, and he did feed himself. During the feeding he
12. looked at me and said, "I bet I can beat you." I said, "I bet you can't." Mrs.
13. Kramer made some remark about how I probably noticed that he was a ter-
14. rible eater and it was really hard to get him to eat. She put the baby in the
15. high chair and started feeding it as rapidly as she had before. The baby had
16. this dismayed look on her face. She kept feeding the baby faster and faster. As
17. soon as she put the spoon in, she put it in again. The baby, toward the end of
18. the feeding, began spitting out the food. She started yelling at her and telling
19. her there was no reason for her to do that. About the end of the feeding she
20. gave her some milk, also forcing the baby. You could hear the baby gulping
21. the milk down. Then she sort of choked, and Mrs. Kramer made a remark
22. like "I bet you think mother is trying to strangle you" and laughing. She
23. thought it was very funny. At the end of the feeding the baby threw up all
24. over her tray. Mother was very upset about the mess and how she made a

25. mess on her dress. She again took the baby out of the high chair without
26. taking the tray off. The baby's foot got caught again. She put her on the floor
27. and began wiping it up and saying that she had gotten it down into the seat
28. by the metal rings where it was hard to clean. This seemed to disturb Mrs.
29. Kramer. She then took a cold cloth and wiped the vomit off the side of the
30. chair.

31. At this time, I went into the house. Mrs. Kramer was still trying to feed
32. Sharon the bottle, and the baby obviously didn't want it. Mrs. Kramer was
33. spanking the baby rather hard and telling her that she had to take the bottle,
34. that she shouldn't do like this. Mr. Kramer at this time was taking a bath. He
35. came out and heard Mrs. Kramer spanking the baby and said, "Gertrudy,
36. why are you spanking the baby? She doesn't want the bottle so don't force
37. her." It seemed to calm things down for a while. Then they finally got into
38. bed, and Mrs. Kramer went into her bedroom and lay down with the baby
39. and told the baby that if she didn't take the bottle she was going to punch her
40. good. Then she put the baby to bed and came in and sat down with her feet
41. up and said that she was very tired and that she was going to bed.

The feeding problem continues to dominate the situation.

1. Mrs. Kramer fed the baby. She alternated between peas and plums. She fed
2. her a spoonful of one and then the other. The baby was gagging and spitting
3. the food out. She jerked her hand one time and caused Mrs. Kramer to spill
4. it, and she said, "Now don't you do that," and she hit her. Then I asked
5. Mrs. Kramer how fights like these had started, and she said that she really
6. didn't think they were fights, they were just disagreements and that she didn't
7. agree with—she wasn't going to let any man get the best of her. "He was al-
8. ways going out," and she didn't think that was right. I asked her how she or
9. what she thought of the home visit. She asked me what I meant. I asked her
10. what she thought of my being there for the home visit, and she said she
11. thought it was all right. She said, "I must have made you feel bad," and I
12. said, "No." She said, "I'm sorry but I am not going to let any man get the
13. best of me." Then I began to think of things she had said about her children.
14. She said she has a feeling that her children get into the trouble in the neigh-
15. borhood. Yesterday some woman was telling her that her little girl hurt her
16. toe—the kids had made a game of stepping on her toe. She told Mrs. Kramer
17. that it wasn't Charlie. Mrs. Kramer said, "Oh, that's a change; it's usually
18. always my kids." Sharon's feeding was rough. It ended in Mrs. Kramer
19. pulling her out. Every time she takes her out of the high chair she gets her leg
20. caught.

It is clear that the observer is finding real difficulty in controlling her feelings and that she feels that the mother is aware of this. She calls to tell me that she feels that she is making a mess of things and that she better get out of the house.

Vignette 6

The observer becomes aware that she is not the only person reacting strongly to Mrs. Kramer. The husband is constantly at war with her and at times seems to set her up for some deflating remark.

1.   Mrs. Kramer's mother said, out of the clear blue sky while we were all sit-
2. ting in the living room, "Did you hear about the 14-year-old girl who sucked
3. her thumb?" It was an article that both Mrs. Kramer and myself had read in
4. the paper, and we had been talking about it. Mr. Kramer said, "That's the
5. third time I've heard about it today," and Mrs. Kramer said, "You know
6. they say thumb sucking comes from emotional problems." The day before she
7. had said it came from a lack of security. He said, "Well, I don't know
8. anything about it, Gert," and then she said, "Maybe that baby has emotional
9. problems." He said, "Maybe you have emotional problems." It made me
10. think of the movie *Gaslight,* in which the husband, through his talking and
11. setting up certain incidents, tries to convince the wife that she is mad and al-
12. most does it. For some reason I thought of this today.

13.   Very soon in the meal the topic of marriage arose. They both mentioned in
14. sort of a jesting way that they used to fight quite a bit. Mr. Kramer said
15. something about the day he got the license. This seemed to amuse them very
16. much. I noticed that all during dinner Freddy's eyes were everywhere around
17. the table, especially on his mother's and father's faces and on mine. He
18. seemed very preoccupied. Perhaps one of the saddest things that happened all
19. day was just another joking remark that Mr. and Mrs. Kramer made. It had
20. something to do with getting away. Mr. Kramer said something about his
21. taking off, and Mrs. Kramer said, "You know what would happen, don't
22. you? You would end up with all the kids in the trunk of your car."

23.   She paged on and there were some pictures of women with fancy hair
24. styles, and she asked me if I ever thought of getting a wig and I said yes, I
25. had thought about it. She said her husband had thought about getting her one
26. but he decided not to. Mr. Kramer flatly denied this. He said he never
27. thought of getting her a wig. She said, "Oh yes he did, oh yes he did." He
28. said, "I did not." He said, "What you really ought to have is a mask." She
29. said, "Why do I want a mask?" At this period there seemed to be sort of a
30. gradual change in Mrs. Kramer's behavior. She didn't seem nearly as ir-
31. ritable and nervous, and she seemed more to be joking with him. She seemed
32. to rather enjoy this kind of sarcastic banter. She giggled and just seemed to
33. become younger. In fact, at one point during the conversation she had her
34. chin resting on the table, and she just acted . . . Then she said something
35. about, she said, "Yes, you said you were going to get a Negro girl," and he
36. said, "Maybe I will." She said, "Well go ahead; maybe she will or you can
37. beat her head and get some money." He said, "What have you done all day?
38. Nothing?" and she looked at me and said, "See what I mean?" Previously
39. she had told me that he would come home and that he would say, "What
40. have you been doing all day? Nothing?" He glanced around and saw that she
41. had cut some roses, and he said, "Who cut the roses?" She said. "I did." He
42. said, "What did you cut the buds for?" Also she asked him if he wanted a di-
43. vorce, and he said, "Go ahead and file." They began arguing about who
44. would take the children, and he said he would, and she said she would since
45. she was the one who had borne them. He asked her how she would take care
46. of them, and she said, "Oh, you would be surprised." She kept insisting that

47. she wanted Sharon. Charlie came in, and she remarked how cute he was. Mr.
48. Kramer asked me if I were married, and I said no. He said, "Take my advice;
49. don't get married." They had been fighting about what she was going to wear
50. tomorrow night. He didn't want her to wear a certain dress because she
51. looked like a blimp. They might launch her tomorrow, he said. She said she
52. wasn't going to wear some suit. The night was filled with this ridiculous
53. bickering—back and forth. It had lost its playfulness of before and neither of
54. them seemed to be amused anymore by it.

The more paranoid elements begin to emerge, and the observer finds herself caught up in some of mother's delusional ideas.

Vignette 7

1. At this time Mr. Kramer said he wanted to go see his mother. Mrs.
2. Kramer said that she didn't owe the woman anything and why didn't he go
3. tonight instead of tomorrow because she didn't want to go. This got into a
4. bickering stage, and she said especially "when she sends spies to spy on me at
5. the school when I have Charlie and Freddy with me, or at the picnic; I don't
6. need those spies; I don't need anything to do with anybody like that." I asked
7. her what picnic and what spies, and she didn't say anything to me. Mr.
8. Kramer had gone out of the room. After a period of time Mrs. Kramer said
9. that she didn't want anything to do with the woman. Apparently she had
10. reported to Mrs. Kramer that someone had seen the children and said, "I
11. heard your kids really acted up at the picnic and at the school." Mrs. Kramer
12. had insight enough to say that kids usually run wild at a picnic and that she
13. didn't need anybody spying around. She said this very definitely looking at
14. me.

The observer finds herself unable to control some of her aggressive feelings, as for example, in the following interchange.

1. I thanked them for the nice day, and Mr. Kramer said he didn't think it
2. had been very nice. He said, "Maybe we will go out for a ride or something
3. tomorrow," and she said, "I'm not going; you go where you want." Then she
4. started talking about how he said she was "nuts" all the time and that she
5. didn't have to take that. She said, "He tells me I'm nuts and I tell him he's
6. nuts." "I don't have to take that." I asked her if she felt nuts, and she said
7. no. Mr. Kramer kept saying, "Why don't you tell her the whole story?" I
8. said, "What's the whole story?"

There is no doubt that Charlie is reacting to the situation between his mother and the observer.

1. After we finished playing with the dirt and we had come into the house, he
2. brought this plate of dirt into the house. I asked him to leave it outside, and
3. he said his mother wouldn't care if he brought it in. She had washed the
4. kitchen floor, and he dumped this dirt on the floor. I said, "*Oh*, Charlie, look
5. what you've done." She at this time was about to feed the baby, so I told her
6. that I would sweep it up. When I was sweeping it up, he came over and

7. kicked his foot out in front of my face. I said, "Don't kick me, Charlie," and
8. then he kicked me. I asked him again please not to kick me, that I didn't like
9. to be kicked; I like him but I didn't like his kicking. He said he "could too
10. kick me." Finally I asked him if he wanted to help me sweep up the floor, so
11. he took the dust pan and held it while I swept the dirt into it. He took the
12. dust pan in the living room and said, "Come in here; we can sweep the living
13. room." I said no, that the broom wasn't used to sweep the living room. Then
14. I found out that he had spilled some dirt by the door, too. Then his mother
15. went out of the room, and he started hitting me and I asked him please not to
16. hit me, that I didn't like to be hit, that it hurt. He was doing this—he wanted
17. me to come outside with him. I told him that I was going to stay with his
18. mom, and he hit me. I said that I didn't think that was the way to ask people
19. to do things. He finally did stop hitting me, and his mother came in and
20. wanted to know what we were talking about, and he said cherries. I said that
21. I was asking him why he was hitting me.

22. He began hitting me with the badminton rackets. He didn't hit me hard at
23. first. I was just lying there and he hit me on the back with one pretty hard. I
24. jumped up rather suddenly, and I said, "Charlie, don't do that," and he got
25. this terrible look of fear on his face and started running toward the door and
26. said, "No." Then I told him that I was going to rest and would see him later.

The other child, Freddy, is also caught up in the malestrom.

1. Mrs. Kramer kept yelling at Freddy from the bedroom to "please finish
2. drying the dishes." Freddy looked at me and said, "I'm sure glad this world is
3. in one piece."

At this point the observer remarks to the supervisor that she feels quite fragmented.

The process of acculturation to the psychotic milieu is clearly different for the two families. Whereas depression is the predominant affective reaction to the first family, anxiety is paramount in the second. Here the observer experiences considerable emotional discomfort from time to time and goes to bed quite worn out. She finds it difficult to escape from the situation and feels as if she has been walled in. The pseudomutual lives of the family members begin to seem isolated and fragmented, as each individual glues himself to some preoccupation irrespective of what anyone else is doing. Life is full of harassment, and everybody at times reaches a peak of frustration that finds vent only in screaming. When the parents are in conflict, the children act like an audience, wide-eyed and voyeuristic. On other occasions, they look as if they are remote from the eye of the storm and enveloped in their own worlds. Desperation periodically seizes the whole family and plunges it into unrecon-cilable antagonisms. The dreams of the observer in contact with an involving psychosis are manifestly concerned with overwhelming forces. They take the form of being suffocated, drowned, or buried alive in the earth and are remarkably similar to those dreamed by the children.

As Winnicott (1965) pointed out, the "chaotic" mother is extremely difficult to live with and "the most difficult kind of ill mother that one can have." She is constantly fragmenting her environment, muddling the family, and creating tremendous emotional havoc. It is hard for children to survive a mother like this, since disintegration constantly threatens whenever she is around. This is precisely what the observer experiences and what she reacts to, often with much internal disturbance.

The Lewis Technique: Focal Interviewing

The focal technique attempts to take parts of the psychotic picture, as it affects a variety of people, and to elicit a total impression of the illness as seen through their eyes.

The T. family is made up of father, mother, and seven female children, ranging from 5 to 17 years of age. Following a severe street accident in which the mother and three of the children had been struck by another car on the express highway, Mrs. T. had developed a psychosis characterized by intense excitement, hyperactivity, hyperassociation, and bizarre delusions. Seven of her ribs had been broken, her teeth knocked out, and her jaw and ankle fractured. Clarissa, one of the daughters, had severe injuries to the arm and leg and was hysterically blind during the period of shock; Cynthia, the youngest, had fractured both her femurs and was in traction for six weeks. Ruth was bruised but unhurt. The father had been driving in a second car with the other four girls, who had all witnessed the accident. The mother's psychosis coincided with her recovery from her physical injury.

Prior to this the family had lived a Victorian life under the patriarchal domination of the father, who appeared to regard the eight females as his exclusive harem. The girls, when not at school, were more or less incarcerated in the house and were forbidden any outings not undertaken by the whole family. The father treated any kind of rebelliousness with physical punishment amounting to crude sadism, and the older girls sensed that he got considerable pleasure out of beating them.

The psychotic crisis completely opened up the family life, which, until then, had been run along extremely conventional and stereotyped lines. This opening up involved not only the immediate illness but also past experiences that had been strongly suppressed. The interviewer is trying to obtain a composite picture of the mother and her illness as seen through the eyes of the family members.

The accident (if accident it was) becomes a historical pointer in the life of the family. Things were different before the accident and they have never been quite the same since the accident. It not only precipitated mother's psychosis but has unleashed a good deal of pent-up feeling. It would seem that before the accident, the mother had for some time vaguely suspected her husband of unfaithfulness but more or less suppressed her suspicions. When she became psychotic, her level of craziness was such and the preoccupation with the infidelity was so intense that the hospital understandably regarded this as a delusion, especially after they had talked to the father.

In the focal interviewing, it becomes apparent that every member of the family has their own ideas about this matter so that the group has become polarized around the question of delusional or not delusional.

Father's report: The day before she was going to come home, she developed a mental shock. She became very excited and irrational and thought that I was a devil, just imagine that! I brought her some chocolates, and she said that it was poison. I ate it in front of her to show her that it did not kill me. When she got home, I did not understand she was crazy at first, and I must admit I treated her roughly, but I wasn't going to have anybody talking to me like that. The worst thing is that she thinks that I am seeing another woman, and I find this hard to take. Here am I working at two jobs in order to pay the doctor bills, and no one gives me credit. All I get are criticisms and accusations. It's hard to take. She listens on the phone and questions the children about my movements. She tries to check up on me. When she was very crazy, I could stand it, but now that she's only a little crazy, I won't. When she argues with me, I don't argue back. I simply tell her that she has to see her doctor and take her medicine or go back into the hospital. And would you believe it, this makes her even more angry.

Martha's story (aged 17): She said that Dad was going with another person. I believed it at first. I didn't want not to believe it. When it all started in the hospital, she wanted us to get rid of everything black in the house, like shoes, clothes, etc. It all had to do with the devil. When she's sick she gets very religious, and we become the seven daughters out of the Bible. Everything is then patterned on the Bible. She would pace back and forth all the time and seemed to have no control over herself. I couldn't stand it and would scream, "Stop it" when she started her walking. It was upsetting all the kids. She would run from one wall to the other and leap off the wall. Then she would sit on the floor and shake and wouldn't listen to us. She is so suspicious of Dad. We have to tell her about every phone call. She found some valentines in a glove case and immediately thought the worst. I get disgusted when she starts with her suspicions. She goes through all Dad's things and examines them very carefully. She collected a lot of evidence against him and hid it somewhere in the house. Then, when she got her shock treatment, she forgot where she had hidden the evidence. It included an account of his outings, his phone calls, the valentines, a photograph, a handkerchief, and many other things. She once took me out with her when she was spying on him. At times I act as if I believe her just to keep her calm, but then she accuses me of playing both ends against the middle. She talks about all this in front of the little ones.

Janet's story (aged 14): When she was in the hospital I noticed the change. It wasn't like her at all. She behaved weird. For example, she suddenly came on Martha as if she were going to kill her, and Martha screamed. She would say that Dad was going out with someone. She found some valentine cards in the glove compartment. He sometimes drives girls home from work, but this is just friendly. He is like that. But she said to me, "Don't tell your father but I think he is going out with someone else." She is always trying to convince us. I didn't want to believe it. It made me mad. I told Dad everything that she told me. She had the valentines as proof against him, and she hid them away. We tried to find them but couldn't. She changes her mind all the time. You can never tell from one day to the next what she is going to say or do. It drives me crazy. I feel so mad at her. She says to Dad, "You want to go and have a good time and I have to stay and work with the kids." When she was in the hospital, Dad took her some candy, but she said he was the devil and would not eat it. She didn't smile and looked at us funny. She said to Ruth, "You have to be a good girl. Don't ever wear black; that's the devil's color." She nearly scared Ruth to death. She took her black ring and threw it out of the window. I get so disgusted with her. At home she would go out spying on Dad and would take Cynthia with her. She took me once. She said that Dad was in a certain house, and we saw that all the shades were down. She said that people pulled the shades down when they tried to hide something. She began hunting for the lady and said that she had found out what she looks like. She would confide in us girls, and when I stopped listening she would say, "There you go, Daddy's little girl!" When she talks, she goes on and on, and I tell her to shut up. I always know when her trouble is coming on, because she starts shaking her foot and won't listen to anyone. She keeps pulling at her hair and behaving like a maniac. I get scared and say, "For God's sake, cut it out. You're driving everybody out of their minds." Poor Cynthia sits there with her wide, scared eyes and a weird stare on her face. Since she does not go to school, she just goes out spying with Mother. I'm so sick and tired of it all. I get so mad I could kill her. At times I wish she would really get so bad that she would go away into the hospital forever. When she did go into the hospital, peace descended on the house, and we were able to sleep and no one was walking about and no one was staring at the ceiling. I slept without any nightmares. Now when she goes to the outpatient department, she shuts up like a clam, and the doctor doesn't see this bad side of her, but we kids see it all. We wish that he would see it like we do. She says, "You kids are turning away from me." When she gets sick, I have terrible tornado dreams.

Clarissa's story (aged 13): "Mama had an accident and it was a shock. She was afraid she was going to die and leave us all alone. She was worried about Dad going with another woman. It could be true, and I think I believe it. She is getting a little better, but Dad keeps arguing with her. He'll say things like, "Well, you don't seem so good today," or "You're doing nothing." He pushes the argument, and she gets mad and depressed. She didn't start it, and yet he actually stares at her as if she was a nut and shakes his head and begins teasing her. I think he is trying to drive her crazy again. He says, "I'll put you back in the pit." She always turns to her religious books when she is upset, and he purposely hides them. He says it's because he doesn't want her to get worse. But she likes to read her books, although there's a lot of things to be done in the house. I think Dad tells lies, and I can't stand people who tell lies. Martha and Jan do the same thing to her. They copy Dad. They tell him everything she does is stupid. It's not true. I think he's been going out. Mom found certain things. You can tell from them that it's true. I also found some things that I could show. I can tell when Mom gets broken all up. She doesn't make any sense anymore. She just gets religious and goes overboard with it. She has a wild look in her eyes and sits and stares and scratches at her scalp and shakes her foot. I also do this. I have some of her habits. I rock a great deal until someone yells at me, and then I stop. Rocking seems to release me and perhaps it's the same for Mom. Then Dad says, "Well, she's going to be a nut again."

Ruth's story (aged 11): Sometimes she gets suspicious that Dad is going out with someone, a lady. When she's out and comes back, she asks us whether he made any phone calls. Most of the time he doesn't. If somebody calls we don't know who it is. He doesn't tell us who it is. He never does. She just assumes that he tells us. If he goes to the store, she thinks he is going to call on his girl friend. I don't think it's true, but no one has asked me about it. They wouldn't ask me. We never really see anyone come, and we always tell the truth. I have never seen him out with a lady. We sometimes go out with her and sit in the car for three hours. We stop outside a house watching, and she doesn't know whether to go in or stay out. We get cold. Sometimes we kids play games like "I Spy." We ask her about going home because we get so tired, but she just sits there thinking. At home I am trying to watch TV, and all she does is walking back and forth because she does not know what to do. We all ask her to stop, but she keeps doing it even after we have gone to bed. Dad says that she doesn't sleep good at all. At night I have very bad dreams like murder and stuff. Sometimes I get murdered, and sometimes one of the other girls, and sometimes we murder each other.

Ada's story (aged 9): Mom had a nervous breakdown, and she keeps talking, and everyone goes out of the room because they don't want to hear about it anymore. When Dad says he is going to take her to the doctors, she goes quiet again, but after a while she goes back to walking from wall to wall. She was so wild she messed up her bed. I don't believe everything she tells me about Dad and about a lady, but sometimes I do. If I cry about it all, it gets on her nerves and she takes away my dolly. I then have bad dreams about someone coming after me and they almost catch me. It helps if I write stories. I wrote a story about my Dad being killed in an accident. Everyone said he had done something wrong, but he hadn't done something wrong and he was trying to get away.

Hope's story (aged 7): My mom had an accident and then she got a nervous breakdown. She was mad at me all the time, correcting me at the dinner table. She clobbered me and put me to bed. She locked me in until supper, and I had to go back afterwards and go to sleep. I was jealous because she went to the hospital and got much better food than we did. I really don't want to have her back because she doesn't let us have any fun. When she is in the hospital, I have dreams of a monster lying on my face, and I can't breathe. I'm always afraid of getting sick myself. When she is sick, I keep thinking all about her and don't get my homework done, and then I get an F. It's funny—when she goes to the hospital, I write stories. One story was about the man and lady who were married but they were getting divorced. The lady was going out with another man, and the daddy was very sad because he worked very, very hard to get money and give the children good things. I also like to pray. I have lots of prayer books. I pray about everything bad becoming good.

Cynthia's story (aged 6): I had an accident and broke two of my legs. We all had to go to the hospital, and I had my legs in plaster. I was crying a lot. When Mom had to go to the hospital again, she was shaking and walking back and forward. She was nuts. I was real scared. We go out during the day and watch. Nothing happens; we just watch. We stay all day in the car, and we just watch. She said to watch for a lady, but I only saw a man with a dog. She said Dad likes a lady. I hate the lady. Why can't she stay in her house? When we come back home, Mom gets mad. Then I get scary dreams. It's always to do with Mom, and I think it's real some of the time, and then when I get up it's not real. I don't know what's a dream sometime because it's like real.

Here we have a vivid picture through the eyes of the family members of psychosis entering a household and disrupting and conflicting it. Depending on their ages, each of the children seem to see facets of the illness that are meaningful to them. The agony sustained by the little group comes out in each of the reports. Clarissa is the girl most closely identified with the mother and most likely, according to our test material, to develop psychosis herself. She is very clearly on the side of the mother, believing her evidence and supplying some of her own. She sees her father as deliberately trying to drive her mother crazy, but she is also aware of the latent craziness in him. The two older girls side with the father, although Martha attempts to play a reconciling role. Janet is openly hostile and sees her mother's disturbance as intentionally provocative. A peculiar psychotic triangulation exists between the mother, the father, and the two older girls, and the mother baits them for being the father's "little women." She frequently hints at incestuous actions, which makes the girls further doubt her accusations against him. The younger ones are also caught up in the delusional conflict but tend to express their own convictions symbolically or indirectly through dreams and fantasies. Two of the children respond to the pressure by storytelling. Ruth is the marginal child, who occasionally sides with the older subgroup but transacts more often with the smaller children. She is generally regarded as heading the younger set, although she shows little in the way of leadership qualities and is ready to take her cues from Ada, who is a much more positive and affirmative child.

When the mother's "delusion" first entered the family, there was a general tendency on the part of the children to believe in it, especially as she accumulated and presented her evidence in a very dramatic and convincing fashion. However, the other aspects of her psychotic behavior gradually began to sap their acquiescence. The father's open contempt for and sadistic teasing of his wife also eroded her reliability as a witness. When she "lost" the material parts of her evidence on her return from shock treatment, the disbelief grew more profound. Her persistent suspiciousness and watchfulness has played a further part in alienating whatever support she had in the children's group. Both Janet and Hope openly express the view that they want to be rid or her. Martha, who tried at first to take a neutral part in the family discussions, eventually joined forces with these two in pushing the case for delusion. Clarissa has rallied the younger ones by presenting her additional evidence and pointing to the fact that the father actually spends very little time with the children (where does he go?) whereas the mother works very hard for them. Ruth, for all her passivity and self-effacing behavior, turns out to be a crucial member of the group, since the younger ones turn to her for guidance, and in her soft way she is more susceptible to Clarissa's unconditional loyalty to the mother than to Janet's hard-nosed hostility. During a period of time the children oscillated anxiously between belief and disbelief. The question was never answered one way or the other but has imperceptibly faded out of the picture until it fails to matter any longer. It is as if they worked the delusion out of their systems as a crucial problem for them at a time when the mother's own suspiciousness was still gaining in intensity. The airing of the delusion within the family circle has undoubtedly played a part in mitigating its impact. Brought into the open through the focal interviewing, it seemed to lose much of its psychotic virulence.

If we examine the protocols from the focal interviewing, it is clear that the interviewer-participant had himself become deeply involved in the truth or falsity of the mother's accusation. During the early stage he had assumed, along with the other experts, that since the mother was psychotic her testimony was likely to be delusional. The older children undoubtedly experienced him as being on the side of reality along with them, and they eagerly corroborated his beliefs. The interviews with the younger ones confronted him with "projective" evidence that he construed in favor of mother's accusations. At this point he began to regard the older children as biased and unduly influenced by the father. The younger ones, on the contrary, were seen as offering naïve, straightforward, untarnished evidence that supported the mother. Later interviews with the father obtained the admission that he had in fact been unfaithful earlier in the marriage but was not philandering at the time of the delusion. The delusion, therefore, had a basis in actuality, and the mother's accusation was both right and wrong. The father's defense was both right and wrong, and the children, in their different ways and to different degrees, sensed both the truth and the falsity of the accusation and the defense in different proportions at different times, depending on the ratio of ambivalence toward the parents. The matter was further contaminated by the father's instability and lack of a firm sense of reality.

Conclusion

These two naturalistic methods of studying disturbed families represent different "strategies of penetration." The holistic approach, as used by Henry, allows one to study the transactional aspects of psychosis as it simultaneously affects the family members. My own modification of this approach is to regard the observer-participant as an additional family member, whose training allows her to introspect her reactions more readily than the actual family members. The protocols reveal how sensitively her reactions can help us to differentiate involving from noninvolving psychoses as they influence family life. In the focal approach, based on the technique used successfully by Oscar Lewis in his investigations of severely impoverished people, the picture of the involving psychosis is built up through partial portrayal furnished by each member of the family. The interviewer-participant allows himself to become part of the subculture and to react to the material, so that the final picture is filtered through his reactions. This approach, again, goes beyond the method used by Lewis and represents a further attempt on my part to make the interviewer, like the observer, an integral part of the interview and the observation, and not a foreign body uncomfortably attempting to camouflage his intrusion into the landscape. It is my belief, from these experiences, that the concurrent studies of families by the living-in and focal techniques, with the additional dimension of observer and interviewer reactions brought into the final account, offer between them a unique opportunity for assessing the impact of endogenous and exogenous factors on family life.

References

ANTHONY, E. J. On observing children. In E. Miller (Ed.), *Foundations of child psychiatry*. Oxford: Pergamon, 1968.

ANTHONY, E. J. The mutative impact of serious mental and physical illness in a parent on family life. In E. J. Anthony and C. Koupernik (Eds.), *The child in his family*. New York: Wiley, 1970.

ANTHONY, E. J. The contagious subculture of psychosis. In H. I. Kaplan and B. J. Sadock (Eds.), *Comprehensive group psychotherapy*. Baltimore: Williams & Wilkins, 1971.

ANTHONY, E. J. Risk, vulnerability and intervention in children of psychotic parents. In E. J. Anthony and C. Koupernik (Eds.), *Children of psychiatric risk*. New York: Wiley, 1974.

FRAZIER, J. *The golden bough*, London: Macmillan, 1949.

FREUD, S. *Group psychology and the analysis of the ego*. (Standard ed., Volume 18). London: Hogarth, 1955.

GOLDE, P. *Women in the field: An anthropological experience*. Chicago: Aldine, 1970.

HARTMANN, H. On rational and irrational action. *Essays on ego psychology*. New York: International Universities Press, 1964.

HENRY, J. *Pathways to madness*. New York: Random House, 1965.

LÉVI-STRAUSS, C. *Tristes tropique*. (Translated by John Russell). New York: Atheneum, 1967.

SCHALLER, G. *The year of the gorilla*. Chicago: University of Chicago Press, 1964.

WINNICOTT, D. W. The effect of psychotic parents on the emotional development of the child. *The family and individual development*. London: Tavistock, 1965.

EXPERIMENTAL RESEARCH

INTRODUCTION

The spirit of experimentation has often been regarded as antipathetic to the clinical approach. It short-circuits Nature's meandering methodologies. The clinician, for many centuries, was a natural healer and went about his business with inexhaustible patience, content to bide his time until the bodily processes shifted in his favor, doing little actively except to facilitate the change. Although modern therapeutic agents have accelerated the mechanism of recovery, he has retained his traditional alliance with nature and still inclines to a general policy of noninterference. The clinical investigator carries some of this attitude with him into the research situation. He may wait for the "experiment of nature" to come his way rather than shape events to suit his own time and convenience.

With the medical model reasserting its position in psychiatry, laboratories have once more entered the field of psychiatric research, and the psychological laboratory is becoming an intriguing annex to many units of clinical investigation. It cannot be claimed that all phenomena are equally appropriate for the use of the experiment. The complexity of the human individual, within his complex ambience, renders many clinical phenomena unsuitable for experimentation. It is often impossible to isolate and control certain significant variables in human life and it may also be questionable ethically.

To obviate some of these problems, techniques have been developed for making use of experimental methods at certain key points in the complex manifold of the clinical situation; that is, the experiment becomes part of a general approach. Clinical experiments are in their very nature complex, often involving a systematic arrangement with rotation of stimulation and groups in order that the weight and nature of various factors may be determined and compared. The more simple type of experiment, in which all but one of several variables are kept constant, can seldom be applied to the behavioral field without oversimplifying the research issue. It is the reductionistic element that often repels the holistically minded clinician. To quote Anderson:

> The experiment takes the complex phenomena of nature, breaks them up into segments, studies the action and relation of the segments, either singly or in combination, and arrives at appropriate generalizations. Thus, every experiment is an abstraction, *since material is pulled out of its individual and characteristic context.* Whatever the method used, the control is deliberate and in a sense artificial.

He goes on to stress the important distinction between statistical and psychological significance, the latter pertaining to the meaningfulness of the relation found and its fit in the framework of existing knowledge.

381

So much experimentation in the psychological field has been justly accused of being simplistic, artificial, trivial, and meaningless that the approach obtained a bad name for itself among clinicians, but the new approach attempts to preserve material "in its individual and characteristic context," to look below the surface, to maintain as natural a setting as possible, and to explore its meaning not only to the experimenter but to the subject. The clinical experimenter is sensitive to all this as well as to the "psychological significance" of what he is doing. He is aware that when the experiment means something to the child in terms of his own personality and experience it adds a special element of "seriousness" to the proceedings. It is this research phenomenon that is pursued in this next chapter.

Reference

Anderson, J. E., Methods of child psychology. In L. Carmichael (Ed.), *Manual of child psychology*. New York: Wiley, 1954.

THE USE OF THE "SERIOUS" EXPERIMENT IN CHILD PSYCHIATRIC RESEARCH

E. James Anthony

All the world is a laboratory. . . . [An actual laboratory] is only a place where one may better set up and control conditions.

—*Martin Fischer*

I think your solution is just, but why think? Why not try to experiment.

—*John Hunter, in a letter to Edward Jensen, 1775*

I love the Fool's experiments. I am always making them.

—*Charles Darwin*

The Nature of the Experimental Method

It may seem somewhat anachronistic that a clinician should be attempting to foist the experimental approach on other clinicians at a time when behavioral scientists are seriously questioning the value of experiment in the behavioral sciences. Kelman (1967), for example, has recently wondered whether it was naïve to expect principles of behavior to emerge from the laboratory rather than from life and whether the more important task for the future was to study the individual systematically in his natural environment. He was not depreciating the experiment as such but seeing it in a better perspective, as a useful adjunct to other research methods and not an end in itself. Near enough the same opinion was held by Brewster-Smith (1969), who maintained that insights can be gleaned from sources other than experiment and that common human experiences should not be underrated in this respect; there is no single

E. JAMES ANTHONY, The Harry Edison Child Development Research Center, Washington University School of Medicine, St. Louis.

royal road to truth, not even the experimental path, and the most promising strategy is to converge upon it from many points of vantage.

Clinicians have traditionally been antiexperimental, but for different reasons. Dalen (1971) has diagnosed their particular bias as a misunderstanding of what is involved in experimentation. Clinicians, he said, admire the elegance of the experimental method and genuinely regret that it cannot very often be applied to their field, since it requires laboratory conditions of artificial simplicity and maximum control of variables that are unobtainable in a clinical setting. This is not the case at all, if one considers the experiment in Popperian hypotheticodeductive terms, with the emphasis not on proof but on refutation (Popper, 1963). In this context experiment implies an active search for disproving facts coupled with the logical construction of testable hypotheses. For this procedure no laboratory is needed. One can practice it anywhere and at any time.

The second misconception is that the unifactorial point of view is a *sine qua non* to the experimental method, which excludes the clinician from its practice on the grounds that clinical thinking cannot be anything but multifactorial. Although complexity adds problems to the experimental approach, diversity in itself is not a hindrance and, in fact, characterizes the nature of experiment in the behavioral field.

A third misconception, with a certain amount of truth to it, is that the experiment is alien to the clinical mind by virtue of its constraints, its artificiality, its dissociation from reality, its irrelevance to the life of the individual, and its all-too-frequent preoccupation with trivial problems. In the past the experimentalist has often reacted to the mind-boggling complexity of human behavior and motivation by denying it, simplifying it, reducing it, or isolating a small part of it, which has lost its significance when dismembered from the whole. The purpose of this presentation is to justify the use of the experiment as a research method in child psychiatry. It is suggested that the clinical experimentalist can approach his subjects with a genuine consideration for their well-being and with an understanding of them in depth. Furthermore, the experiments that he devises can have as much subtlety, sophistication, and seriousness as the therapeutic situation and can manifest as much flexibility and imaginativeness.

The fourth and last misconception is that the intellectual organization of the clinician is so intricate, amorphous, and unquantifiable that no mathematical techniques exist for organizing his type of data. Feinstein (1967) has pointed out ways in which the clinician's data can be organized without loss of meaning and cites Piaget for his use of a nonnumerical, symbolic system of analysis.

Feinstein goes even further than this. He indicates how important it is for clinicians to become clinical scientists or at least to take some steps in this direction. The field has too much to lose if they exclude themselves from it for any of the reasons put forward. According to him, "There is no invention, apparatus, or possible substitute from other fields for the clinician in this venture. No one else than the clinician is in the possession of the knowledge of the problems or of the needed skills. No one else than the clinician is in the position to make the necessary observations, therapeutic experiments, and the consequent studies of prognosis, humanely and precisely, needed for the transformation." The next step, to the experiment, is not a large one. Clinicians are constantly experimenting unsystematically without being aware of doing so, and it is high time that they become more self-conscious of their experimental work, so that they can pursue it more systematically and scientifically.

The child psychiatric researcher who is looking for an experimental approach with which to supplement his more usual observation and interview procedures will need assurance that the method in question satisfies these criteria of significance, relevance, naturalness, meaningfulness to the child, awareness of the child's developmental status and environment, and, above all, seriousness.

The Emergence of the "Serious" Experiment

Experimental psychologists, prior to the 1920s, must be held responsible for much of the antagonism felt by clinicians toward the experimental approach. They showed no interest in real-life problems or in the dynamics of human motivation, spending all their time collecting facts that had little relevance to the human condition. When they did approach complex behavior problems, they made use of simplistic solutions to generate simple laboratory procedures, from the results of which they drew simple-minded conclusions. Then, in the 1920s, a young psychologist arrived on the scene and opened up new perspectives on the kind of problems with which experimentalists ought to be concerned. Years later he described this larger context as follows:

> The psychologist finds himself in the midst of a rich and vast land full of strange happenings: There are men killing themselves; a child playing; a child forming his lips trying to say his first word; a person who, having fallen in love and being caught in an unhappy situation, is not willing or not able, to find a way out; there is the mystical state called hypnosis, where the will of one person seems to govern another person; there is the reaching out for higher and more difficult goals; loyalty to a group; dreaming; planning; exploring the world; and so on without end. It is an immense continent full of fascination and power and full of stretches of land where no one ever has set foot. Psychology is out to conquer this continent, to find out where its treasures are hidden, to investigate its danger spots, to master its vast forces, and to utilize its energies [Lewin, 1940].

Had these words been spoken by a psychoanalyst they would have occasioned no surprise then or now, but issuing as they did from the mind of an experimentalist, they represented the beginning of a new era in psychology. It was one part of the revolution that disturbed and defined the first half of the present century. The dozen of American psychologists toward the end of this period summed it up in the following words: "Freud, the clinician, and Lewin, the experimentalist,—these are the two men whose names will stand out before all others in the history of our psychological era. For it is their contrasting but complementary insights which first made psychology a science applicable to real human beings and to real human society [Tolman, 1947]."

One would have thought that clinicians would resonate strongly to all this, but the surprising fact is that although they have continued to incorporate Freud into their daily clinical work, they have chosen to ignore Lewin almost to the point of complete neglect. The clinical experimentalist, however, cannot afford to pass by and disregard the only concepts and methods that can help him to explore the here-and-now of actual experience in a scientific way. The thinking that went on behind such experimentation is well worth examining more closely.

The Lewinian Type of Experiment

There are three concepts formulated by Lewin that help with the definition of the real-life experiment: landscape, life space, and seriousness.

Landscape is referred to in the first article that Lewin wrote (1917), in which he described how the appearance of the landscape is transformed as a soldier moves from the base to the front line or, as he put it, from the peace landscape to the war landscape. The physical environment begins to look radically different because the needs of the soldier are different with respect to safety, food, possessions, comfort, and boundaries. It is incongruous to use "peace things" in a battle area or "war things" at the base. The transformation cannot be attributed simply to an awareness of increasing danger, since it is experienced as an objective feature of the landscape. The background is constantly supplied and re-created by the needs that activate the individual in the foreground.

The *life space* he defined as the total psychological environment, which the individual experiences subjectively, and it includes all that exists for the person, such as needs; goals; unconscious influences; memories; beliefs; political, social, and economic events; and, in fact, anything that might directly affect behavior. All these act as interdependent factors within the life space and come under a system of tensions and forces. To describe what happens within the space, Lewin made use of a nonquantitative geometry, just as Piaget was later to make use of a nonquantitative algebra to delineate the operational thinking of the child.

In Lewinian terminology, it is possible to conceptualize the experiment as a specialized field in the here-and-now within the life space of the individual, surrounded by an ambient landscape stretching beyond the experiment in both time and space. The child in the experiment can be considered as a complex energy system activated by needs and psychic tensions that propel him in different directions. The specific quality of this type of experiment is that it is "serious" in its implications for the child and consequently likely to be taken seriously by him. The field of experiment has a certain time depth that includes both the reality and the unreality of the psychological past and the hopes, aspirations, expectations, wishes, and daydreams for the psychological future. However, it is the here-and-now element that most influences behavior.

Lewin defined *seriousness* as a characteristic of those experiments that bridge the gap between life and laboratory. It is, therefore, coterminous with the personality of the individual in the experiment and is "lifelike." Although the experiment simulates the life experience, it is not by any means an exact replica of what is found in life. Critics had questioned how serious the laboratory experience could be because, they said, it offers only a faint substitute for the natural event and moreover brings about no profound alteration in the individual's way of life. For both of these reasons, they said, the study of motivation in the laboratory is inconceivable. Lewin emphasized that the purpose of this serious experiment is not to replicate the real-life situation exactly, since nothing new can be learned from that, but to set up analogous but controlled conditions in which to study the natural laws involved in the responses. The lesser intensity of the laboratory reaction does not negate the possibility that the same laws are in operation, nor does it imply a lesser capacity to reach into the core of the personality. The serious experiment is one that is taken seriously by the subject, is reacted to *as if* it were a real *life event*, and is relevant to his personality and past life.

Luria's Extension of the "Serious" Experiment

Luria (1960), the Russian experimental psychologist, was much influenced by Lewin's attempt to introduce "seriousness" into the laboratory and thus to extend its pertinence to real life. What Luria seemed to be aiming at was the establishment of an experimental "neurosis" through the setting up of some sort of conflict within the experiment. According to him there are three possible conflicts inherent in any experiment: a conflict over input and whether to accept it; a conflict over response and whether to give it; and a conflict over the connection between the two, which he termed the "conflict of the setting." The coupling of stimulus with response raises, in the mind of the subject, the question of appropriateness. If these conflicts are resolved, the child becomes motivated—and "serious." In cases in which children have sustained a previous traumatic neurosis, a threat of punishment can precipitate a disorganization of behavior that not only affects the experimental response but is also carried over into ordinary life. Luria thus added another criterion to the concept of the "serious" experiment, which is the continuation of the laboratory effect after the child has returned to ordinary life.

Levy and the Phenomenon of "Release"

Levy (1938) devised a type of "serious" experiment in which feelings that have been bottled up within some past traumatic situation can be "released." The therapeutic experimentalist familiarized himself with all the details of the stressful event and then set the stage to simulate, to a certain extent, what had taken place on that occasion. He himself played the role of prompter and furnished the situation with additional resonances when they were required. In this role Levy called himself the "property man."

In order for the experiment to work, certain conditions had to be satisfied. The stimulus had to be precisely evocative so that the real-life event was systematically explored to identify the various components that had contributed to the trauma. Furthermore, in order for the "release" to be effective, a recent intervening event must have occurred so that the child was still in a state of reverberation. When abreaction occurred, the effects went beyond the experimental situation in helping to improve the emotional adjustment of the child. The technique was especially efficacious in helping the inhibited child to express aggressivities bound up with such experiences as sibling jealousy (Levy, 1936), parental divorce, or a death in the family. By means of these ingenious procedures Levy opened the way to further developments in the elaboration of the therapeutic experiment that had the double advantage of providing treatment and at the same time of producing important research data.

Although Levy inclined toward psychoanalytic explanations to account for his empirical findings, his results can easily be interpreted in terms of Lewinian psychic dynamics or field theory, in which a system under tension attempts to find ways and means of releasing the contained energies and thus equalizing this state in relation to neighboring states. Tension releasing and the problem of unreleased tension were built into the theory.

Further Developments in the Construction of "Serious" Experiments

It was characteristic of Lewin's approach to the experiment that he encouraged his students to explore the basic concept of seriousness rather than to seek for exact quantitative measurements. As a result, "seriousness" was investigated more ingeniously than rigorously, with an appreciable gain in experimental freedom. Zeigarnik (1927) made her classic contribution in discovering the preferential recall of uncompleted tasks, and the finding was added to by Ovsiankina's (1928) demonstration that as long as the need was not satisfied and the tension remained unreleased, the tendency toward spontaneous resumption persisted. Another important real-life problem investigated by Mahler (1923) dealt with the everyday question of substitute satisfactions and the extent to which one kind of activity could be replaced by another. What she found was that "real" substitutes, or substitutes based on action, had more replacement value than unreal substitutes, such as walking or thinking. Unfortunately this experimental approach to the problem of sublimation was never followed up, although the significance for the clinician is very apparent. However, Sliosberg (1934) did continue to study the effectiveness of substitutes in terms of make-believe versus realistic situations, such as the reactions of little children to the replacement of chocolate cookies by cardboard pieces of the same size and shape in real-life and in play situations. It was shown that only after the child's needs had been satisfied was he able to make the transition to a lesser degree of reality. Another of Lewin's students, Dembo (1931), studied the genesis of frustration and anger and their relation to the field forces at work in a situation. Her approach was similar in many respects to Levy's. She first searched for ways to generate anger in an experimental situation and explored the context of recent angry episodes reported by her subjects. Her working hypothesis stated that if a person tries to reach a goal and is frustrated in spite of his best efforts, he becomes angry. This hypothesis led to the investigation of so-called "barrier" behavior. She discovered that different individuals responded to obstacles in quite different ways: some exploded angrily; some became irritable; some turned to substitute activities; some tried fantasied solutions; some became utterly unrealistic; and some gave up altogether.

Dembo, in this pioneering work, realized the concept of "seriousness." Why did the children, as they obviously did, take the experiment so seriously (or to put it in the framework of Lewinian theory, why does the force vector, working on the subject, direct it toward a certain valence?). The situation was taken seriously because it was an interesting one for the child, because it was one that involved him personally, because he had already committed himself to it and to the experimenter, because it was not unlike some of the situations he had often had to face in his past life, and because failure was a difficult pill to swallow. The experiment was a serious one because it was lifelike and was so conceived by the children, because it did create a conflict situation that was similar to others in real life that the children had encountered, and because the conditions had generated an intense need that strongly affected the structure of the life space.

It is at this point that the clinical experimentalist becomes dissatisfied with the limitations of the Lewinian approach. His clinical drive will not rest until he has found out why the different children react in different ways to the same frustration. The ahistoric Lewinian thinking, in its devotion to the here-and-now, tends to overlook the real-life fact that children come to the experiment with a long history of idiosyncratic responses behind them and that even the fact of "seriousness" is a function of the "seriousness" they have experienced in the past. To some extent this drawback in the Lewinian approach has been rectified by more recent clinical experimentalists, such as Beller (1959), who has attempted to link the frustration–aggression experiment with the history, personality, and parenting of the child. Another example is the work of Murphy and her co-workers (1956) in their well-known developmental study of normal children. The child brought with him into the experiment a unique and distinct personality with a specific temperament. He entered a "miniature life situation" with a dossier that represented a nearly complete record of his growth and development. In addition to ego-blocking experiments designed to provoke frustration and hostility, ego-gratifying experiments were also used in which the child was allowed to run the show and give commands and as a result was able to discharge a large amount of pent-up aggression.

The clinical development of the "serious" experiment was carried a step further by Frenkl-Brunswick (1949) in her study of prejudiced children, in which she attempted to relate the personality development of the child to his laboratory behavior. In her exploration of the family she found that these children tended to be the offspring of authoritarian parents who, in general, treated them sadistically, inflexibly, and unlovingly. Hypothesizing from real life and personality structure, she contrived a series of "serious" experiments in which she predicted that the prejudiced, as compared with the free children, would be characteristically rigid and unable to shift their perspectives, readjust their preconceptions, tolerate ambiguity, or accept differences with understanding and equanimity, and the results tended to support most of these predictions. Unfortunately the untimely death of the investigator brought this fascinating study to a premature conclusion.

Piaget and the "Serious" Experiment

There are close similarities between the way in which Lewin brought psychodynamic problems into the laboratory and the way in which Piaget made use of a "clinical method" (meaning by this something derived from clinical practice) in his experimental work with children. The two men shared the same flexible attitude about the experiment: it was something that could be shaped to explore their theoretical ideas. They would not submit to its classically stringent demands; it had to bow to their requirements. Both Lewin and Piaget have been accused of manipulating the experiment to suit their own systems. Both transposed fragments of real life into the experimental mode with the intention of accumulating relevant knowledge and creating a science applicable to real human beings. Both were well aware that they were using the experiment in a special way for a special purpose. In Lewin's words, "To proceed beyond the limitations of a given level of knowledge, the researcher, as a rule, has to break down methodological taboos which condemn as 'unscientific' or 'illogical' the very methods or tasks which later on prove to be basic for the next major progress [1927]." Piaget, from his side, felt that the experiment itself had to be investigated and understood, since it, too, was an integral part of human development: "If we wish to consider the assembling of knowledge solely by experiment, we can justify this only by seeking to analyze what the experiment is [1971]." To this one would like to add the phrase— still outside the consideration of both men—"and to analyze what the experiment means to the child."

Piaget demonstrated over and over again that the value of experiments lies not only in proving or disproving but in probing, in trying out something. The word $\pi\epsilon\iota\rho\alpha$ (peira), from which the term experiment is derived, had in its ancient connotation the global meaning of trying out something.

> A four-and-a-half-year-old girl was being put through some experimental procedures devised by Piaget. In attempting to guage the quality of her pre-operational thinking, she was asked to predict the outcome to certain situations: where would one place an object in relation to a light in order to produce a shadow on a screen? Would a penny or a cork float or sink in water? She gave the matter careful and sober attention, and then said, "Why don't we try it out and see what happens!"

Here the little girl was dealing with the experiment in the original sense of the term and not in its subsequently acquired meaning of predicting, testing, and verifying. Both Piaget and Lewin made use of the experiment as an exploratory tool.

Piaget's experimental setup was not an *Ernstsituationen* according to Lewin's understanding of the term. The child's personality was not captured deeply by the process, and conflict was not at the heart of the experiment. For the child it could be an intriguing but bland experience; his emotions were not generally aroused, and he rarely made any attempt to leave the field. (It is difficult to conceive of the well-brought-up Swiss child walking out on the experimenter even under the very frustrating conditions of the Lewin experiment.) The Piaget experimenter is essentially nomadic. He sets up his laboratory in any school willing to loan him a room. The apparatus that he carries with him is relatively simple for the complex epistemological problems that it is expected to solve. The material is homemade, inexpensive, and familiar to the child. He can manipulate it at will and is expected to "think aloud" as he does so. When the experimenting is concluded, an interrogation follows. The child is questioned closely about the procedure and his method of going about it. Although the following schematization is not included in the instruction, in practice the experimental period can be roughly divided into three phases. In the first a working research alliance is established with the child, and any anxieties that he may have about the situation are set at rest. During the second phase the child is allowed to experiment with the material according to the instruction given him at the beginning. In the final phase the experimenter conducts a friendly inquiry in which every answer provided by the child is given serious consideration however wide of the mark it might be. It, therefore, fulfills one aspect of the "serious" experiment: it takes the child seriously, and it follows him seriously into whatever cognitive flights he chooses to embark on. This is where Piaget's wizardry as an experimenter showed itself in the verbalization induced by the conditions. No other child experimentalist has been able to use questioning so artfully in the service of experiment as the Swiss psychologist. His interrogation distinguishes his method from experimental approaches that shy away from the pitfalls of suggestion, persuasion, and playful imagination to which "conversational research" is a ready prey. But in the hands of its author, it is a creative instrument. "It analyzes down to its ultimate constituents the least little remark made by the young subjects. It does not give up the struggle when the child gives incomprehensible or contradictory answers but only follows closer in chase of the ever-receding thought, drives it from cover, pursues and tracks it down until it can seize it, dissect it, and lay bare the secret of its composition [Claparède, 1926]." Even after he modified the experimental situation to include the actual manipulation of objects, Piaget continued to use the method of free conversation that is governed by the questions put but that follows the direction indicated by the spontaneous answers. The two procedures work well together. "Conversation with the child is much more reliable and fruitful when it is related to experiments made with adequate material and when the child, instead of thinking in the void, is talking about actions he has just performed [Piaget, 1971]."

Here then are the different elements of "seriousness" that various researchers have considered essential to this type of experiment:

1. It brings real life into the laboratory in terms of "life space" and "landscape," and the subject reacts to it *as if* to a real-life situation (Lewin).
2. It generates feelings comparable to those in real-life situations, and the behavior of the subject may follow the same patterns as it does in real life (Dembo).
3. Because of the conflict created by the experimental conditions, the resulting disorganization of behavior may persist in the form of an "experimental neurosis" (Luria).

4. Conversely, pent-up feelings from past, real-life, traumatic situations may gain release in the experiment (Levy).

5. The "serious" experiment thus becomes a "miniature life situation," to which the subject brings the "dossier" of his past life (Murphy).

6. The personality may so determine the outcome of the "serious" experiment that experimental responses can be successfully predicted from the knowledge of personality characteristics (Frenkl-Brunswick).

7. To gauge the "seriousness" of the experiment, one must understand the underlying process, and to understand this, one must question the subject; the "knowledge" of the experiment can come only from him (Piaget).

The only other circumstance outside real life that brings together a similar complex of "serious" elements is that of the therapeutic situation, which, since it has been studied for a longer period in depth, provides a useful structure for considering the "serious" experiment.

A Therapeutic Model for an Experimental Approach to the Psychopathology of Childhood

It would appear almost inevitable, and certainly understandable, that today's clinician would attempt to infuse an element of mutuality into the experimental situation, since psychotherapy is currently much absorbed in considering the role of the therapist in the therapeutic situation. This attempt may or may not be an offshoot of Heisenberg's pointing out that the observer's influence cannot ever be excluded from the field of his observation, but a similar type of awareness is growing in both treatment and experiment.

There is a decided trend among some scientifically oriented therapists to regard their field of endeavor in experimental terms: on the basis of past history they diagnose the patient and construct, as it were, a working model of his present capacities. From then onward they test out a series of hypotheses by feeding interpretations into the situation and then determining the outcome. The therapeutic-experimental style is somewhat loose and flexible, but it is often followed through with a great deal of imagination. The clinical experimentalist must also cultivate his scientific imagination as much as his scientific methodology, since ideas do not emerge inductively from facts, as the older position assumed from the time of Bacon, but are first imagined and then verified empirically. The contemporary philosophy of science, as evident in the work of Popper, is making it abundantly clear that the work of the experimentalist consists chiefly in putting forward and testing theories and that this is in essence an hypotheticodeductive method, meaning that a hypothesis can be empirically tested only after it has been advanced. Without research ideas one is out of business even before one can begin. Theories are, to quote Popper (1963), nets to be used to "catch the world," and, scientifically, all that can be done is to make the mesh finer.

The research strategy behind this view lies somewhere between naturalistic, correlational studies and the "true" experiment that is designed in terms of dependent and independent variables, involving maximum artificiality and control, and purporting to expose some lawful relationship or causal statement in a probabilistic framework in which the design eliminates all but one of several predictions. The intermediate form of experiment admits an *ex post facto* strategy in which the probabilistic causation cannot be inferred from the results. Moreover, the independent variable is chosen "after the fact" or without direct experimental manipulation. The experimentalist begins with groups that are initially different in some respects and then proceeds to treat them differently. In this approach he can converge on causation only by a series of contrasting studies. However, as with "true" experiments, he must make a careful attempt to control extraneous variables by not carelessly imposing unwanted variations on the experimental procedure.

This type of experimentation is clearly less alien to the clinical point of view, especially if one is prepared to add "parameters," as in treatment, to bend the method to his specific requirements. Two further additions have helped in the construction of the therapeutic model.

The Individual in the Experiment

Although Lewin had vitally concerned himself with the depth of the encroachment of the experiment on the personality of the subject, his ahistoric point of view precluded the same close attention to individuality. It was left to Kelly (1955) and his followers to stress the crucial importance of individual experience and "the irretrievably interpersonal nature of each person's system for organizing and making sense of himself and the world around him," which, of course, includes the experimental situation in which he is placed. This view implies that experimentation, however seriously conceived, will remain "stilted, sterile, and frustrating" unless due acknowledgement is made to the uniqueness of the person. It is as important to find differences, disagreements, and exceptions on the individual level as on the group level and to accept the unpalatable fact that findings sometimes may not be repeatable because the individual is in a constant process of change. Although this approach sets a ceiling on the generalizability of the experiment, it has the advantage of extracting general properties as compared with the aggregate properties obtained when the focus is on group differences. The latter focus frequently represents little more than the superficial study of a number of individuals at the same time.

The therapist is made acutely aware of this discrepancy when an outside investigator, bent on evaluating therapy, amasses large groups of patients who fail to show aggregate improvements based on four-point scales of progression, the rich and complex individual gains being swallowed up in the statistical process. In the therapeutic model of experimentation, emphasis is placed on the quality and quantity of the individual responses.

The Influence of the Experimentalist on the Experiment

One of the most potent, covert, systematic, and extraneous variables introduced into the experiment is the bias of the experimentalist. It generally operates to confirm his expectations—as Rosenthal apparently demonstrated (Rosenthal and Jacobson, 1968)—particularly if he begins with powerful preconceived notions. Unfortunately Rosenthal's own experimental work on the experimentalist's bias has come under fire, intriguingly enough, for the same reason. He began with a powerful preconceived notion that powerful preconceived notions tend to bias judgment.

However, Rosenthal's assumption has been explored more systematically and fully by Friedman (1967), who carefully examined Powdermaker's and Frank's view that the scientific discussion of any method should include considerable detail about the observer: the role he plays, his personality, and other relevant facts concerning his position and functioning in the environment in which he is working. Friedman described the experimentalist as "a much neglected stimulus object, full of hidden biases" and pointed out that if he is responsible for the setting up of the experiment, a representative design demands that he too be sampled. Friedman also pointed out that in experimental textbooks the experimentalist, rather like the psychoanalyst in the analytic situation, is considered a nonperson, the experiment a nonsituation, and the experimentalist–subject encounter a noninteraction. This assumption has been demonstrated to be untrue in the therapeutic situation, and it is being currently negated in the experimental situation. Friedman expects that the future experimentalist will become increasingly conscious of his own position in the situations that he contrives and aware of the inevitable interpenetration of the experimentalist and the subject. Friedman detects evidence that this is already very much in the making in that recent analyses of the experiment are attempting to make the mutual interaction much more explicit.

The Essence of the Therapeutic Model

As mentioned earlier, many leading therapists have pointed to certain similarities in the experimental and the therapeutic situations. For example, Hartmann (1959) spoke of psychoanalysis as a "quasi-experimental situation," Kris (1947) of its "experimental design," and Kubie (1956) of the way in which "under controlled conditions" the therapist produces certain deliberate and calculated interventions that could be looked upon "as working hypotheses to be tested by certain implicit or explicit predictions."

Because of his background the clinical experimentalist is a peculiarly sensitive instrument in the experimental situation. Before coming to it he has already enhanced his awareness of what goes on not only in the subject or in the setting but also in himself. He is, therefore, ideally suited to conduct the "serious" experiment. His only drawback, as Dalen (1971) has pointed out, is that he never quite shelves his primary motive of helping people or his personal view of the subject. Furthermore, because as a clinician he is a consumer rather than a producer of knowledge, his orientation is inclined to be eclectic and multifactorial, which, at worst, may render him diffuse and paralyzed by his inordinate sense of overdetermination. However, if one's aim is to bring something of real life into the laboratory, then he is indispensable for this purpose. His ability to establish a strong enough therapeutic alliance to withstand the wear and tear of therapy will be reflected in a research alliance that encourages the subject to remain fully motivated until the end of the experiment. His therapeutic background will also enable him, like Piaget, to pay meticulous attention not only to the outcome of the experiment but to the process of development through its various phases. He will be interested in the subject's evaluation of the purpose and meaning of the experiment as well as his assessment of the "hidden agenda" of the experimentalist and what the experiment means to him. The clinical experimentalist must be equally aware of what both he and the subject bring to the experiment and what he and the subject hope from the experiment. The subject is constantly alert to finding out the latent purpose of the experiment and helps to fulfill it or demolish it. In dealing with the experimental demands he may manifest as many defenses as the patient does in the therapeutic situation, and he may defeat the experimentalist by regressing, escaping, perseverating, ritualizing, and dedifferentiating, all of which reactions must, in the soundly designed, "serious" experiment, be brought into the total picture and used in the service of the experimental method.

The following representation schematizes the various aspects of the model, although to complete it one should add the "landscape" to the "life space." As Riessman (1962) has indicated, the experiment is a social situation. The experimentalist–subject dyad is not an island of interaction separated

from the mainland of the everyday environment but a place to which both pro-
tagonists carry their entire interpersonal repertoire. The nearer the experiment is to real life, the more does it reflect life tendencies and the more
does it gain what Lewin referred to as "life value." However, all these factors
complicate the field immeasurably, and, as Luria (1960) has pointed out, the
clinical experimentalist, as compared with the physicist and the chemist, must
acknowledge certain limitations: even with the best-designed experiment, he
had to admit regretfully that a great many of the facts that he analyzes lie beyond his control and are incapable of being recorded and that he does not by
any means have access to all the processes involved. In the "serious" experiment he can construct the phenomenon under examination to only a
minimal extent, and there is no "transference behavior" that enables the
therapist to judge how closely the current conflict replicates the original one.
Lewin brought real-life reactions into the experimental situation, and Luria
took reactions in the experimental situation out into real life, at least for a
transient period. The big question that arises is whether, as in analytic
treatment, the earlier event can be reproduced in the experiment, so that the
subject responds with the same intensity as he did in the past. In other words,
is there an experimental neurosis comparable to the transference neurosis, or
does the brevity of the experiment make it impossible for such a neurosis to
build up?

The difference is between a transient reaction to the experiment, as in
Lewin's model, and a more stable affective disturbance, extending beyond the
temporal and spatial borders of the experiment, as in Luria's model, or an
emotional replay transferred from earlier times, as in Levy's model.

In summary, the experiment becomes a "serious" business like therapy
when a certain number of conditions are satisfied: when the outside world is
brought into the laboratory, complete with "landscape" and "life space";
when conflict is created within the situation; when the past is transferred into
the present, and the individuality and uniqueness of the subject as an in-
constant and variable respondent are recognized; when the mutuality of the
experimentalist and the subject views the former as an integral component inside the experiment; when the "natural history" of the experiment is seen to
unwind in a logical fashion from its inception to its conclusion; and when the
experimentalist retains the feeling that he is experimenting not *on* but *with* the
individual. The total picture is saturated with subjectivity, and the true experimentalist might well complain that "seriousness" has ruined the experiment
and rendered it unworkable. The "serious" experiment can be objective,
however, in the best sense of the term, which does not necessarily include a deliberate distancing by the experimentalist. To quote Popper (1963), "If scientific objectivity were founded upon . . . the individual scientist's impartiality or
objectivity, then we should have to say goodbye to it." Thankfully, we do not

have to say "goodbye" to it, simply because we have tried to analyze and understand all the ingredients that feed into the very complex milieu that we call the experimental situation.

The "Serious" Experimental Approach to the Psychopathology of Childhood

Since the "serious" experiment proved successful in the further elucidation of the child's dynamic, psychological responses, one might anticipate that it would be equally effective in clarifying certain enigmatic features of childhood psychopathology. Maladjustment seems to have a more individual quality than adjustment, but this may well be a clinician's fallacy, since the largest share of his experience is with maladjusted individuals. In an aggregate type of response, this individuality threatens to be lost. It is the business of the experimentalist to extract from the individual whatever can be generalized across other individuals as well as to consider his uniqueness, for example, his inconsistency, his feelings toward the situation, and his reactions to his own responses. The patient-subject, like the normal subject, develops his own strategy for dealing with the problems of life, experiments with the situations confronting him, makes his own predictions, and establishes his own controls. These are the "research activities" of everyday life and are primarily directed at "making sense" of the predicaments in which he is placed. The experimentalist has to learn that when he is experimenting, the subject is also experimenting, and that in order to obtain the most out of the experiment, it is important to set up some sort of dialogue with the subject before, during, or after the experiment. In the literature this dialogue is often termed a "conversational model of inquiry," in which evidence and proof can be jointly examined by the dyad in the experiment.

To set about constructing a "serious" experiment in clinical research, one must first make a detailed examination of the "landscape" and the "life space." He can often do this best by investigating the family in the natural setting of their home to discover the serious elements in family living that involve and influence the child to the extent of making him symptomatic and deviant. It is from these family studies that the "landscape" of behavior emerges. When the "landscape" is sampled as it unfolds over time in a given family, it becomes clear that different children may experience it in quite different ways.

The "landscape" represents the different environments during childhood as perceived psychologically by the child. As with Lewin's soldier, the individual's responses are to a great extent determined by his conception of the landscape. Thus he sees, does, thinks, and feels in a certain way when in the "peace landscape" and quite differently when exposed to the "war landscape."

The landscapes of development do undergo actual changes during development, but it is the individual's perception of these landscapes that causes the greatest variability. Thus the same landscape may be experienced differently by different children in the same family. The major problem arises when the individual passing from one landscape to another becomes unable to shake off the earlier influence and thus begins to respond incongruously, for example, to a "peace landscape" *as if* it were a "war landscape." This incongruity means in Lewinian terms that the time perspective, the state of expectancy, and the degree of reality are carried relatively unchanged into the new life space, so that the past begins to affect the here-and-now. This analysis represents an extension of field theory to embrace a concept not unlike that of psychoanalytic transference, and it is extremely doubtful whether Lewin would approve of such an extrapolation. However, using such an extrapolation furnishes the life space of the "serious" experiment with a connection to earlier child-rearing events, without which much of the "seriousness" would be lost.

When I began my own experimental approach to the psychopathology of childhood more than 20 years ago (Anthony, 1957, 1958, 1959, 1960), I was unaware of Lewin's earlier work. My construction of the experiment was originally modeled on Piaget, but since the samples involved clinically disturbed subjects, the critical element of "seriousness" almost immediately entered into consideration. The construction of "serious" experiments thus began prior to my knowledge of Lewin's fundamental work in the area. In a series of clinical studies my basic premise stated that child subjects who had experienced certain intense situations in the past would tend to reproduce this experience in the experimental situation in much the same way as they did in the therapeutic one. This premise related "seriousness" to replication and suggested a therapeutic model for experiment.

Early Studies Involving the "Serious" Experiment

A sample of 76 encopretic children of both sexes, ranging in age from 6 to 12 years, was divided into two groups, in one of which the soiling had been continuous since infancy, while in the other it had appeared after a period of continence. Investigation revealed that the continuously soiling child was more frequently a dirty child in other respects, coming from a generally dirty family that was burdened with every conceivable form of social problem. The child's messiness was an integral part of the family's messiness and appeared to be ego-syntonic. Both child and family displayed a high tolerance for dirt and dirty behavior, and both were singularly lacking in feelings of guilt and shame. The mother in these families tended to be neglectful and *laissez-faire,* making little or no effort to train or discipline her children. In contrast, the dis-

continuous soiler turned out to be the compulsive child of an equally compulsive mother, who was overcontrolling in her maternal behavior and inhibited
in her emotional life. The child, in turn, was constricted, constrained, and
inundated with shameful anxiety. The mother's training philosophy was rigid
and punitive, and the child reacted to dirt with the same abhorrence as the
mother.

The "serious" experiment focused on the child-rearing history, on the
mother–child interaction, and on the reaction of disgust. It was predicted that
if the children were exposed to fecallike material, the discontinuous soilers
would show a marked aversion reaction, which would differentiate them significantly from the continuous soilers. The testing was carried out under
quasi-therapeutic conditions as near to the procedures of play as possible. A
perceptual battery was constructed in which each subtest involved separate
sensory modalities. The stimulus range was from pleasant to unpleasant (as
judged by adult responses) on a 7-point scale, with extreme attraction and re-
pulsion poles and a neutral response at 4. All cases were exposed to the
pleasant end of the spectrum first. In addition to verbal responses, motor and
autonomic components of behavior were also noted. In one case vomiting
actually occurred, and gagging was not infrequent. The hypothesis was
generally supported but much more strongly in the case of subtests using near
sense modalities, such as smell, taste, and touch, as compared with subtests
using distant receptors. The olfactory reaction discriminated best, the tactile
next, and sight and sound less effectively. A strong aversion reaction was
associated with a discontinuous type of encopresis, coercive toilet training, a
long period of bowel continence before the onset of dysfunction, and marked
reaction formations with respect to dirt. The weak aversion reaction was
associated with a continuous type of encopresis, neglectful toilet training, and a
persistence of infantile coprophilic interests and behavior.

The "serious" experiments in this study were based on the evocative capacity of sensations for reactivating forgotten memories. In the comparometer
experiment I devised, the subject matched two circles, one of them fixed and
the other capable of being made larger or smaller by manual adjustment. This
was the manifest experimental task, and during the first phase the research
alliance was established as the experimentalist and the subject both endeavored
to make the perfect match. During the second phase photographic content related to standard toilet-training procedures was introduced into the fixed
circle. It was hypothesized that resonances from the past, in the form of
shame, disgust, or pleasure, would cause the discontinuous soiler to underesti-
mate the disturbing content as a "perceptual defense" and for the continuous
soiler to overestimate the stimulating content. In the third phase the children
were questioned on the experience in terms of their understanding of it and its
meaning to them. This phase tended to confirm the findings of the second

phase: those who contracted the circle described its content as "dirty," "bad," "wicked," etc., while the circle expanders giggled a good deal or laughed with excitement or amusement as they described the content as "funny" and asked to be shown it again.

In the word-association experiment words with excremental significance were alternated with neutral words, and autonomic reactions (galvanic skin responses) were simultaneously recorded. In the discontinuous soilers, not only were the reaction times significantly prolonged, but the first excremental word that was uttered tended to set an inhibition on further behavior, so that even responses to neutral words underwent restraint. The autonomic reactions mirrored these responses and also differentiated the two groups. With the most effective differentiators (the olfactory and tactile experiments), aversion and attraction were directly and immediately manifested. In these exposures the coprophilic and coprophobic reactions were more prolonged, and one child vomited some time after he had left the experimental environment.

A control group, in which there was no symptomatic disturbance of the excretory functions and no history of disturbed or difficult toilet training, gave reactions that fell between those of the two symptomatic respondents. For all the children, whether in the experimental or in the control groups, the procedures met the criteria of "seriousness." Seriousness was also demonstrated in other ways. Some of the children were in treatment, and it was reported that the experiments stimulated a great deal of affect, a recrudescence of early memories, and the production of dreams in which the experimental content was only very thinly disguised. Table 1 summarizes the results obtained.

In my next experimental study, of sleep disturbances (night terrors, nightmares, and sleepwalking), the concept of "seriousness" was derived from

TABLE 1
Strong Aversion Reaction for Different Sensory Modalities

Perceptual battery	"Continuous" type (%)	"Discontinuous" type (%)	Level of confidence (%)
Smell	7	90	0.3
Color	17	14	Not sig.
Touch	21	53	1
Sight[a]	43	67	10
Sound[a]	37	60	10

[a] Long reaction time in (the word association subtest and underestimation in the comparometer test have been interpreted as aversion tendencies.

Murray (1933), who focused on the "landscape and its prelude to the 'serious experiment.'" When his daughter had a weekend house party in the country and invited four friends, all aged 11, Murray "landscaped" the program as follows: motoring through the countryside ("normal pleasure-invoking circumstance"), followed by the assessment of 30 photographs of men and women abstracted from *Time* magazine on a 9-point scale ranging from goodness to badness, followed by a game of "murder" ("fear-invoking situation"), followed by a retest from the photographs. On the night of the murder game one of the girls, Jane, woke the household in a state of great fear and declared that she had seen burglars; after careful investigation this event was attributed to an hypnopompic hallucination. Two of the girls believed the story, and two were skeptical. The two believers refused to sleep in their own bedroom and insisted on adult supervision and night lights. In the retest the difference between the susceptible and the nonsusceptible group was marked, the former judging the faces as much more malicious than before, while with the latter the reverse was true. For some months later Jane continued to suffer from nightmares about burglars. The weekend events are summarized in Table 2.

Murray's explanation of events threw some further light on the "serious" experiment. According to him the activated fear following the game continued to reverberate over the whole period of time, mobilizing an "active, unconscious imagery" that was then projected onto the material provided. The susceptible girls were clearly more fearful, more emotional, more suggestible to the contagion of fear, and possibly more liable to undergo a partial dissociation of the personality.

In the sample of sleep-disturbed children Murray's findings were essentially confirmed. The Rorschach test disclosed latent anxiety in the group susceptible to night terrors and nightmares, and any attempt to replicate the frightening situation of sleeping and dreaming tended to bring about a manifest increase in fearfulness. When asked to relax, facing a blank screen and imagining a dream to be taking place, the susceptible children became almost too tense to cooperate, even though in the subsequent interrogation they recalled the spontaneous appearance of frightening images, some taken from dreams of the previous night, and some apparently re-created on the spot from an internal reservoir of "bad images." Another factor that added to the "seriousness" of such experimental exposures was the strong eidetic tendency that existed in many of the susceptible children. It was difficult for them to break away from the image once it was implanted. This difficulty was demonstrated in their responses to the Jaensch cards, especially those with a threatening content, when the subjects anxiously shook their heads in an effort to shake off the disturbing experience.

With autistic children (Anthony, 1958) my attempt to construct a "serious" experiment was less successful than in my experiment with encop-

TABLE 2

A Weekend Country House-Party (after H. A. Murray)

The events	Jane	Mary	Lou	Jill	Nan
Motoring in country First project-photo test (av. rating per photo)	Enjoyed 7.00	Enjoyed 5.40	Enjoyed 5.13	Enjoyed 5.53	Enjoyed 7.27
The game of murder (2 games)	Victim and murderer	"Frightened to death"; "so scared"	Afraid	Enjoyed	Enjoyed
Hypnopompic hallucination of burglars	+	—	—	—	—
Belief in its verity Refusal to sleep in room	Complete belief Complete refusal	Inclined to believe Complete refusal	Inclined to believe Complete refusal	Disbelief Occupied room	Disbelief Occupied room
Sleep response (suggestibility)	Search for burglars under bed and in toilet, demanded night light and adult visits; voices low "so burglars can't hear"			Dropped off soon and slept peacefully	
Second photo test	7.80	6.47	6.01	5.33	6.67
Difference in rating	+0.80	+1.07	+0.94	-0.20	-0.60
Personality predictions (hostess)	Susceptible	Susceptible	Susceptible	Nonsusceptible	Nonsusceptible
Later sleep disturbances	Nightmares (burglar content)	—	—	—	—

retic children. The tendency of autistic children to withdraw fundamentally hampered the process of serious consideration. It was difficult to involve the children in the experiment unless strong rewards were in the offing. I again used the "serious" approach effectively in a study of children with a symptom of micropsia (Anthony, 1960). In the neurotic variety of subjects manifesting this unusual symptom the conflict was often very evident and quickly transferred to the experimental situation. The fact that these children diminished the size of a threatening object by means of a "perceptual trick," which is a very "primitive," "organic" maneuver, indicated that they were in some way deficient in traditional coping and defense mechanisms. Confronted with an experimental situation in which the perceptual expectations of largeness, smallness, nearness, and farness were reversed or confused, the subjects actually underwent confusion and on a few rare occasions actually had an attack of micropsia. In the interrogation of the third phase the subjects often demonstrated primitive misunderstandings regarding perceptual constancy. An approaching object was, they insisted, actually becoming larger, and they would even insist that it not be brought too close.

In the family relations test (Anthony and Bene, 1957) a "miniature life situation" was created in the laboratory. The subject was invited to pick a family from a group of representations and to become this family over the period of the experiment. They were placed around him (see Figure 1), and with the help of small cards with "feelings" that were both positive and negative written on them, he was asked to distribute them among the various members of his "family." The "feelings" were of various sorts: there were those that he had for his family and those that he imagined they had for him; there were good and bad feelings coming to him and emanating from him; there were special feelings that he had for himself ("me" feelings); and there were feelings that could not be fitted in in relation to any of the family members and had to be put, defensively, into a "Mr. Nobody." (See Figure 2.) The subject often entered into this situation with a great deal of interest. The fact that the "feelings" disappeared into the "bellies" of the figures (as they do in real life) without giving any evidence of piling up against the "feeler" had a certain face-saving and anxiety-mitigating influence. The test represented a "serious," complex family study that could be completed in about 30 minutes and offered a vivid picture of the degree of involvement of different members of the family, the ambivalence felt toward them, the defenses operating against strong family feelings, the amount of narcissistic feeling, and the general sense of acceptance or rejection. In the interrogation the child often added meticulous details to validate some of the feelings that he expressed in the test situation, and some subjects actually underwent a catharsis. Others, following the experiment, treated the figures in an almost counterphobic way.

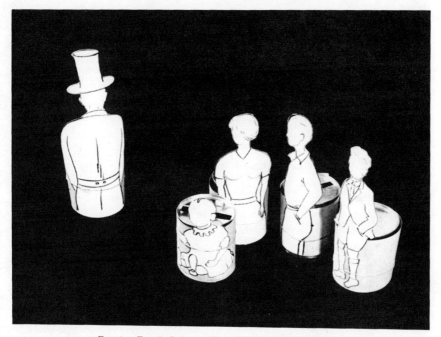

FIG. 1. Family Relations Test (F.R.T.) (Bene-Anthony).

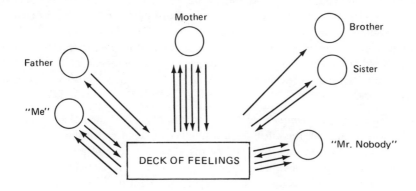

POSITIVE (To and From) "This is the person I love...."
"This is the person who loves me...."
NEGATIVE (To and From) "This is the person I hate...."
"This is the person who hates me...."

FIG. 2. Family Relations Test (F.R.T.) (Bene-Anthony): ambivalence score (+/−), involvement score, defense score ("Mr. Nobody"), self-preoccupation score ("Me").

Recent Work with the "Serious" Experiment

In my recent work with children of psychotic parents (Anthony, 1971) the preliminary exploration of the family situation was made through a series of overlapping family studies and culminated in a week of living in by an observer. These investigations led not only to a vivid appreciation of the psychotic "landscape" during periods of both remission and relapse, but they also helped us to understand the meaning that different psychotic phenomena had for different children within the family. It was possible, although only very crudely, to plot the response of a particular child on a continuum of "seriousness," which then allowed the construction of a large number of "serious" experiments. Many of these were discarded eventually, after experience had indicated that they lacked a critical level of "seriousness." These naturalistic studies of the family in the home setting[1] illustrated the wide variety of ways in which the psychotic parental behavior affected the children, inclining them toward the overlearning of pathological responses, the imitation of abnormal behavior, identification with sick roles, and adaptation to the system of disordered thinking, feeling, and communicating. The expectation was, therefore, reasonably high that at least some of this influence might carry over to the experimental situation. The assumption was that children in the "subculture of psychosis" would be faced constantly with incongruities in the feelings expressed toward them, with irrational paranoid feelings directed toward them for which they could find no cause, with confused communications that often said one thing and meant another, and with the misunderstanding of natural events, which were then misinterpreted in magical terms. We assumed that these incongruities of feeling, thinking, communicating, perceiving, and relating would be present in different degrees in different cases and would be experienced in different degrees by different children.

Four "serious" experiments, varying, however, in seriousness, are discussed here.

The Affect-Discrimination Experiment.   The experimental task for the child was to identify the affect from a number of facial expressions presented photographically and then to correlate the affect with one of a number of affect-provoking situations. The "landscape" to which the child had been chronically exposed was one of several types met with in the psychotic milieu, that is, the parental affect was flat, unstable, incongruous, unpredictable, or excessive. Subjects from such environments might possibly have difficulty in diagnosing the affect or in placing it correctly in the right context. (A normative study had been carried out in the schools through the elementary grades, and there was, therefore, enough data to indicate the best response at a

---

[1] See "Naturalistic Studies of Disturbed Families" by E. James Anthony.

particular age.) In terms of "seriousness," the experiment was generally taken very seriously by both the subject and the experimentalist, but the connecting up with the affect disturbance in the home both currently and in the past was not so evident, nor was there any striking affecting response from the subject. Yet the test did discriminate significantly between children of psychotic and children of nonpsychotic parents. A number of children demonstrated extreme responses in making gross errors in judgment, and these for the most part fell into the group in which the parents had been classified as hebephrenic, process, noninvolving, or low-performance types. The difference between this special group and the control subjects reached the .01 level of significance. Although no catharsis was observed during or after the experiment, some of the children appeared vaguely disturbed by the experience but were unable to verbalize the reason during the inquiry.

The Benevolence–Malevolence Experiment.   This experiment was based on the assumptions of naïve psychology systematically advanced by Heider (1958). The child tends, even more than the adult, to construct a common-sensed psychological viewpoint that stands him in reasonable stead for all practical purposes in everyday life. Where this viewpoint is inclined to fail is in novel or unusual situations, in which past experience is of no help. An encounter with a stranger in a strange environment may overtax the resources of the child's naïve understanding and compel him to fall back on guidelines derived from parental attitudes and behavior. In the experiment the subject was confronted by a stranger presenting two sets of objects: one set, by childhood standards, was attractive, delectable, and need satisfying (a seductive combination of toys and candy), while the other, by childhood standards, was repulsive, unpleasant, and uninteresting and had no functional purpose. Two questions were then put to the child: Which of the two sets of objects is the stranger likely to offer you? If the stranger has to choose between giving himself one of the objects and offering the other to you, which object would you expect to receive? For the average control child from "an average expectable environment," there was not much doubt about the first question. The strangers of the world were collectively regarded as benignly disposed toward children and motivated only by good wishes and intentions. The same anticipated benevolence determined the average child's response to the second question. It was again tacitly assumed that adults, as a collective, tend to place the child's welfare ahead of their own. It was difficult for any child in the 7–12-year range to admit that ignorance of the stranger's background and credentials made it impossible for him to predict the stranger's intentions. He could not admit having insufficient information to reach a valid conclusion. Both normal and disturbed children attempted, therefore, to make conjectures. The experiment did not significantly differentiate the children of psychotic

TABLE 3
The Strategems of Naïve Psychology

	Benign to stranger	Benign to child	Malevolent to stranger	Malevolent to child
Stranger's choice for child only	−	+	−	0
Child's choice for stranger only	+	−	0	−
Child's choice for himself only	−	+	−	0
Stranger's choice between himself and child	0	+	+	0
Child's choice between himself and stranger	0	+	+	0
Stranger's choice for himself only	+	−	0	−

parents as a whole from the children of nonpsychotic parents, but it did elicit some extreme individual reactions and abreactions from some of the children. This small group had parents who had been hospitalized *more than once* with paranoid schizophrenia and were from the lower social class. The difference from control subjects was significant. Within the inquiry the basic mistrustfulness of these children was clearly demonstrated. As a group they insisted that they could not depend on people nor trust them and that unless they were very careful, they nearly always got "the dirty end of the stick." In their dismal picture of the human condition adults often ruthlessly exploited children for their own selfish ends. Certainly for this type of child the experiment had a moderate degree of "seriousness." (See Table 3.)

The Double-Bind Communication Experiment. The communication to which the child was exposed in this experiment was not a "double-bind" in the Batesonian sense. The two contradictory communications came not from the same parent but from two parents or, rather, two parental voices, a male voice and a female voice. The male voice delivered a set of instructions into one ear of the subject, and simultaneously a female voice offered an opposing set of instructions to the other ear. In the first part of the experiment the child was instructed to ignore the male voice and to respond only to the female; in the second part of the experiment the instruction was reversed; and in the third part the subject was told that he was free to respond to whatever voice he chose. On theoretical grounds one would expect the experiment to have a high degree of "seriousness" for two reasons: ambiguous and confused communications are thought by some to be a generating factor in schizophrenia; the inability to screen out unwanted stimuli and to attend to wanted stimuli is also felt to be a crucial generating factor. Several responses can be made: the subject may respond only to the female voice whenever he hears it, or only to the male voice; or he may respond to part of the instruction from one voice and to part of the instruction from the other voice (mixed response). The findings did not differentiate the main aggregate groups, but a number of individual respondents gave a significantly high number of mixed or no responses, and these subjects were found to come with a greater frequency from chaotic, disorganized, confused, and confusing families. In the inquiry they seemed unable to cope with conjunctive sentences containing more than one idea, a failure not related to low intelligence or to race, although the black children showed significantly more "mixed" responses than the white children when social class was controlled. Some of the subjects whose parents showed an involving psychosis scored better than average, and in the subsequent inquiry it was found that they organized and ordered their daily lives by setting up small islands of their own within the general disorganization of the family. Disturbed children from all groups did worse than nondisturbed children, but the differences did not reach an acceptable level of significance. (See Tables 4 and 5.)

The Broken-Bridge Experiment. In this experiment a concrete representation of a Piaget "open-ended story" was presented in serial form to

TABLE 4
Double Communication (Normal Subject)

Runs	1st Experiment father deciding		2nd Experiment mother deciding		3rd Experiment free choice	
	Father items	Mother items	Father items	Mother items	Father items	Mother items
1	+	−	−	+	−	+
2	+	−	−	+	−	+
3	−	+	−	+	+	−
4	+	+	−	+	−	+
5	+	+	−	+	+	−
6	+	−	+	−	−	+
7	−	+	−	+	−	+
8	+	−	−	+	+	−
9	+	−	−	+	−	+
10	+	−	−	+	+	−
Totals	8	4	1	9	4	6
Mixed responses	2		0		0	

the subjects so that a certain dramatic effect was obtained. Pictures told of a couple of children who were stealing apples from a tree in an orchard; the farmer came out, saw them, and chased them. They ran across a somewhat old and dilapidated bridge that broke under their weight and precipitated them into the water. The crucial question put to the children raised the possibility of what Piaget referred to as "immanent justice," the notion that retribution for crime pervades the very substance of the universe: Would the bridge have broken when the children were running across if they had not been stealing the apples? The test was also one of magical thinking. As a group the experimental children did better than the control children, and the most disordered of the experimental children did the poorest as a group. The experiment had many of the characteristics of "seriousness": it captured and maintained the children's attention, and they considered the question posed with great care and attention, as if important issues depended on their answers. One of the factors that made this test "serious" was the moral question raised. Some of the children became almost obsessively preoccupied with goodness and naughtiness, even to the point of meting out additional punishment for the wrongdoing. (See Table 6.)

There seemed to be ample evidence that the peculiar developmental environment in the home tended to invade the different experimental situations to a greater or lesser degree. The subjects appeared to respond to the experiments as if they were relevant, meaningful, natural, and important, although the in-

TABLE 5

Double Communication (Experimental Subject—Psychotic Mother)

Runs	1st Experiment father deciding		2nd Experiment mother deciding		3rd Experiment free choice	
	Father items	Mother items	Father items	Mother items	Father items	Mother items
1	−	+	−	+	−	+
2	−	+	+	+	−	+
3	+	+	−	+	+	+
4	−	+	+	+	+	+
5	+	+	+	+	+	−
6	−	+	+	−	+	+
7	+	+	+	−	+	+
8	+	−	+	+	−	+
9	+	+	−	+	−	+
10	−	+	−	+	−	+
Totals	5	9	6	8	5	9
Mixed responses	4		4		4	

TABLE 6
The "Serious" Experiment

Experiment	Degree of seriousness	Difference
1. Affect discrimination test	Low	Psychotic > control Involving < noninvolving[a] (0.05) Disturbed > nondisturbed Black > white
2. Benevolence–malevolence test	Moderate (older) High (younger)	Psychotic > control Involving > noninvolving[a] (0.01) (Paranoid mothers, 1+ hospitalization) Disturbed: nondisturbed Black > white Low S/E: high S/E
3. Double-bind communication test (Limited Sample)	Moderate	Psychotic > control Involving > noninvolving[a] (0.05) Black > white[a] (0.05) Disturbed: Nondisturbed Low S/E: HIGH S/E
4. Broken-bridge test	Low	Psychotic > control[a] (0.05) Involving > noninvolving Black > white Disturbed > nondisturbed Low S/E > high S/E

[a] Indicates significant difference.

quiry was not always able to elicit reasons for this "serious" assessment. The more "serious" the experiment, the more likely was behavior to disorganize, to regress, to become "silly," and to be accompanied by appreciable affect. For reasons that appeared to have little to do with the difficulty of solving the problem built into the experiment, the subject might become incompetent, distractible, withdrawn, or engaged in a whole variety of nonsolutions of every sort. A clinical criterion for regarding a given experiment as "serious" might be the symptomatic response engendered by the situation.

Conclusion

The making of the "research alliance" is an integral part of the "serious" experiment, and without it the experiment is very likely to fail. Murphy

(1956), one of Lewin's students, has stressed the flexibility of the whole procedure and its dependence on the judgment of the child's attitude from moment to moment. She pointed out that "as is the case with most projective techniques, it is more important to keep these intangibles as constant as possible than it is to maintain a misleading objective control over less relevant but measurable variables such as time, position of the subject, etc." She also emphasized the importance of establishing a workable research relationship:

> Let us consider, for example, the attitude of a child at the beginning of an experimental session. It is essential to make each child feel as completely at ease as possible, but to do so the experimenter may find it necessary to use very different techniques with each child. He may be fairly aloof with one, he may put his arm around another, or try to induce another to laugh before he starts the experiment. The exact procedure and the time involved must necessarily vary and much obviously depends on the judgment of the experimenter, since his task is not to follow a fixed experimental plan, but consciously and skillfully to manipulate a situation while keeping certain major ends constantly in view.

Murphy insisted that the experimentalist must be a "friendly, familiar, and unthreatening person" and that none of the experimental procedures should ever be attempted until the child has become acquainted with him. In the first phase the experimentalist talks freely with the child and attempts to reduce the child–adult distance as much as possible. He must also give the child time to "warm up" and familiarize himself with the situation, and an easy, casual relationship is paramount in achieving this. Following the experimental session Murphy feels that it is useful to observe the child's subsequent behavior outside as well as his attitude toward the experimentalist the next time that he encounters him.

Forty years ago Adolph Meyer expressed the opinion that all human functioning must eventually be brought within the scope of natural science. It is only recently that experimental work has entered the psychiatric field, and it is still to a large extent looked upon as an alien procedure. The child psychiatrist is still chary of the experiment as a possible threat to his young patient, and when he goes in search of knowledge, he still tends to follow the traditional research pathways. In this presentation I have endeavored to demonstrate that the experimental mode need not be harmful nor degrading nor divorced from reality nor trivial nor nonsensical if one comes to understand that "seriousness" can play as much of a role in the experimental as in the therapeutic situations. I have frequently reiterated throughout this chapter that what matters is the attitude of mind of both the subject and the experimentalist, and this attitude must go beyond the superficial. The clinical experimentalist has constantly to bear in mind the words of Pasteur in his address to the academic youth of the Soviet Union: "While you are studying, observing, and experimenting, do not remain content with the surface of things."

References

ANTHONY, E. J. An experimental approach to the psychopathology of childhood—encopresis. *British Journal of Medical Psychology,* 1957, **30,** 146–175, 1957.

ANTHONY, E. J. An experimental approach to the psychopathology of childhood—autism. *British Journal of Medical Psychology,* 1958, **32,** 1.

ANTHONY, E. J. An experimental approach to the psychopathology of childhood—sleep disturbances. *British Journal of Medical Psychology,* 1959, **32,** 1.

ANTHONY, E. J. An experimental approach to the psychopathology of childhood—micropsia. *Psychiatric Research Reports,* 1960, **13,** 63–99.

ANTHONY, E. J. A clinical and experimental study of high risk children and their schizophrenic parents. In A. R. Kaplan (Ed.), *Genetic factors in schizophrenia.* Springfield, Ill.: Charles C Thomas, 1971.

ANTHONY, E. J., and BENE, E. A technique for the objective assessment of the child's family relationships. *Journal of Mental Science,* 1957, **103,** 541–555.

BELLER, E. K. Exploratory studies of dependency. *Transactions of the New York Academy of Science,* 1959. **21,** 414–426.

BREWSTER-SMITH, M. *Social psychology and human values.* Chicago: Aldine, 1969.

CLAPARÈDE, E. Introduction to *The language and thought of the child* by J. Piaget. London: Routledge, 1926.

DALEN, P. One, two or many. In A. R. Kaplan (Ed.), *Genetic factors in schizophrenia.* Springfield, Ill.: Charles C Thomas, 1971.

DEMBO, T. *Der Anger als dynamisches Problem. Psychologische Forschung,* 1931, **15,** 1–144.

FEINSTEIN, A. R. *Clinical judgment.* Baltimore: Williams & Wilkins, 1967.

FRENKL-BRUNSWICK, E. Intolerance of ambiguity as an emotional and perceptual personality variable. *Journal of Personality,* 1949, **18,** 108–143.

FRIEDMAN, N. *Psychological research: The psychological experiment as a social interaction.* New York: Basic Books, 1967.

HARTMANN, H. Psychoanalysis as a scientific theory. In E. Hook (Ed.), *Psychoanalysis, scientific method and philosophy.* New York: New York University Press, 1959.

HEIDER, F. *The psychology of interpersonal relations.* New York: Wiley, 1958.

KELLY, G. A. *The psychology of personal constructs.* New York: Norton, 1955.

KELMAN, H. C. Human use of human subjects: The problem of deception in social psychological experiments. *Psychological Bulletin,* 1967, **67,** 1–11.

KRIS, E. The nature of psychoanalytic propositions and their validation. In S. Hook and M. R. Konvitz (Eds.), *Freedom and experience.* New York: Cornell University Press, 1947.

KUBIE, L. S. The use of psychoanalysis as a research tool. *Psychiatric Research Reports,* 1956, **6,**

LEVY, D. Use of play technique as an experimental procedure. *American Journal of Orthopsychiatry,* 1933, **3,** 266–275.

LEVY, D. Hostility patterns in sibling rivalry experiments. *American Journal of Orthopsychiatry,* 1936, **6,** 182–257.

LEVY, D. "Release therapy" in young children. *Psychiatry,* 1938, **1,** 387–390.

LEWIN, K. "Kriegslandschaft." *Zeitschrift für Angewandte Psychologie,* 1917, **12,** 440–447.

LEWIN, K. *Gesetz und Experiment in der Psychologie.* Berlin: Weltkies-Verlag, 1927.

LEWIN, K. Formalization and progress in psychology. *University of Iowa Studies in Child Welfare,* 1940, **16,** 3.

LURIA, A. R. *The nature of human conflict.* New York: Grove Press, 1960.

MAHLER, V. Ersatzhandlungen verschiedenen Realitatsgrades. *Psychologische Forschung,* 1933, **18,** 26–89.

MURPHY, L. *Personality in young children.* New York: Basic Books, 1956, Vol. 1.

MURRAY, H. A. The effect of fear upon estimates of the maliciousness of other personalities. *Journal of Social Psychology,* 1933, **4,** 310–329.

OVSIANKINA, M. Die Wiederaufnahme von unterbrochener Handlung. *Psychologische Forschung,* 1928, **2,** 302–389.

PIAGET, J. *Psychology and epistemology: Towards a theory of knowledge.* New York: Grossman, 1971.

POPPER, K. R. *Conjectures and refutations.* London: Routledge, 1963.

POWDERMAKER, F., AND FRANK, J. *Group psychotherapy—Studies in methodology of research and therapy.* Cambridge, Mass: Harvard University Press, 1953.

RIESSMAN, F. *The culturally deprived child.* New York: Harper & Row, 1962.

ROSENTHAL, R., and JACOBSON, L. *Pygmalion in the classroom.* New York: Holt, Rinehart and Winston, 1968.

SLIOSBERG, S. Zur Dynamik der Ersatzes im Spiel und Ernstsituationen. *Psychologische Forschung,* 1934, **19,** 122–181.

TOLMAN, E. C. Memorial address on Kurt Lewin, delivered at the Annual Conference of the American Psychological Association, 1947.

WHEWELL, W. *History of the inductive sciences.* 1837.

ZEIGARNIK, B. Über Behalten von erledigten und unterledigten Handlungen. *Psychologische Forschung,* 1927, **9,** 1–85.

THE ONTOGENESIS
OF THE
INVESTIGATOR

INTRODUCTION

What can one say about the prodigious productivity of Bender over these many years? Judging from this scientific autobiography, it would seem as if every stage in her training had made a relevant contribution to her final emergence as a neuropsychiatric investigator. The inevitability of this development leads one to conclude that from very early in her career she must have had an intuitive understanding of where she was going, of what she wanted to do, and of how she would go about doing it. Her research strategies have been quite characteristic, and it is possible to typify her style of investigation as "Benderian" since many of her leading students have displayed it to some extent. In essence it is a straightforward, pragmatic approach involving careful psychiatric and neurological examinations, the use of special tests like the famous one that bears her name, the assessment of family background, and the follow-up. It is this last link in the research sequence that constitutes perhaps her major procedural contribution. The follow-up study is a sobering experience for clinicians and many are loath to put their narcissism on the line and risk their diagnostic and prognostic reputations. Bender is too much of an investigator to allow such false pride to intrude upon her work. She is very ready to check on her postulates.

Another admirable attribute is Bender's willingness to learn from others and to transmit what she has learned to others. All of us in academic child psychiatry would take pleasure in the thought that we have passed on to our students many of the good things that we have received from our teachers, but unless our talents are many, we are often left in greater debt to the past. Bender has repaid her past teachers in good measure by incorporating some of their key concepts into her general theory. She remains very appreciative of those who taught her and even married Schilder, perhaps the most gifted one among them, dedicating herself to exploring many of his seminal ideas. It was Gesell, however, who helped her to "wrap it all up" in a coherent developmental picture. By any standards her contribution has been monumental and much of it is already in the textbooks.

The fact that Bender is fundamentally a neuropsychiatrist who uses a medical model has led the more dynamically oriented to look less appreciatively at what she has had to offer, but if psychiatry continues along its present psychobiological path, her output may well go on record as providing some of the basic underpinning for our discipline. What is too often overlooked is that she has not been unaware of cultural, social, or psychodynamic factors but has chosen to emphasize brain function in the understanding of the child since it has been so obviously neglected by almost everyone else.

Lourie's clinical and organizational skills have tended to draw attention away from his quietly and steadily pursued research career. At each step of his professional growth he has carried out investigations that have reflected his age and stage of development. Much of his research is therefore, "phase-specific."

Unlike others who have first embarked on research at a much later date, as a young investigator, Lourie, like Freud, was able to build his research experience on a sound biological basis, and subsequently, like Freud, he felt free enough to take off into less tangible spheres. His speculations, like his analyses, have never become "wild," since he has always been able to maintain a sound, common-sense view of nature and life and to keep at least one researching foot firmly on *terra firma*. His psychoanalytic background is reflected in much of his work but neither Freud (nor Maslow for that matter) can be held responsible for his humanism, his honesty, his balanced judgment, and his wry sense of humor. These must have been derived from his physician father, whose adopted name itself must have communicated a blueprint to his son for scholarly integrity and reliability. These attributes are still sufficiently uncommon in the higher professional reaches to render their owner indispensable.

So useful has Lourie been to his country and to the world at large that the demands on his services have been constant both at national and at international levels, and as a result precious time has been taken from his career as a researcher. This may have been unfortunate for research but very fortunate for world mental health. One simply has to recognize that he is not the person to be confined within a single laboratory, a single project, a single hospital, or even a single country. He is a much-wanted man who has given very generously of himself. I have always regarded him as an ideal person with whom to be shipwrecked on a desert island because he is practical, inventive, speculative, dependable, friendly, and a born raconteur. He would also be invaluable in setting up a sound research department on the island!

A CAREER OF CLINICAL RESEARCH IN CHILD PSYCHIATRY

LAURETTA BENDER

With hindsight I can say that my career as an investigator in child psychiatry started when I was at the University of Chicago studying premedical and medical courses and pathology from 1918 to 1923. I worked in the pathological laboratories of H. Gideon Wells studying the blood of tuberculous guinea pigs and learning the methodology and philosophy of research (Bender and DeWitt, 1923–1924).

C. Judson Herrick and the Evolution of the Central Nervous System

My medical studies in neuroanatomy brought me to C. Judson Herrick, who investigated and taught the anatomy of the central nervous system from the point of view of evolution, embryology, and development. Years later he summarized his life work in a book, *The Evolution of Human Nature* (1956). To him I owe the concept of the living brain as a stage in transit in evolution and the mind as a function of the brain as well as motility. He said, "Motility is the cradle of the mind. Mentation arises within behavior and primarily for the advancement of its efficiency [p. 240]."

Dr. Herrick saw development as an extension of evolution and as self-regulating and goal-directed. He also taught that every human action and every human experience is a biological event. He said, "Many puzzling features of the part played by the cortex in regulation of behavior are explained by evolutionary history [p. 418]." The individual's life pattern is determined by endogenous inborn characteristics modified by his environment and experiences.

LAURETTA BENDER, Clinical Professor of Psychiatry (Retired), Columbia University Medical School, New York.

Samuel T. Orton and Strephosymbolia

I transferred to the State University of Iowa in 1923 to complete my clinical medical studies and to continue my studies in neuropathology with Samuel T. Orton, professor of psychiatry.

It happened that he had just started his work on a new project, the first in this country on reading disabilities or dyslexias in children. I was made a member of a mobile mental hygiene clinic, that traveled from school to school in a semirural community in Iowa to study children who were not achieving adequately in their schoolwork (Orton, 1928).

Dr. Orton, did important pioneering work (1937). He spoke of specific difficulties in acquiring language skills in these children, delineating reading, writing, and spelling difficulties and relating them to developmental disturbances in cortical dominance, left–right-handedness, -eyedness, and -footedness, and the learning of language skills. He noted that these children tended to reverse letters, numbers, syllables, or whole words. Thus he used the term *strephosymbolia* ("twisted symbols"). He also noted difficulties in spatial orientation.

The term *congenital defects* in language acquisition was already in use in the literature, but Orton felt that this term tended to overstress the inherent difficulties and to underemphasize the many environmental factors, such as methods of teaching and emotional and social factors, and he preferred the use of the term *developmental disorder.*

Orton ascribed many of the sensory confusions, especially the visual ones such as the reversals of letters and groups of letters, to the confused cortical dominance. He described a failure of the elision of the memory images or engrams from the nondominant side of the third level symbolic of the sensory cortex. Thus he saw a failure of association between the presented visual stimulus and its remembered concept. He was convinced that such disorders should respond to treatment "if we become sufficiently keen in our diagnosis and . . . clever enough to devise the proper training methods to meet the needs of each particular case [1937, p. 200]."

Though my actual work with children was delayed for nearly ten years, my interest in the problem of developmental delays in language skills in children was continuous throughout this time.[1] Meanwhile I recalled Herrick's teachings and saw the maturational lag in the acquisition of language skills as an evolutionary problem related to the recent acquisition, in humans, of language and symbol formation, with dominant handedness for the use of tools and pen and pencil related to cortical dominance (Bender, 1957a). The rate of maturation in affected children is variable in the timing and also

---

[1] This was perhaps in part because Dr. Orton had recognized that I was such a case, partially self-corrected but still retaining every feature of confused cortical dominance, with reversal tendencies, left–right and other spatial disorientations, and difficulties in all language skills.

between different functions such as visual, auditory, and proprioceptive perception, and motor control in the poorly dominant hand.[2]

Phipps Clinic of Johns Hopkins Hospital and Adolf Meyer

I went to Phipps Clinic of the Johns Hopkins Hospital as a research associate with Adolf Meyer in the fall of 1929. Adolf Meyer talked about the organism as a whole and psychobiology: "man as a psychobiological integrated biological unit." He emphasized the life experiences and reactive patterns or working adjustments (the ergasias) in mental illness and de-emphasized the biological factors. He expressed concern that if a biological basis was emphasized, residents in training would not try to treat their patients by urging a better adaptation to their life problems.

He did not accept psychoanalysis, saying that he was not convinced of the unconscious. Nevertheless he arranged for the teaching of every school of thought to his staff. Therefore he had as a visiting professor for three months of 1930 Paul Schilder, a Viennese psychiatrist, neurologist, and psychoanalyst.[3]

Paul Schilder

Paul Schilder had a view of life's constructive processes in integrating body functions, neurological processes, mind, psychology, and social relationships in a reality-related and goal-directed fashion. Much of our work later together at Bellevue was done with children, of which he said:

> The principle of constructive psychology can help in a deeper understanding of the child [which] can only be understood as a continuous process of trial and error [leading] to construction and configuration as a basis for action. . . . Behavior difficulties . . . are an interruption of this constructive psychological process. . . . The approach to childhood problems is a definite dynamic and constructive one. The

[2] Graduating in medicine from the State University of Iowa in 1927, I was sent, on a Rockefeller Traveling Fellowship, to Amsterdam, Holland, hopefully to study developmental and evolutionary problems of the central nervous system with Professor G. van Rijnberk (physiology), Professor B. Brouwer (pathology), and Professor C. U. Ariens Kappers (anatomy). I was made content to study the cerebellar control of the vocal cords in dogs, as the professors decided (Bender, 1928). I learned a great deal about the cerebellum, about research methodology and scientific writing, and about the wonderful Dutch people, especially those with whom I worked. When I returned from Holland, I had a psychiatric residency at Boston Psychopathic Hospital.

[3] From the second day of January 1930, when I first met Paul Schilder in the Phipps Clinic, he became the man of my life. We worked together those three months, and in the fall of 1930 I followed him to Bellevue Psychiatric Hospital in New York City. We were married in 1937 and had three children. We continued to work together until his death in 1941. After his death I collected all his writings on children and developmental problems in Paul Schilder, *Contributions to Developmental Neuropsychiatry* (1964).

child is seen as a growing organism with definite problems of maturation. . . . Great stress however should be placed on the living situation and emotional problems of childhood life as these are continually modifying the developmental process. The development of the child is seen in accordance with the general
principles of psychoanalysis as an emotional interdependence between the parents,
the surroundings of the child and the child itself [1940].

Paul Schilder also innovated skills for studying all the neuropsychiatric, communicative, and social functions through his inimitable capacity for direct observation of behavior, motility, etc., and through his verbal interviews, in which he explored fantasy material, description of pictures, comics (then new), and movies. He also used spontaneous art productions of patients, through which he explored perceptions, thought processes, emotions, and relationships to reality, objects, and other persons. Finally, he had a capacity to collect such data, analyze them, and hypothesize his own "constructive psychology," which is more than integrative psychology. It includes integration but also im-plies an open-ended construction that is goal- and reality-directed.

Schilder developed conceptual frameworks to explain these data, some of which were concerned with research in child psychiatry. In this he accredited me as a co-worker.

1.   The body image is a total, integrated gestalt of all of the individual's perceptual and social experiences. It is never static. It is in a continuous state of construction. It matures as the child matures and is affected by any distur-bances in maturation. It regresses with any disorganizing process. The drawing of a man was found by us to be a projection of the body image (Bender, 1940; Schilder, 1950).

2.   Soft neurological signs were first noted by Schilder in the manneristic features of adult schizophrenics, not quite neurological in significance. Later in children we saw them as maturational lags especially in patterned behavior sometimes called reflex, such as the postural patterns, oculomotor patterns, vestibular-tonic patterns, cortical dominance, and right–left orientation in space (Schilder, 1964).

3.   He early emphasized the importance in the vestibular organization in relation to tone, motility, and relationship to reality (through the gravity of the earth) and to interpersonal relationships (Schilder, 1942).

4.   He explored the tonic neck-righting attitudes and whirling motility in development and in the maturational lags of children in whirling and in flying fantasies, as well as in the religious ecstasies of adults.

Visual Motor Gestalt Test and What It Demonstrated

While at Johns Hopkins Hospital (1929–1930) I started work on the Visual Motor Gestalt Test (VMGT) (Bender, 1938). In the beginning I used mute, regressed, autistic schizophrenic women at the Springfield State Hospital, whom I was studying at that time. I asked the patients to copy figures that I had adapted from Max Wertheimer's studies on gestalt psychology. He had asked normal adults to describe their perceptual experiences (Wertheimer, 1923, 1938). My method revealed that it was possible to demonstrate many principles in the evolution of development and regression of perceptual-motor experiences other than the *"gute Gestalt,"* which Wertheimer described. Thus I concluded that there was a "suggestion of development in the visual motor patterns . . . that the more primitive sensory motor patterns are dependent on the principle of constant motion which seems to be largely whirling movement in a vortex in a clockwise or counterclockwise direction with an associated radiating directional component and with a tendency to emphasize the horizontal plane [1938, p. 24]." Most of the basic principles of the genesis and maturation of the visual-motor gestalten experienced were determined at this time. But many finer elaborations were developed later on normal nursery school children, public school children, children in institutions for the retarded, and disturbed children in clinics and wards of psychiatric hospitals, such as Bellevue, as well as many adults. Studies were also made on normal adults to explore optic imagery whish, which emphasized the evidence of movement in imagery. Tachistoscopic studies revealed the significance of time in the development of a visual-motor gestalt in each individual experience and in the maturation of visual-motor gestalten in developing children.

The VMGT was finally evaluated as one of maturation in visual-motor *Gestalt* functions and of deviations in maturation especially due to biological developmental and organic factors in children and to organic pathology and regression in adults.

A later statement (Bender, 1970c) summarizes the principles of maturation of visual-motor gestalten in children as follows:

1. Vortical movement, biologically determined, in the optic field, gives rise to the most primitive visually perceived forms, such as circles and loops.
2. The movement always present is vortical and directional, clockwise or counterclockwise.
3. The horizontal plane is first emphasized as directional, dextrad or sinistrad.
4. If these action patterns are controlled or inhibited, globes, circles, and arcs are constructed.
5. These forms organize the visual field into a foreground and a background.
6. Boundaries between the forms are delineated.
7. Verticalization arises concurrently with maturation of the body image as the postural model shifts in the young child from the prone to the upright posture.

8.   Crossed lines and diagonal or angular formations are a later level of maturation, usually occurring between six and eight years of age.

In spite of my training in research methodology, I had none in psychology. This has called forth considerable criticism from many researchers and an effort to correct the defects, as they see them, in the VMGT. There have been many efforts to make rating scales and scoring systems that can be applied to the test with statistical validity (see Tolor and Schulberg, 1963). All of these methods diminish the significance and value of the test (Bender, 1938). They fail to take into consideration the essential global nature of the gestalt function, the inseparableness of the perceptual and motor constituents, and the inherent nature of maturation in all mental, personality, and organismic functions, including the gestalt function of the personality as a whole. These are living abstractions and cannot be reduced to concrete parts without the sacrifice of the total concept and value of the test.

Follow-up Study of Schizophrenic Women

My main assignment the year I was at Phipps Clinic was to start a follow-up study on schizophrenic women who had been observed and diagnosed at Phipps Clinic and who had been transferred to Springfield State Hospital of Maryland. The study covered the years from 1913, when Phipps Clinic opened, to 1929, when I was there. I continued the study in 1956. This was 26 to 43 years after the women's initial admission to Phipps Clinic—26 years after my first follow-up and after I had had 20 or more years' experience in child psychiatry (Bender and Hitchman, 1956).

My study included the making of life charts, which Adolf Meyer had developed to emphasize the life experiences, both biological and environmental, from birth to the ultimate outcome of the individual.

From the point of view of child psychiatry, this study was significant for showing many of the same characteristics in these adult and aging schizophrenic women and a lifelong continuity of a pattern starting in childhood, adolescence, or early womenhood that we later saw in children at Bellevue and followed into adulthood (Bender, 1973b).

Bellevue Adult Services, 1930–1934

In 1930, I followed Paul Schilder to Bellevue Psychiatric Hospital and the New York University Medical School. The first four years I worked with adult patients of the great variety that Bellevue has always cared for. My major responsibility was clinical, but I had the opportunity to continue my gestalt studies on the great variety of adult psychiatric and neurological conditions. I also continued my gestalt studies with children in the community.

Neuropathological Studies

During these years I also had the opportunity to carry on neuropathological studies through the courtesy of the pathology department of New York University and the Neurological Institute of Columbia University, where Samuel T. Orton was then an associate.

These studies were made on patients who died in the psychiatric wards of Bellevue Hospital and who were studied psychiatrically and neurologically by Paul Schilder and me before death. We were especially interested in patients who succumbed to alcoholic encephalopathy (Bender and Schilder, 1933).

Clinical studies demonstrated regressive phenomena, such as startle reactions, sucking and grasping reflex activity and groping with both the mouth and the hands, asynergia, clouding of the consciousness, sleep disturbances, hypersensitivity to pain, muscular rigidity with resistance phenomena, and athetoid and rhythmic movements of limbs. Vegetative disturbances were impressive, with emaciation, erratic temperature curves, sweating, and pellagralike changes in the skin. Some who recovered, while in remission regained functions at higher levels of organization and lost regressive features.

We found that the neuropathological lesions occurred in those parts of the brain and cord that were bathed by the spinal fluid and were most severe where the spinal fluid flowed least freely, especially in the ventricular system and submeningeal spaces. The gray masses along the ventricles and the base of the brain seemed to be selected electively and characteristically by marginal and ependymal and invasive and productive gliosis with underlying proliferative vascular lesions.

These pathological studies acquired increasing interest as the newer studies on damage to the central nervous system of the human fetus and newborn infant have shown a similar distribution of lesions in the periventricular areas, particularly in the subependymal germinal matrix, with infarction and hemorrhages into the underlying gray matter in the premature infant with hypoxia or before birth in association with prenatal asphyxia (Banks and Larroche, 1962; Towbin, 1970).

In term infants hypoxia leads more often to subdural cortical damage resulting from stasis thrombosis. This damage may prove to be more serious, but it occurs less often. These findings have been determined, of course, in fatal cases.

There is evidence that the more frequent lesions to the central nervous system recognized after birth are due to "latent processes having origin prenatally and may be well advanced prior to labor. Attention is focused on the occurrence of precocious destruction of cerebral germinal matrix as a factor in enigmatic development of organic mental retardation or cerebral palsy . . . and other neurologic defects associated with prematurity [Towbin, 1970, p. 541]." These other defects are related to respiratory and cardiac difficulties, poor tone and irritability, or visceral and autonomic dysfunctions.

Infants damaged in periventricular areas show varying degrees of motor or mental retardation. Even milder damage results in maturational lags with ultimate normal or near-normal motor and mental development but with clinical signs of minimal brain damage, such as soft neurological signs and features referrable to periventricular disorganization, including vegetative functions.

Later (Bender and Anderman, 1965) I studied blind children with retrolental fibroplasia, who were sent to Creedmoor State Hospital because they were thought to be children with autism, since they were essentially nonfunctioning and untestable with psychological testing. Careful studies of the mothers' histories of pregnancy and the development histories, of behavior, neurological and physical development, and of response to treatment indicated early fetal damage leading to premature expulsion of the fetus and hyperoxia in incubators at a critical period in eye development, which caused the retrolental fibroplasia. Thus they were organically defective as well as blind.

Bellevue Child Psychiatry, 1934–1956

In the fall of 1934 I took charge of the children's service of Bellevue Psychiatric Hospital of New York City. But before this Paul Schilder and David Wechsler had been making studies on the children that contributed to my thinking. These are collected in Paul Schilder's *Contributions to Developmental Neuropsychiatry* (1964). Of special interests were studies on "The Child and the Symbol" (1938) and "The Psychology of Language" (1936), "Children's Attitude Towards Death" (1934), "Children's Concept of the Inside of Their Body" (1935), and "The Psychological Implications of Motor Development in Children" (1937).

From 1934 to 1956 in the Bellevue Hospital of New York City and from 1956 to 1969 in Creedmoor State Hospital of the New York State Hospital system, I had the privilege for over 35 years of functioning in public facilities caring for a wide range of early developmental and reactive behavior disorders in children and adolescents, including neurological, psychiatric, intellectual, learning, and social-emotional problems; of investigating and using many methods especially applicable to the examination and observation of children; of exploring many different therapeutic methods and spontaneous adjustments; and of following many patients through to institutions.

The Brain-Damaged Child of the 1930s

It was assumed in the 1930s that most of the children in residence were disturbed because of some form of brain damage, such as encephalitis, and that they had a rather poor prognosis. Indeed the ward had been opened in 1920 to accept children who were thought to have a postencephalitis syndrome following encephalitis lethargica and to send them to Kings Park State Hospital, which had also just opened a ward for the chronic care of such children (Gibbs, 1930).

Viral Encephalites, 1934–1940

The epidemic encephalitis (lethargica) that followed World War I produced conditions in both adults and children throughout the world that resulted in studies that were considered the epitomy of brain damage (Von Economo, 1931). It was from the studies of children with such conditions that the concepts of organic hyperkinesis, asocial psychopathic behavior disorders, and brain driveness arose. The epidemic also lead to belief in the progressive nature of such disorders and the hopelessness in the prognosis of all brain-damaged children.

At Bellevue between 1934 and 1940 I was able to recognize and differentiate 11 children who had a history of encephalitis lethargica between 1920 and 1926, 5 cases of acute viral encephalitis, type undetermined, 4 cases with disseminated encephalomyelitis due to measles, 11 cases of pertussis encephalopathy, and 24 cases of Sydenham's chorea,[4] all with associated emotional or behavior disorders. This was a total of 55 cases from over 4000 children observed in the ward during the same period or an incidence of less than 0.15 percent. Thus these viral encephalites were a rare cause of disturbance in children sent to a city observation hospital at that time (Bender, 1942c).

But we learned a lot from these children.

Encephalitis Lethargica in Children

The 11 cases of encephalitis lethargica showed a remarkably similar clinical picture and course. They had a recognizable acute illness between four weeks and four years of age. This was followed by an apparently latent period before sequelae symptomatology was noticed or became disturbing. This lapse of time, however, may have been due to inadequate observation in the preschool years.

---

[4] At that time the cause of Sydenham's chorea with rheumatic fever was not known and was assumed to be due to a virus. Since then the significance of repeated streptococcus infections has been verified.

In all cases the condition proved to be progressive. There were disturbances in (1) motility, (2) oculomotor and pupillary control, (3) perceptual
maturation, and (4) personality reactions.

1.   The motility disorder was entirely extrapyramidal, with a variety of
Parkinsonian features and choreiform motility of the hands. There were also
some cerebellar features. In most cases these neurological features were not
recognized until the age of eight or nine years, when the child was referred
from schools for examination. One child from an intelligent family with a
private pediatrician noted choreiform features from infancy. The motility
disturbance increased into adulthood and finally crippled the individual.

2.   A constant feature was the progressive oculomotor and pupillary
disturbances, including strabismus, nystagmus, poor convergence, pupillary rigidities, irregularities, and inequalities. These findings were also first recorded
at eight or nine years, when the children came to Bellevue.

3.   The impulse disorder seemed to be basic to the behavioral problems.
Paul Schilder (1951) ascribed this to the striapallidal substantia nigra system,
which is also the area involved in the motility disturbance. Our understanding
of what an impulse is is not clear. I have thought that the problem is one of
patterning or organizing the impulses and not one of increase or diminution of
impulses. Furthermore, the patterning of the impulses is related to the perceptual patterning and is therefore a gestalt function.

4.   The difficulty in the patterning of the perceptual-motor functions was
apparently first explored at Bellevue in these early years (the 1930s) with the
use of my VMGT (1938), the Goodenough draw-a-man test, and the patterned perceptual tests from the Stanford-Binet. Tests dependent upon spatial
orientation, visual and auditory memory, and baragnistic sense were generally
failed. This work was done by Florence Halpern at Bellevue (Bender, 1946a,
p. 163).

The inability to draw a man at the level of the child's mental age was
present in all of these children (Bender, 1940). This inability was looked upon
by Paul Schilder as an inperception of the body image and was based on perceptual difficulties related to the child's own body functions and structure as
well as visual perception. It also represented difficulties in organizing all of his
perceptual experiences and resulted in inadequate body image, self-image, self-
identification, and social orientation.

Otherwise the children's intellectual capacities were normal, with IQs
ranging from 68 to 129. There was no deterioration. There was, however, a
considerable discrepancy between the verbal and performance scores. One
boy's verbal IQ exceeded the performance by 40 points at nine years and by 37
points at 20 years, when the verbal IQ was 129 and he was no longer able to
function out of an institution because of his severe motility disorder, with
athetoid and Parkinsonian features and oculomotor disturbances. Sleeping

sickness had been diagnosed at eight months in 1920 and he was a conspicuous hyperkinetic, asocial behavior problem as a child. His drawing of a man was never better than a seven-year level.

Hyperkinesis, in my opinion, was secondary to the perceptual problems of these children and to their inability to get gratification from perceptions, from contact with the world of reality, or from their drive to experience reality in perceptual experiences of the world, their own bodies, their body images, and their self-images. Hyperkinesis, therefore, was due to their poorly patterned motor-perceptual experiences and impulses. Thus we see the touching, grasping, biting, destructive, abusive, and sexual activities. These also represent immaturities and are often associated either with depression and mood swings, especially in adolescence, or with the opposite, periods of flatness, dullness, and inactivity.

Acute Viral Encephalitis

During the same period (1935–1939) we observed five children following an acute viral encephalitis of undetermined type. No two were alike, they had a variety of neurological signs. All improved in adolescence and none progressed.

Disseminated Encephalitis with Exanthemata

During this same period we observed four cases of disseminated encephalitis with measles (one also had chicken pox). These cases presented a variety of clinical pictures and progressions. Some cases had catastrophic cortical destruction with or without convulsive states, which could become fatal. In two cases remission occurred at puberty, followed by apparent complete or partial recovery.

Pertussis Encephalopathy

Pertussis encephalopathy, which probably consists of a diffuse viral inflammation with hemorrhagic areas due to the convulsive coughing, was seen in 11 children. This was in the 1930s, when pertussis vaccination was not available. This was often a most crippling disorder and often demonstrated motor disabilities, convulsive disorders, and intellectual deterioration, as well as behavior and personality disturbances. There was evidences of focal pathology in almost any part of the brain, and frequently air encephalograms showed that the ventricular system enlarged. The prognosis was poor.

Sydenham's Chorea[5]

Sydenham's chorea with rheumatic fever was seen by us in 24 cases at this time. Children—usually from a poor background—were sent to us from the community as behavior problems without knowledge of their chorea or rheumatic fever. Others were transferred to us from pediatric services as known cases of rheumatic fever because they were unmanageable in open wards owing to their bizarre, panicky behavior, especially at night. Often they had been diagnosed as schizophrenic. Neurological examination always revealed chorea of more or less severity, and evidence of endocarditis and other features of rheumatic fever were either present or related in the history.

These children responded remarkably well to fever treatment in their chorea, in other rheumatic features, and in their behavior. They were sent out, usually to convalescent care, as very much improved. They were considered one of our most favorable therapeutic results.

Unfortunately a follow-up study did not confirm this success (Keeler and Bender, 1952). We were able to follow 20 of these 24 patients after they were 22 years of age. We found that only 3 had made a good adjustment; 6 had made a fair and 11 a poor adjustment. Six had subsequent attacks of rheumatic fever with chorea, 2 had died, and 7 had shown subsequent evidence of neurological disorders, apparently secondary to the rheumatic fever. However, an important factor in the adjustment failures appeared to be preexisting poor home conditions, low IQs, previous encephalitis (3 cases, possibly 4), schizophrenia (2 cases, possibly 3), reading disability, and behavior and personality disorder. Furthermore 6 cases that had repeated psychometric studies showed a dropping off of the IQ, indicating an organic deterioration.

Pyogenic Encephalomyelitis

From 1935 to 1939 thirty children were observed in the Bellevue children's ward with behavior disturbances and a history of meningitis, pneumonia, mastoiditis, osteomyelitis, or carbunculosis at an earlier age (Bender, 1942a). It should be recalled that there were no antibiotics or vaccines against these conditions at that time. Still, these conditions were relatively uncommon since 30 cases among 5000 children observed at the same time is an incidence of less than 0.10 percent.

The children with pyogenic encephalitis showed a variety of symptoms, depending on the type of the infection, the localization and severity of the process, the age when the child suffered the acute illness (3 months to 9 years in this series), and the age when the child was observed (5 to 12 years). The meningococcus infection tended to localize at the base of the brain and to in-

[5] See the footnote on p. 427.

vade the ventricles. The ear and mastoid infections tended to involve the adjacent areas, the basal ganglia, the eighth nerve, and the cerebellum. Pneumococcus encephalitis secondary to pneumonia, osteomyelitis or carbunculosis, being blood born to the brain, produced more diffuse sequelae. The behavior disorders or poor school application, restlessness, etc., were most evident in the early school years. After this the behavior disorders and the neurological signs gradually improved, especially during puberty and early adolescence. Many of the patients seemed quite normal thereafter. Others showed a subsidence of hyperkinesis and mood swings that permitted a subdued adjustment at home or in an institution.

The clinical signs were less severe than those seen in the children with encephalitis lethargica and were not progressive. There were extrapyramidal, choreiform, or cerebellar adventitious movements, especially in the hands. There were some oculomotor and pupillary disturbances, most often only poor ocular convergence. There were often respiratory irregularities. There were discrepancies between the drawing of a man (body-image imperception), the visual-motor gestalt drawing (VMGT), and other perceptual-motor tests as compared to the verbal scores on the Stanford-Binet. There was restlessness, hyperkinesis, distractibility, and asocial behavior as the children grew older.

Also the children that we saw had suffered from disturbed or actually depriving early family life. Furthermore, in the 1920s and 1930s, when infections in children could not be specifically controlled or treated, it was customary for the sick baby, after a long period in the hospital, to be sent for months to a convalescent home where he could not be visited. This grossly depriving experience often seemed as significant in the cause of the psychopathiclike behavior as the inflammatory process in the brain.

Burn Encephalopathies

A burn encephalopathy appeared to account for a postencephaliticlike course with neurological patterning, perceptual disabilities, and personality problems in seven children observed at Bellevue and followed into later life (Bender, 1943). Severe burns may be fatal after a period of convulsions and coma. Other children with severe cortical damage and dementia necessitate institutional care. The seven children sent to Bellevue ran a course similar to those with a pyogenic encephalitis. They tended to improve in adolescence, losing their neurological signs. Some lived relatively normal lives, while others seemed dull and flattened emotionally and became dependent in institutions or at home. There was also often an emotional body-image problem when the scar left by the burn was disfiguring. Again there was often a history of a poor family life and disturbed parents who may have battered or neglected the child, which accounted for the burn in the first place.

General Statement on Postencephalitic Behavior Disorders

As a result of our observation of these children in Bellevue in the 1930s, we were able to point out the importance of careful neurological examination that differentiates between pyramidal and extrapyramidal defects and regressive cortical damage. We had to learn that impulse disorders, hyperkinesis (or hypokinesis), and distractibility were secondary to perceptual-motor disorders and body-image defects, which can be tested by my VMGT and the drawings of a man. We also learned that the home background appeared to be a common factor in contributing to the child and decompensating from whatever brain damage he may have suffered. Longitudinal studies indicated that viral encephalites, Sydenham's chorea, and pertussis encephalopathies appeared to be progressive more often than the encephalites associated with pyogenic infections. In the latter both the behavior disorders and the neurological signs often cleared entirely in adolescence and allowed for normal adult adjustment, though some children seemed emotionally flat, dull, and dependent. It is possible that this occurred more often if the child had too much custodial, institutional care.

The most important factor in a favorable prognosis seemed to be a supportive family experience before the illness, with already well-established normal personality traits and the absence of other biological handicaps, such as mental deficiency, epilepsy, earlier encephalitis, or latent schizophrenia.

Head Traumas

A 10-year study (1934–1944) of 86 children (0.175 of the total of 5000 children observed at the same time) who had a history of severe head injuries was made by A. A. Fabian and me (1947), and earlier studies were made by Blau (1936) and Bowman and Blau (1943). Our criteria included a definite history of a severe head injury followed by a period of unconsciousness, X-ray evidence of a skull fracture, bleeding into the spinal fluid or from one of the head orifices, and definite neurological signs. The children were 1 to 15 years of age on admission, which was a few days to 10 years after the injury. Fifty-seven percent of the children had X-ray evidence of skull fracture.

Accidental falls from heights, usually out of windows, predominated for the children under five years; being struck by automobiles in the street was more common after five. The peak age for head injuries was five to six years. Boys were 92 percent of the total.

It was found that clinically recognizable mental deficiency, epilepsy, organic brain disease, or psychoses existed prior to the head traumas in 25 percent. Of the remaining 65 apparently normal children, 33 or 51 percent had had two or more major accidents, and nine or 15 percent had had three or more before the designated head injury, suggesting accident proneness.

The family patterns were strikingly similar. Twenty-seven of the children (41.5 percent) had one or both parents chronically addicted to alcohol. The parents of another 27 children were known by records to be mentally abnormal—with the first group, a total of 83 percent of the whole group. The combination of a sadistic father and a masochistic mother was common. Siblings were also known to have accident proneness or other behavioral or personality problems. The head-injured children were known to have often been battered by parents or older disturbed siblings. Strong sadomasochistic behavior patterns accounted for the most characteristic family profile.

In another part of this group some acute responses to recent head injuries were also observed. These children showed a sudden regression to infantile behavior, with an enormous amount of anxiety, real terror, and what was called "naughty behavior." In a week or 10 days they recovered. One child during this time lost considerable of his academic skills and tested like a retarded dyslexic child but regained all his skills in a few weeks. All subsequently recovered and did well. They all happened to come from good homes.

The chronic behavior disorders observed by us at Bellevue several years after the accident were thought at that time to resemble the postencephalitic behavior disorders and to have a bad prognosis, especially for those who developed convulsive disorders after the injury. It was thought by both their schools and their families that some children had regressed mentally after the injury. But testing showed that this was not true and that the children were functioning academically at a less mature level because of hyperkinesis.

The overactivity and infantile behavior, included in some cases with actual grasping, groping, touching, destructiveness to objects, sucking, biting, attempts to put every object in their mouths, and devouring, progressed to all sorts of asocial behavior as the children grew older. This of course is closely similar to postencephalitic behavior and to the clinical picture of alcoholic encephalopathy. It lead to the speculation that the major pathology in the brain was vascular disturbance at the base of the brain. Occasionally there was a focal disorder such as a slight paresis of one hand, but this could be dealt with specifically since it belonged to the "periphery of the personality" (Schilder, 1931) and need not be related to the more diffuse personality problems. Otherwise the child needed help in reducing anxiety and building defenses and in repatterning and organizing impulses, perception, learning skills, and behavior to meet social demands and to give satisfaction to the child himself.

Actual follow-up after 10 years showed that the majority of these children were doing remarkably well. Ultimate successful adjustment was less related to the severity of the trauma or to the neurological signs than to the degree of normality of the child before the injury, to the adequacy of the home both before and after the injury, and to the effectiveness of the subsequent academic program for the individual child (Bender, 1946a).

Minimal Brain Damage

Minimal brain damage as a discrete condition resulting in a diagnosable clinical state with many common problems in developing children was a concept growing out of these early experiences with grossly brain-damaged children. Minimal brain damage was found to occur in children with a history of defect, injury, or inflammation of the brain *in utero*, prenatally, or perinatally and during the first two or three years of life. It has seemed to fit the picture resulting from damage to the subependymal germinal matrix and periventricular areas described by Banks (1962) and Towbin (1970) in surviving children. Of course a child with more severe or extensive structural damage to the brain any time during the developmental period will have developmental problems and clinical signs of both gross and possibly focal pathology, as well as all of the signs of minimal brain damage.

The common problems that add up to the clinical syndrome include maturational lags in any or all of the cerebral functions, soft neurological signs, poor organization in impulses and in perception, immaturity in body image and self-concepts and self-identity, diffuse anxiety, dependency and clinging, and immature personality. There is also, however, a tendency toward later acceleration in maturation and reorganization of impulses and perception, toward building defenses against anxiety—the best of which are obsessive compulsive traits—and often toward becoming essentially normal by adolescence. Nevertheless, this problem underlies many of the developmental and behavior problems of children and also contributes to the personality characteristics and sometimes the problems of adults. The therapeutic needs of the child are for a longer period of maturation; he needs more dependent mothering and other interpersonal experiences, and he needs specific help or tutoring in any area in which the maturational lags and poor patterning accentuate any existing problems, such as language or motor skills or inadequate parent–child relationships.

Some of the above-mentioned concepts need elaboration.

Maturational lag is a concept I developed during my years at Bellevue as an outgrowth of Herrick's teachings, my own experiences with learning disabilities with Orton, and my subsequent experience with developmental disorders. It is a much more functional and dynamic process than mental defect or mental retardation. It indicates a lack of differentiation of patterning (as envisaged by the embryologists) in the development or maturation of perceptual-, mental-, and reflex-motor patterning, so that the child functions more immaturely in some or all areas. The chief characteristic is a less mature level of patterning in perceptual, mental, motor, and also visceral and autonomic behavior. There is no structural defect, no function is lost or defective, and maturation will continue, if slowly, and may even tend to acclerate after puberty. Maturational lags occur most specifically in minimally brain-damaged children, children with learning disabilities, and schizophrenic children (Bender, 1950).

Soft neurological signs as described by Schilder (1964) are related to the maturational lag. Included are signs of immaturity or poor organization in the patterned behavior of postural responses and neck-righting attitudes (Teicher, 1941), oculomotor and pupillary responses, tone responses to vestibular stimuli, and cortical dominance with right- and left-sidedness and right–left orientation disorders.

The diffuse anxiety that occurs in brain-damaged children has been best described by Phillis Greenacre (1941). She postulated a predisposition to anxiety as a physiological tendency that is due to an organic stamp of suffering related to brain damage at or near the time of birth. She emphasized the heightened basic anxiety arising from the frustration due to the damaged organization of the individual and the inadequate neurotic defenses. She saw as a result the facile identification with and mirroring of the mother and other objects in reality and the weak relationship to reality. Her observations were made on some of the adults she treated psychoanalytically but have proved to be similar to the experiences that we observed directly in the minimally brain-damaged child.

It is finally postulated that minimally brain-damaged children, whatever other problems they may have, have the common problems of (1) difficulties in patterned behavior in motor, perceptual, and emotional-social areas, with a tendency toward maturational lags and specific difficulties in body image and self-identification; (2) poorly patterned diffuse anxiety with inadequate defenses; (3) a greatly increased need for human support or mothering for a longer time than the nondamaged child; and (4) a compensatory tendency toward accelerated maturation, self-healing, and building of defenses, especially in adolescence.

That perinatal brain damage is common to many developmental problems in children has been confirmed by many studies, such as those of Knoblock and Pasamanick and their co-workers (1960). Later, when I was working at the Creedmoor State Hospital, Gloria Faretra and I (1972) studied the histories of children whom we had seen together at the Creedmoor State Hospital's children's service and whom we had seen individually in private practice and in a child guidance clinic for evidence of damage during pregnancy, perinatally, or in early infancy. We found that approximately 66 percent had histories of complications during pregnancy, birth, and early infancy. Our study included children with schizophrenia, brain damage, and behavior problems. The number diagnosed and the number with perinatal complications were similar for the three clinical facilities, and the number of perinatal complications was also remarkably similar for the three diagnostic groups.

Paul Wender's (1971) concept of minimal brain dysfunction (MBD) includes these disorders, but also all of the other problems of childhood except the grossly defective, organic, and psychotic disorders.

Deprivation Syndrome in Children

In the 1920s and 1930s, when it was believed that all brain-damaged children ran the course of the postencephalitic syndrome with a progressive psychopathic behavior disorder and would not respond to any form of treatment or training, it was also believed that any child that presented a pattern of asocial, psychopathic, nonneurotic behavior was undoubtedly brain-damaged even though there was no confirmatory history or neurological signs. Our Bellevue experience, however, convinced us that we could diagnose the brain-damaged child and differentiate the different types. It further showed that not all brain-damaged children progressed into a chronic neurological and psychiatric disorder but that many spontaneously remitted, especially in adolescence, and lived relatively normal adult lives. Most of the children who did not so improve were found to have experienced severe emotional and social deprivation in infancy and early childhood.

We soon were aware that we were observing many children who presented a picture of infantile asocial hyperkinetic behavior but without a history of infantile illness or any neurological signs. However, they had had the common experience of early emotional deprivation, because they had been institutionalized as dependent infants, had been moved about among many foster homes, or had experienced serious breaks in the mother–child relationship in the early years of childhood.

I reported the first case of this type in 1935 and made other reports through the years (1946, 1947, 1950, 1959). Many others have written important contributions to the subject, such as David Levy (1937), Lawson Lowery, (1940), John Bowlby (1944, 1951), R. A. Spitz (1945), and William Goldfarb (1943, 1945, 1955).

In my 1935 report I indicated that if loving maternal care is interrupted at an early age or never provided, the personality becomes arrested at the infantile level and the child may develop what I called a "psychopathic" behavior disorder. This individual retains an infantile personality. He is insatiable in his demands for love and attention. He is a behavior problem as a child and in constant conflict with society and the law as an adult. He lies and steals and is undependable in his work. He is promiscuous in his love life and lacks a sense of value for a love object inasmuch as he did not experience a dependable love object at the critical infantile period. He does not experience anxiety even at the prospect of losing a love object. He does not develop neurotic defenses. He is fearful of the abuse of others. The majority of children of this type whom we have seen were foundlings and children who have been cared for in homes or institutions for infants from the earliest infancy. The institutions in the 1920s and 1930s were faced with the problem of controlling cross-infections and this contributed to further isolation of the infants. The importance of personal and affectional care of the infant or "tender loving care" (TLC), as well as protective nursing and pediatric care, was not recognized (Bender, 1935).

In 1947 I described the characteristics of the psychopathic behavior disorders of children resulting from early social and emotional deprivation as follows (1947b):

1. The personality remains retarded at the infantile level without anxiety or any defense mechanisms. There is no capacity to feel guilt and develop neurotic defenses.

2. The primary defect seems to be an inability to identify or to form human interrelationships. There is a lack of awareness of object relationships and of love.

3. There is a defect in language development and in the conceptualization of abstract or social concepts. There is a failure in communication except to meet personal needs (Goldfarb, 1955).

4. The defect in the concept of time is of special theoretical interest and of significance in explaining some of the child's personality difficulties. It appears that we develop our concepts of time from the passage of time in our earliest love relationships, remembering past satisfying contacts in feeding, etc., and anticipating future ones. The psychopathic child does not remember the past, he does not learn from past experiences, he does not anticipate the future, and he has no future goals. He cannot be motivated to control his instinctive drives, impulses, or needs for future satisfactions. There is a somewhat similar defect in spatial concepts. Thus even when he is momentarily related to a person, he loses the contact as soon as the person is absent.

5. Rhythmical mood swings may appear in adolescence, apparently related to biological and instinctual drives that can not be controlled or patterned.

6. There develops in the older child a mirroring, imitative, "as if" quality of behavior. His inherent drive to be normal can find expression only

by his copying the behavior of others. Psychopathic lying and confabulation is common, while the inner fantasy life is rather sterile.

7. The personality defect appears to be unmodifiable by any treatment program after the period of deprivation in early childhood has passed. However, several follow-up studies have indicated that some individuals can carry on a prolonged period of satisfactory adjustment if during adolescence they can find or be placed in a satisfactory dependent position with some kind of mother figure, e.g., in a marriage, in institutional employment, or in the marines. The latent-age child is best cared for in the protective environs of a benign institution where he can imitate the behavior of other normal children.

Behavior Disorders with Aggression and Delinquency

In the early years at Bellevue, before we had clarified the diagnostic categories in the psychiatric problems of the children that were sent to us, we made studies of various behavior categories or syndromes and later follow-up studies to determine the outcome. These studies were collected into two books, *Aggression, Hostility and Anxiety in Children* (Bender, 1953), and *A Dynamic Psychopathology of Childhood* (Bender, 1954).

Children's Idea of Death

Meanwhile, in 1934 Paul Schilder and David Wechsler studied children's attitude toward death (Schilder, 1964). They concluded that children under the age of 12 do not believe that death is something that lasts because the child's own deprivations are usually not lasting. This fact makes it easier for the child to wish for the death of others and to speak of killing without guilt. For the child death consists primarily of the idea of deprivation and is reversible. Death does not appear to him as the natural end of life. It is the result of the hostility of others. The child is a realist. He knows what he sees. Children say that the dead cannot move or breath and that they are buried in the ground.

Suicidal Preoccupations and Attempts in Children

In 1937 Paul Schilder and I studied 22 children, 6 to 15 years of age who had been observed at Bellevue between 1930 and 1934 and who had fantasied, threatened, or attempted suicide. They were followed up for 13 to 17 years until 1951 (Bender, 1953; Schilder, 1964).

We found that these children had reacted to an unbearable situation with an attempt to escape through suicidal preoccupations or attempts. But it must also be remembered that the younger children did not have the idea that death was final. Mostly these unbearable situations consisted of deprivations of love. At least the child assumed that the love was not sufficient for his needs, which in some cases were especially great because of an organic disorder or earlier social deprivation.

The suicidal attempt also constituted a punishment of the persons depriving the child of love and a plea for a greater amount of love. In some children whose parents had died, the suicidal preoccupations also represented an attempt at reunion with the love object. Suicidal attempts following disappointments in love in young adolescents were also attempts to reach the love object, which in the final analysis was always the parents.

In the subsequent career of these children it became progressively evident that they were threatened increasingly by turmoil within themselves or in the family that became progressively more difficult. Four had mothers who were psychotic, epileptic, or antisocial with sexual misdemeanors and all of whom became more violent and negligent of the child until institutionalized, thus breaking up the home. One boy had a father who was severely paranoid with ideas of death for himself and for the boy and who finally committed suicide, leaving the child homeless. Three children were themselves developing schizophrenic psychoses including a preoccupation with death and two boys had poorly controlled epilepsy. Several were inadequately cared for in foster homes after the death of or abandonment by their parents; several had poor intelligence, minimal brain damage, poor academic opportunities and adjustment, inadequate homes, and disturbed parents.

In no instance in the course of the 14 years of the study when all were adults did any of these individuals kill themselves. Later they either tended to direct their aggression against the environment in asocial and delinquent behavior or suffered emotional and intellectual flattening and, in many instances, accepted refuge in institutions.

Children Who Have Killed Others

My experience with aggressiveness in children is best demonstrated by a presentation of the case material on children I have known who have actually caused the death of another person. If the psychoanalytic theories were correct, instances of children causing a death should not be uncommon. But in 35 years of psychiatric practice in New York City and New York State, I was able to collect only 34 cases of children under the age of 16 years who had apparently been responsible for a death. All cases were followed up at least 5 years to 25 years after the homicidal incident (Bender, 1973a).

By 1945 eight children had been observed at Bellevue who were held responsible for a death (Bender, 1953; Bender and Curran, 1940). The conclusions were overwhelming, the death was always accidental and unexpected by the child. Neither had the child any concept of the irreversibility of death. The death occurred because the victim happened to be in the path of the activity that was initiated by the child and was unintentionally fatal. The child then responded with a severe depressive grief or mourning reaction. His life pattern changed critically from that point. He tried by every means in fantasy and by acting out to deny the act and its consequences, the death of the victim and its irreversibility. He might even attempt to repeat the whole experience in order to prove that it could not have happened. These children needed long periods of careful psychiatric care to ameliorate their emotional disturbance and protect them from repeating the experience.

In 1959 (Bender, 1959d) and again in 1969 and 1973 (Bender, 1959b, 1969a, 1973a) I reported more extensive studies on 26 additional boys and girls to the age of 16 years who had caused a death. The conclusions this time were that a constellation of factors is always present when a boy or girl causes a death. There has to be a disturbed, poorly controlled, impulsive child, a victim who acts as an irritant, an available lethal weapon, and always a lack of protective supervision by some third person who could stop the fatal consequences.

In the total of 34 cases of death-causing children studied psychiatrically, some combination of the following factors was found: (1) organic brain disease with an impulsive disorder, an abnormal electroencephalogram, and/or epilepsy in 15 of the 34 cases; (2) schizophrenia with preoccupations with death and killing in the pseudoneurotic phase of younger children or with antisocial paranoid preoccupation in the pseudopsychopathic phase of the adolescent children in 13 of the 34 cases; (3) compulsive fire-setting in 13 cases; (4) defeating school retardation with reading disabilities in 13 cases; (5) extremely unfavorable home conditions and life experiences. As indicative of the last factor, 6 children had one or both parents and a sibling who were mentally ill in a hospital, and two children had observed their father being killed, one by the mother. The IQ range was 18 to 127 (mean 87). There were four with an IQ below 70.

The mode of death in the younger children was by fire (6 children); drowning (5 children); pushing off a height (3 children); and choking (1 child). The deaths by fire and drowning were all purely incidental. The child's subsequent severe depression and grief-ridden reaction required psychiatric care. Nevertheless, of these 15 young children—10 years old and under—7 were schizophrenic and 3 were grossly defective with developmental brain damage. The 5 involved in a drowning were all fire setters. They had all been known to threaten to kill before the drowning. None were free from family, social, and personal disorders of grossly damaging degree. Multiple deaths (of 2 and 3 people) were caused by drowning and fire.

The 19 older boys, ages 11 years through 15 years, caused deaths by stabbing with sharp weapons (7 boys); by repeated blows with a heavy object (6 boys); and by shooting (6 boys). Four younger boys, aged six, eight, and nine, are included in these categories. This group showed the most pathology, with clinically recognizable schizophrenia, epilepsy, and/or significant brain damage diagnosed in all cases.

The psychodynamics of the prepuberty child after he has caused a death is that he does not believe that he was able to kill or that death is irreparable, and he attempts by fantasy and acting out to prove that it is not possible. An adolescent makes an effort to deny both guilt and feelings of guilt for his part in the act that caused the death and to claim amnesia or other repressive defenses. Both are usually misunderstood and dangerous. Eight of the boys who had caused a death were afterwards still threatening to kill whenever they were frustrated. Several expressed fear of their own ability to kill. Sixteen of the 34 boys and girls, because of their early disturbed behavior, had had a psychiatric evaluation before the incident that led to the death. Five boys and one girl had been reported as very dangerous.

We are faced with the problem of determining why there is not more violence committed by the "potentially dangerous" recognizable by psychiatrists. The low incidence reenforces the concept that a constellation of factors is required: endogenous pathology; an unfavorable social environment; an irritating victim; a lethal agent; and a lack of protection.

In such a psychiatric evaluation of known child and young adolescent killers there is no place for the psychoanalytic concepts of universal inborn aggressiveness or death instincts or death wishes, as formulated by Freud and many of his followers. Through all these studies emphasis was placed on the data that gave evidence that murderous hostile aggression is not a normal pattern of behavior for children. It occurs infrequently as a result of disorganizing pathology, both endogenous and environmental, in a constellation of factors, so that the death occurs without the intent of the child but as an unexpected occurrence.

Normal Drives in Child Development

I have postulated the following normal drives in child development:

1. An inherent drive for normality, determined by biological maturation, patterned with a direction toward a goal, and never completely blocked or diverted by any pathology within the child or in his outer world.

2. An inborn capacity to relate and identify with other humans, such as

the mother, and thus experience love, social relations, communication, and language.

3. An inborn capacity for fantasy, symbol formation, and projection in all experiences, and an ability to communicate these experiences, thus reconstructing and mastering the outer world with creativity (Bender, 1948).

Therefore, destructiveness and hostile aggression in a child is a symptom complex caused by developmental pathology, which disorganizes the normal constructively patterned drives so that inadequate gratification leads to frustration (Bender, 1948).

Deviant Sexual Behavior in Children

Deviant sexual behavior in children was studied by myself and coauthors at Bellevue, with follow-up studies to adulthood (Bender, 1954, 1968) and a later study by myself at Creedmoor (Bender, 1964).

In the 1930s a child would be sent to the New York City psychiatric observation ward at Bellevue from children's courts or other agencies when suspected of having had sexual experience with an adult. Twenty of these children, from emotionally poverty-stricken homes of the underprivileged social classes of the city, were observed and proved to be essentially normal. They were mostly children with learning disabilities, especially in reading, doing poorly in schools that did not meet their needs. They appeared to have sought adult attention and affection and were attractive children whom adults found too readily available, if not seductive. However, once the relationship had run its course, had been discovered, or had been replaced by a more normal relationship, the child showed little interest in the adult and certainly did not value him as a love object.

The treatment program of choice, after the child was removed from the inadequate home and sex partner, was protective supervision through early adolescence either in a good school-type of institution or in a supervised foster home. Appropriate reading tutoring was essential. It was learned that sexually stimulated children are specifically responsive to pharmacological therapy, especially Benzedrine, which tends to suppress the awakened sexual sensations and preoccupations and results in an amnesia of the experiences.

In adulthood 10 were found to have made a good, stable social adjustment. Only 1, a mental defective girl, had continued with sexual promiscuity. They seemed none the worse for their childhood sexual experiences or their court and psychiatric hospital experiences.

Five of the children observed at Bellevue in these early years were different. They were confused about their sexual identity and immature in psychosexual development. They had sexual experiences with partners of the same sex who were similarly confused. They were all schizophrenic and became schizophrenic adults.

The 16 children seen at Creedmore State Hospital in the 1950s were sent there because they were mentally ill and unable to function satisfactorily as children in the community. They were chosen for a special study because their histories indicated that some time before the age of 13 they had had sexual experiences.

All but 2 of these children were schizophrenic. Nevertheless, their case histories present significant material for the discussion of personality dynamics, especially as they are related to deviant sexual behavior.

The disorganization of family life in this group of children was remarkable. In no instance had the child remained with both parents in their home, nor had any child had any consistent care from one adult. A series of men frequently played the role of stepfather. Sexual identity was never clear, and the child himself could play the role and accept a partner of either sex.

The child was often exposed to a great deal of sexual activity in the home by family members and outsiders so that he almost saw sex as normal behavior and a way that adults got attention, excitement, and fun. Furthermore, he himself was neglected, abused, and left to his own devices for attention and affection. Sexual activities, carried out on his own initiative, usually did not take place until puberty or adolescence, when his sex drives and his tendency to act out his inner impulses became strong enough.

Incest was a frequent pattern to which these children were exposed. Fantasied incestuous experiences also presented a challenging problem. It was not always possible to determine if in reality the child had had the sexual relations he claimed with parents or parent surrogates or had fantasied them. Our child patients were for the most part schizophrenics, to whom fantasy comes more readily and if often retold as reality or maybe, in puberty, acted out realistically.

Summary on Aggressive, Disturbed, and Delinquent Children

Summarizing my experience with aggressive, delinquent behavior disorders in children after 20 years with New York City children at Bellevue (Bender, 1957b) and after 12 more years with the New York State Hospital system (Bender, 1968), I concluded that there are always multiple factors that contribute to the behavior of any child with a problem that requires professional attention. Furthermore the multiple factors always occur in certain constellations of social-cultural patterns and individual pathology.

1. Distortions occur in the dynamics of personality development in children who in earliest childhood or infancy are grossly deprived, neglected, or abused or otherwise traumatized by adults who are themselves disturbed or inadequate.

2. Conflicts arise from the cultural ideology that equates masculinity with aggression and activity and that drives inadequate and deviate boys to assert their manhood by violence or frustration. On the other hand, constitutional or genetic factors are most important in the higher incidence of boys than girls in all categories of developmental and behavioral disorders before puberty. The male develops less smoothly than the female until adolescence, apparently because of the gene pattern (Bender, 1968).

3. Problems in minority groups arise from economic, social, and educational underprivilege, poor home conditions, and the more frequent lack of two parents. There also appears to be higher incidence in perinatal pathology because of the poor health of the mother prior to and during pregnancy and because of poor medical care for the child before birth and during infancy.

4. Learning difficulties in our highly competitive culture and educational system are known to exist in more than 50 percent of all problem and delinquent boys.

5. Organic disease, especially of the brain and usually "minimal brain damage," increases the problems of maturation, mental and personality functions, and identifications and heightens all of the other problems.

6. Schizophrenia, latent or mild or more active, appears to be present in an increasing number of delinquent children as we become more adept in our diagnostic measures, in evaluating life and family histories, and in studying longitudinal views of the whole career of individuals, at least those who are referred for psychiatric attention. I have shown that psychopathic behavior in the adolescent is often the defensive pattern of a schizophrenic condition (Bender, 1959d, 1971a).

To the extent that some of these factors may be considered environmental, they operate only as they affect the life pattern of the individual from earliest infancy on and become woven into the life pattern and the personality. The factors that may be considered endogenous are important only to the extent that they interfere with the individual's capacity to cope with the problems they create and to live creatively in his life situation. Many individuals with these problems are able to form defenses against them, compensate for them, or find ways of using them productively.

Certain it is that the totality of all individuals who have some or all of the above factors far exceeds the incidence of delinquency and mental illness. Some combination of these factors, or severity of them, and certain patterns are required before the child decompensates and becomes disturbed, delinquent, or psychotic.

Learning Disabilities

Learning disabilities in language skills, such as dyslexia has interested me since my work with Samuel T. Orton in 1923, as I have stated. At Bellevue it soon became evident that this was a very common problem, especially among the boys with every category of problems. Fifty percent of the nonretarded boys to the age of 12 years and 75 percent of those of 12 to 16 years were severely retarded readers or nonreaders. This was also reported to be true in all services for disturbed or problem boys, whether court, institution, or outpatient facility. At the same time it was estimated that 5–15 percent of all public school children were so effected (Bender, 1958; Peeke, 1945).

Many studies were made on the children with reading disability at Bellevue (Bender, 1957a, 1958; Schilder, 1964) and later also at Creedmoor State Hospital (Bender, 1970c). My Visual Motor Gestalt Test was found useful in the study of such children, since it showed immaturities and maturational lags both in form and in directional and spatial orientations and configurations. The total test tends to be less well organized, with mobile features often having both dextrad and sinistrad and clockwise and counterclockwise orientation. Vertical and horizontal directions are interchanged. More primitive configurations occur. Open forms are closed.

It is indeed remarkable that at five, six, and seven years the tonic neck-reflex dominance of motility should be controlled while right–left-hand dominance, right–left orientation in space, the oblique-diamond gestalt structures in visual motor performances, and reading readiness all tend to become established. A retardation or lag in one of these areas is usually associated with a lag in all and is predictive of a lag in the learning of language skills (De Hirsch et al., 1966).

It was found that many children, mostly boys, showed a variable combination of the following features:

1. A slower maturation of language skills, with a wide variety of possible patterning but most often a difficulty in learning to read at the usual age.
2. A slower maturation of neurological patterning revealed in the developmental history of motor skills, "soft neurological signs" and motility awkwardness, and often hyperkinesis.
3. An uneven pattern of intellectual development on standard IQ tests, if repeated several times, and an interest variability.
4. Poor establishment of cortical dominance, left-handedness, or "mixed" dominance, with right–left confusion in spatial and directional orientation.
5. Body-image concepts that also show maturational lags and human figure drawings that are immature, especially in younger children

(Silver, 1952). On the other hand, Paul Schilder and I (Bender and Schilder, 1951) found a compensatory ability to make remarkably good art production in children who responded quickly to tutoring and to improved environmental support.

6. Immature personality development and exaggeration of any other personality problem.

7. Often a history of similar difficulties in any or all of these areas in some other member of the family.

8. Reading disability predictable in the preschool period given the presence of the above features, which are essentially problems of maturational lags (Bender and Yarnell, 1941; De Hirsch *et al.*, 1966; Gesell and Amatruda, 1947). Early recognition and treatment may ameliorate later academic and personality problems.

9. Acceleration of maturation, or self-healing. This is usually uneven, so that such children may eventually show high compensatory functions in other areas than the area of the maturational lag, or even in some of the areas of language skills, but still remain characteristically handicapped in other areas, such as left–right orientation, mirror writing or reading, motor awkwardness, etc.

Dyslexic children usually respond very well, even remarkably well, to appropriate tutoring by a tutor who can also relate to and motivate the child, unless the personality has been too severely traumatized by defeatist attitudes or there are associated organic or intellectual defects. Schizophrenic children with dyslexia respond especially well to sympathetic tutoring, which promotes maturation in both the learning skills and schizophrenic disorganization (Goldberg, 1952). The reading skill, however, may be essentially autistic and may exclude an equivalent understanding of content.

Some special features in the conceptualization of these children were emphasized in my studies. These features undoubtedly arise in connection with the maturational lags, the gestalt function, and the right–left orientation in space and direction, as well as in the visual and auditory function of language skills.

These children often show a marked abstractiveness that contributes to interference in the learning of specific or concrete concepts. It is documented in the early psychological testing by high scores in abstract functioning or in the VMGT by the tendency toward free movement of objects and poor differentiation of background and foreground. Overtrained children sacrifice these capacities with obsessive-compulsive rigidities and concreteness in learning skills. It may be a real sacrifice or may be seen in those individuals who compensate with mathematical skills.

Conceptualization of time as well as space is often different in these children (Bender, 1973*b*; Goldberg, 1952). Concepts are based on percepts that are derived from circular movement, which is dextrad or sinistrad and clockwise or counterclockwise. Children with poorly established cortical dominance may be confused by this movement. Telling time by a clock or by a calendar is therefore often a problem.

There are also problems in the understanding of past, present, and future. The memory of past events is poorly organized in dyslexic children. It has been realized that individuals do not remember the processes of learning to speak or to read and write language. Children who learn these skills late or are still in the process of learning them often show a surprising inability to recall, even from day to day, and certainly from a more remote past, the procedure itself, what it is about, or the relationship of the people associated with it.

Congenital Aphasias

There has been a trend, especially in the 1950s, toward considerable concern about congenital or childhood aphasias. Like each new diagnostic concept it has been enthusiastically accepted to explain mental defects, congenitally or traumatically determined; deaf-mutism; infantile autism; and other deviations in child development.

Studies of the children at Bellevue who most closely resembled cases that might be called aphasia were made by Stella Chess (1944). She found that they all had factors of maturational lags. Half of the group became adult schizophrenics, one died as a result of a progressive neurological condition, and two could not be located on the follow-up and may well have become compensated.

My whole experience with many thousands of children at Bellevue, many of whom were followed into adulthood, did not afford one case that could be considered a case of aphasia other than the maturational learning lags in language or schizophrenia. Roberts (1958) has shown that organic brain damage before two years of age, even to the cortical areas (which later were found to function for language, or at least if damaged in adults tend to cause aphasia), does not result in any form of aphasia in children, provided the damage is not so extensive as to cause a general mental defect.

Childhood Schizophrenia

In 1934 we diagnosed the first case of childhood schizophrenia in Marty, a six-year-old boy (Bender, 1939). The diagnosis was subsequently confirmed and he has been followed into his forties in our recent follow-up studies (Bender, 1973b). Soon an increasing number of children were recognized as schizophrenic. Since our early research interests at Bellevue were in clinical and treatment studies, our early reports of schizophrenic children appeared as case studies in a variety of papers on these subjects (Bender, 1937, 1939; Bender and Paster, 1941; Bender and Schilder, 1940, 1941).

Ten years later (1949–1951) follow-up studies on schizophrenic children were made on the children in these various reports [as controls.] Then 25 percent of the children who had not been recognized as schizophrenic were found to be so in other agencies and institutions that saw them later (Bender *et al.*, 1952).

My first brief definition of childhood schizophrenia was published in 1942 in *The Nervous Child*. This journal also contained papers from Bellevue by Jack Rapoport and Frances Cottington: a report on 20 schizophrenic children who were treated with intensive psychoanalytically oriented psychotherapy and a preliminary report on Metrazol-convulsive therapy, respectively.

In 1947, having diagnosed and studied more than 100 children with schizophrenia, I more adequately defined childhood schizophrenia as disturbed behavior occurring in every area of functioning in the child, i.e., homeostatic, vasovegetative, motility, perception, conception, affect, and interpersonal relationships. I saw anxiety as the basic reaction to lack of organization of patterns in these areas. Defenses against the anxiety led to a great variety of secondary neurotic symptomatology, often seeming to dominate the clinical picture. I dwelt on the variety of vasovegetative disorders; the characteristic motility such as hand mannerisms and whirling, which seemed to be immaturities; the dependency and "cohesiveness" or "melting" in relationship to the adult; and the impulsiveness with "darting" and running away and the almost ticlike grimacing. The psychological problems involved self-identity; body boundaries; body image; distortions in perception; language and thought disturbances; and social problems, especially the difficulties in family relationships with mother, father, and siblings (Bender, 1947).

Gesell's Embryology of Behavior

Meanwhile Arnold Gesell had published his *Embryology of Behavior* (1945), which gave me new insights and the opportunity to pull together many disconnected observations. He described the embryology of behavior as evolving through five areas of interweaving patterns.

1. The autonomic or vasovegetative areas or homeostasis was found to be unpatterned in fetal infants, only gradually becoming patterned as the infant matures. In schizophrenic children there is often a continuing failure in balancing, integrating, or patterning of the primary functions under homeostatic control, including the cardiovascular system, the gastrointestinal system, the excretory system, and general growth, allergic responses, metabolic

processes, and responses to illnesses. The "wisdom of the body" is immature. Secondary stress and anxiety are experienced as a result.

2. Sleeping and waking as associated with states of consciousness are unpatterned in the fetal infant. Schizophrenic infants often do not develop the normal pattern of sleeping and wakefulness; they sleep too much or are awake too much. The infant and child is often stuporous. Fluctuation in the states of consciousness, even to the severity of atypical convulsive phenomena, has also been often observed.

3. Respiratory patterns are acquired only after birth, and survival is threatened if there is difficulty in such patterning. Gesell regarded respiration as the most crucial behavior for integration as well as for regulatory purposes as the infant matures. Respiration is incorporated into expressive behavior, and under the direction of the cerebral cortex it becomes the instrument of speech. Respiration, feeding behavior, and language are closely interwoven in the functional embryology of the individual. Respiratory difficulties, often associated with so-called "allergies," gastrointestinal dysfunctions, and other homeostatic disorders, are among the distressing problems of schizophrenic children. Thought disorders, dysarthric problems, mutism, and other language problems are of course typical of schizophrenic children, especially autistic children.

4. The patterned tone of both striated and unstriated muscles is a response to the perception of gravity, the first perceptual experiences *in utero,* which evolves and matures with the vestibular system and from which are evolved perception of time, space, and reality and the awareness of the self and the relationships of objects. In the schizophrenic child all these functions remain immature, fetal, and plastic. The immature tone in all muscular systems is one of the reasons why the child does not react appropriately to any stimuli or relate to objects or other persons.

5. Action patterns or patterns of motor activity arise from the tonic neck-righting responses observed by Gesell as the basic embryological pattern for all bodily activity. Normally tonic neck-righting responses dominate behavior only through the first weeks of postnatal life, and the whirling on the longitudinal axis to the postural testing ceases at six or seven years. In the schizophrenic child, however, these immature responses are retained, often into adult life, or appear again with schizophrenic decompensations. Then they are associated with excessive whirling motility or mannerisms, as well as fantasies of flying into space or religious ecstacies. These, too, increases the anxiety.

If one wishes to explain the disorders and symptoms of schizophrenic children by reference to one mechanism in the body, one could best choose the vestibular apparatus. Many researchers have confirmed that schizophrenic infants and children show immature vestibular, tonic, postural, and neck-righting responses, with general immaturity or maturational lags (Rachman and Berger, 1963). Barbara Fish and M. Alpert (Fish, 1959, 1971; Fish and Alpert, 1963) made a study of the neurological development of infants born to schizophrenic mothers and were able to observe "deviations in the state of consciousness, vestibular function, motility and muscular tone as early as the first day of life and continuing into the early months of infancy." They called attention to Lorente de No's experimental studies (1933), which related these functions to the reticular formation, and they suggested that the deviate tonic responses of these infants was related to the dysfunction of this system.

Considerable important research work has been performed on the vestibular function in the development of children and especially in relation to schizophrenia (Colbert *et al.*, 1959; Fish and Alpert, 1963; Pollack and Krieger, 1958).

Plasticity

In the late 1940s I developed the concept of *plasticity* as a characteristic of the schizophrenic pathology in children (Bender, 1966). The concept is derived from embryology. It refers to primitive, undetermined, and undifferentiated patterning, especially in those areas of functioning most recently acquired, most actively evolving in human evolution, and characteristic of those brain functions most specifically human. Plasticity is the basis of the maturational lags. In learning disabilities the language areas are more specifically involved. In schizophrenia it may be the reticular formation, though it has to be admitted that this a hunch only.

Szentagothai (1961) speaks of the "inherent plasticity, or better, manifold potential specificity in the different reticular mechanisms" and discusses the "plasticity of function in the reticular system."

Plasticity appears to be the specific characteristic of every area of function in the schizophrenic child: vasovegetative homeostasis, motor activity and development, perception, conception, language, thought, affect, social relations, and defensive responses to the similarly affected anxiety. There are no boundaries to any functions, or ceilings, and therefore there is a continual interplay of opposite potentialities, so there may be accelerations as well as regressions. Some schizophrenic children are immature, inhibited, apathetic, mute, withdrawn, and autistic; physically asthenic, puny, sickly, without object relationship, concretistic in thinking, and poverty-stricken in fantasy life. Others are the opposite: precocious in physical development, overactive, with exaggerated intellectual brilliance and creativity in fantasy, abstract in thinking, verbally or graphically productive, invasive in identification, and facile in neurotic defenses. Most have various and variable combinations of these traits. This variability accounts for the great variety of clinical symptomatology in childhood schizophrenia.

Structured Research

Some research based on hypotheses to be proved or disproved developed in the research teams I was able to have with NIMH funding from 1949 to 1951 and from various staff associates who have been interested in my point of view over the years. For example William Helme, in a structured research project (Bender and Helme, 1953), made a quantitative test of my hypothesis employing my diagnostic criteria on a follow-up of schizophrenic and nonschizophrenic groups of our child patients. He confirmed (1) that childhood schizophrenia is characterized by disturbed regulation of maturational processes; (2) that the dominance of tonic neck-reflex motility exemplifies the maturational lags; (3) that the lack of segregation in physiological and psychological systems is basic; (4) that to some extent this lack pervades all areas of functioning; and (5) that plasticity characterizes the disorder. The term *dysmaturational function* was suggested and taken up by several of my associates (Caplan, 1956; Freedman, 1954; Rabinovitch, 1951).

Barbara Fish examined infants at 1 month in a well baby clinic or those born of schizophrenic mothers at birth, and she followed those who seemed vulnerable up to 15 years. She found that she could detect those who later became schizophrenic

> by applying Bender's criteria to a random sample of infants which provided direct corroboration of her concept that the schizophrenic child is distinguished at an early age from his non-schizophrenic peers by specific biologic signs of disordered maturation. Furthermore, later development illustrated the features predicted by Bender, namely (a) overall plastic patterning of development in all areas; (b) immature homeostasis; (c) early torporous states; (d) moluscous muscular tone and immature postural and motor activity [1959, p. 22]. (See also Fish, 1971; Fish and Alpert, 1963.)

The Course of Schizophrenia Through Childhood

The course of schizophrenia in children has many variations but also some predictable patterns. For one thing, the schizophrenic child becomes the schizophrenic adult, following through a life course of schizophrenia, latent, in remission, or decompensated into any of several different clinical forms. Every schizophrenic child is unique and always remains unique. Also the pattern of maturation will be modified by the counstitutional endowment and the total organismic response to the plastic embryonic features of the schizophrenic process and to the responding anxiety and its defenses. The various epochs of the child's life course will show features typical of the maturational problems of each epoch. Boys and girls show different features in relation to their different maturational characteristics (Bender, 1969*b*).

Infantile autism as first described by Kanner (1943) is typical of the infantile period, with its tendency toward extreme loneness, inability to relate to people, desire to preserve sameness in the environment and daily routine, and inadequate language development or "pseudodefectiveness." The plastic fetal physiological disorders have been described by Fish (1959). Many of these children may persist in this pattern of physiological inadequacies; withdrawal from all stimuli, persons, and life itself; and evident or apparent mental deficiency throughout their lives, perhaps complicated by some form of organic defect or damage. Boys exceed girls about 5 to 10 times (Bender, 1959a, 1969b).

In some autistic children there is a tendency for neurotic defenses to develop rapidly in the three- to six-year period. Other children have an apparent onset of schizophrenic features at this age with sterotyped rhythmic activities, compulsions, obsessions, phobias, clinging dependency, and disturbances in habit pattern and in language, in speech and fantasy material, in body-image concepts, in body boundaries, and in object relationships. The picture is often that of a symbiotic psychosis, described by Margaret Mahler (1968), in which the developing schizophrenic child can not resolve the problem of separation from the mother.

Schizophrenic girls are nearly equal in number to schizophrenic boys at this age. The girls are often dramatically psychotic between about four and eight years of age. They may however remit in latency, accepting a symbiotic relationship with the mother with some neurotic defenses, an almost exaggerated femininity, shyness in other relationships, and adaptability to academic programs. After puberty they often become disturbed again with psychosomatic, sexual, and ideational problems. Psychotic episodes may occur and continue into or recur in adulthood, when more women than men need professional care for schizophrenic decompensations.

Boys are different in early childhood. They are babyish and generally immature and inadequate, with puzzling discrepancies in various areas of maturation and behavior. They are shy, fearful, and anxious and have some poorly organized neurotic defenses. They adjust poorly to family, school, and peers. The differential diagnosis between schizophrenia and retardation or minimal brain damage (which is often also present) is difficult.

During latency there is a rapid increase again in the number of boys diagnosed as schizophrenic as compared to the girls. Here we see the typical childhood psychosis. There are a tonic neck-reflex dominance of motility (whirling on the longitudinal axis), impulsivity, grimacing, and mannerisms. Homeostatic and psychosomatic disorders may occur. There is poor muscle tone. There is an inadequate or inappropriate response to pain. There is patent anxiety. There is rich fantasy life. There are introjected fantasied objects (Bender, 1970b; Rapoport, 1944) that direct the child's behavior and impulses. There are distortions in the body image. There are preoccupations with flying, with spatial and temporal distortions, with identification problems including gender identity, with death, and with other forms of annihilation for the self and others. All kinds of neurotic defenses may develop into the picture of a pseudoneurosis. At this age psychotic children may be dangerously assaultative, wander away aimlessly, try to fly from heights, set fires, be brutal to smaller children, and experiment with death.

At puberty (from 10 ½ years of age) many boys (about two-thirds of those in the follow-up study, Bender, 1971a, 1971b) who have been psychotic may have more or less adequate remissions, either spontaneously or, hopefully, aided by treatment: biological, drug, milieu, or psychological. The puberty spurt in maturation is enough to give many schizophrenic boys the best period in their lives and the opportunity to live in the community, to catch up with their education, and often to have their previously established diagnosis of schizophrenia denied.

Some of the ambulatory schizophrenic boys develop pseudoneurotic features of various levels of severity. Others develop antisocial behavior with paranoid attitudes leading to pseudopsychopathic features (Bender, 1959d, 1971a). These patterns may persist into adulthood, or these boys may develop any of the other adult forms of schizophrenia.

Follow-up Studies of Childhood Schizophrenia

One hundred children, 2 ½ to 12 years of age, were observed at Bellevue Hospital between 1935 and 1952, were diagnosed as having childhood schizophrenia, and have been subjects of several follow-up and other individual studies (Bender, 1953, 1954, 1959d, 1973c). A current follow-up brings them to the age of 22 to 46 years, with a mean age of 30.3 years. There were 80 boys and 20 girls (Bender, 1959d, 1960a, 1969b, 1970a, 1973b; Bender and Faretra, 1972).

When classified by onset, 32 of the 100 children had an onset with infantile autism in the first two years of life; 27 were symbiotic from the second or third year of life; 28 had an onset in mid childhood, 3 ½ to 6 years; and 13 had an onset at puberty, 9 to 11 years.

When classified by outcome, 63 of the 100 are in institutions for the mentally ill or mentally retarded and are chronically disabled in various degrees. Thirty-seven, or one-third, are in the community and have been there for more than 2 years up to 30 years.

The diagnosis of schizophrenia in adulthood has not been confirmed in six cases. Three individuals proved to be basically organically impaired and are properly diagnosed as mentally deficient with organic brain disorders. Autistic behavior in early childhood may occur with organic brain disorders and mental deficiency. Autism does not improve the prognosis. Two individuals have diagnosed psychosis with encephalitis, but they have all the characteristics of also having been schizophrenic, both in childhood and in adulthood. One man has been diagnosed as a psychopathic personality. He was a typical childhood schizophrenic who partially remitted in puberty and developed psychopathic features in adolescence, becoming an inadequate, dependent paranoid at 28 years of age.

The studies of cultural, socioeconomic, and ethnic background and family patterns did not yield a sufficient number of cases to confirm any of the theories of an environmental factor in the etiology (such as "schizophrenogenic," "refrigerator," highly intelligent, or having depriving parents), though there were examples of all these. Every kind of home was represented. The cultural pattern reflected the social situation in New York in the 1930s and 1940s, as well as the ability of concerned parents and agencies to find help for these deviant children.

Social studies of early family life did indicate determinants that appeared to be related to the defenses that some of the more capable were able to make in adolescence, whether they were pseudopsychopathic or pseudoneurotic, and whether the ultimate adjustment was one of antisocial turmoil or passive dependency. The family patterns showed a significant degree of pathology in the parents and suggested the kinds of homes from which children might be referred and to which they might be returned. However, these family patterns did not seem to influence the etiology or the adult outcome.

The data on heredity show 215 mentally ill relatives; 86 were psychotic and 129 had personality disorders sufficiently severe to require social or medical attention. Recent researchers (Ketty, 1970; Rosenthal, 1970) have referred to these as the schizoid part of the "schizophrenic spectrum." In this group of 100 patients, schizophrenic from childhood, 17 subjects had 24 psychotic siblings and 17 had 24 personality-disordered siblings (some patients had more than one mentally ill sibling), for a total of 34 percent. There were also 15 psychotic mothers and 25 mothers with personality disorders (40 percent) and 7 psychotic fathers and 36 fathers with personality disorders (43 percent). The recent genetic studies accept F. Kallman's estimate, cited in Heston (1970, pp. 252–253), that 45 percent of each class of first-degree relatives is in the "schizophrenic spectrum." Polygenic and diasthetic stress theories are probably acceptable because, although genetic factors are necessary, other factors, probably environmental, are important in the etiology of schizophrenia.

My own study (Bender 1973c) of the family histories of 50 of these schizophrenic children and 50 controls showed that the schizophrenic spectrum comprised 39 schizophrenic relatives for the schizophrenic patients and no schizophrenic relatives for the controls. The schizophrenic patients also had 50 percent more sociopathic, neurotic relatives. However, the nonschizophrenic problem children had 50 percent more neurotic and inadequate personalities among their mothers.

In childhood schizophrenia I have found stress or the environmental factor to be an organic one occurring *in utero*, perinatally, or in early childhood. Of the 50 children of this type with the earliest onset, 34 percent had, in addition to their schizophrenia, organic disorders that dominated the clinical picture throughout life; none of these could be kept out of an institution. An additional 42 percent had in their histories perinatal pathology that was seen as precipitating the schizophrenic decompensation; 8 of these made a dependent social adjustment in adulthood. This accounts for 76 percent of the early autistic schizophrenics with decompensating organic factors. Eight also had convulsions in childhood or adolescence and 8 died between the ages of 22 and 44 of convulsions or inadequate cardiac and visceral functions.

Of the 50 children whose onset came after infancy and without autism, 3 had organicity that dominated their life pattern, 46 percent had perinatal pathology precipitating the childhood schizophrenia, and an additional 6 showed pathology after 5 years of age but before the onset of their schizophrenia. Of these 50, 19 made a social adjustment as adults, and 3 had convulsions (one of these ultimately died as a result).

Thus 70 percent of the total group had histories or clinical evidence of organicity affecting the brain that accounted for the onset of an early schizophrenic decompensation. There were still 30 percent for whom we had no history or clinical evidence of organicity but who ran a similar course of schizophrenia. Our histories were undoubtedly inadequate, and it may be that factors in early development and a reported uncomplicated birth might have been stressful in some very vulnerable cases.

The characteristic features of the young schizophrenic child are primitive plasticity, maturational lags, and neurophysiological disorganization, especially as noted in the research of Barbara Fish (Fish *et al.*, 1966).

Some interesting data have come from the psychometric tests that were repeated frequently for many of these subjects from early childhood to adulthood. Of the 37 who made a social adjustment as adults, only 2 (as small children with autism) were ever untestable (on one test each), and only 3 others scored below 50 percent on IQ tests at some time in their lives. These 5 and all the others have tended to develop intelligence between the IQ levels of 70 and 100 through most of their life. Six have demonstrated superior intelligence on tests and 3 have acquired college degrees.

There was a tendency for a remarkable stability of IQs over the life span in these schizophrenic individuals, while at the same time they showed variability between verbal and performance scores and an intertest variability. The verbal scores were usually higher. There was no evidence of deterioration due to schizophrenia. Some patients were out of contact and untestable for years, as adults, but if they came in contact again, some because of the recent use of psychoactive drugs, they again achieved IQ scores on a variety of tests comparable to their functioning in childhood or adolescence. However, reality testing and ability to function independently were often not commensurate with their verbal intelligence scores.

In general those 63 subjects who have become chronically institutionalized have had low intelligence scores. None have maintained above-average scores and the majority have clustered around the borderline level. Those children who were most autistic—lacking in language development and untestable on psychometric tests—tended to remain at a low level. Variability in testing was shown in these subjects, as it was in the subjects with higher IQ and better adjustments. Drops in IQ occurred when patients dropped out of contact or when there was an organic deterioration, especially when it eventually led to death. Most impressively, there was a tendency for IQs to rise moderately, especially in adulthood, even for those subjects who were in institutions. Recent drug therapy may have contributed to this improvement.

The 37 individuals who are in community-living represent every level of adjustment: 1 man, who is now 37 years old and in a regressed dependent state, has been cared for by his dedicated mother since she removed him from Bellevue at the age of 11 because his father died in a mental hospital; 3 of them are college graduates, 2 of whom are successful professional men. The 5 men with the most superior intelligence were all symbiotic in early childhood.

All are recognizable as schizophrenic, and all are dependent in varying degrees on psychiatric guidance or treatment, agency support, or unusual family support or other social support.

Twelve have been out in the world since they left Bellevue in childhood. Their parents have been dedicated and had the means to place them in private or parochial schools, sanitoria or residential treatment, or other special programs.

Ten adolescent boys were able to leave institutions between the ages of 14 and 19, apparently because of adolescent remission during which their mental conditions changed. About half were recognized as asocial, with court and training-school records. Two are adjusting as homosexuals. For the most part, their employment is only partial.

In the last 10 years, since the state mental institutions have been using the psychoactive drugs, the activity programs, and the open-door policy with frequent home visits and discharges, an interesting group of 16 individuals has left the hospital after reaching 20 years of age. Not more than 3 are fully employed. Three of these are women, 2 of whom have had illegitimate babies.

Of the 63 who are still in institutions, 35 have been continuously hospitalized, until the present time or until their death. Twenty-seven of these had an onset with infantile autism and had, for the most part, complicating organic factors, including convulsions in 8 cases. All of them had psychotropic drug treatment, as well as anticonvulsive drugs when needed.

Seventeen of these 63 institutionally adjusted patients are women, 7 of whom were home for a few years during the latency period of childhood to mid adolescence. This is the period when girls who are autistic or symbiotic in early childhood have spontaneous remissions.

Twelve boys were out of mental institutions in various states of remission for at least two years during adolescence. This remission is typical of boys, who may also develop pseudopsychopathic and pseudoneurotic features before they settle into their adult pattern, either with sufficient defenses to carry them in the community or with psychotic or regressive features that require their hospitalization.

The hospitalized adult who has been schizophrenic from childhood shows every type of psychotic state. Many are regressed to low levels of functioning and are doubly impaired if they have organic disorders and convulsions. But many are typical adult paranoid, catatonic, and disturbed psychotics.

Conclusions

Childhood schizophrenia, including autism, is an early decompensation in a genetically vulnerable individual. It is caused by organic stress *in utero,* perinatally, or in early childhood. It lasts throughout the person's life, with a variety of clinical features during different life epochs and perhaps dominated by the original decompensating organic condition. Remissions in affected children often occur spontaneously at puberty in boys and during latency in girls. About one-third of the cases studied have a favorable prognosis to make a social but vulnerable and dependent adjustment in the community. Treatment with psychoactive drugs and energetic socializing programs, even in adulthood, may increase the number who make a social adjustment. Many other treatment measures may stimulate maturational lags during development and help to establish coping mechanisms in episodes of decompensation, but these measures do not seem to change the life course.

The concept of childhood schizophrenia that I have developed is as follows. It is a psychobiological entity determined by an inherited predisposition and precipitated by an early physiological or organic crisis and a failure in adequate defense mechanisms. It persists for the lifetime of the individual, but it exhibits different clinical or behavioral or psychiatric features at different epochs in the individual's development. These features are related to compensating defenses. Anxiety is a core problem and calls forth a multitude of defense mechanisms, which sometimes dominate the picture. We see autistic (Kanner, 1973) and symbiotic (Mahler, 1968) features in infancy and early childhood, psychoses in mid and late childhood, remission in puberty, pseudoneurotic and pseudopsychopathic features in adolescence, and a wide range of regressive and psychotic conditions in the adult.

The specific features of childhood schizophrenia are a developmental lag and an embryonic plasticity, with a lack of differentiation of pattern formation and of boundaries in various areas of functioning, i.e., the autonomic area, the motor area, perception, cognition, affect, and social behavior. Resulting psychological problems are concerned with disorientation in identity, time, and space.

Treatment

Throughout the years of my research work with problem children, treatment has always played an important part. My focus has always been on the individual child both when he was being observed in the hospital setting and after he left the hospital.

It is not possible to elaborate here on the treatment programs that were investigated and to some extent checked by follow-up studies without doubling the length of this contribution. However I have recently evaluated treatment of the children I have known over the years in a chapter entitled "Prescription for Treatment in Children" for the revised edition of *The American Handbook of Psychiatry* (1975; see also Bender, 1952).

In general, I can say that many kinds of treatment help children to cope with the numerous problems they usually have and help them to use their own normal resources and defenses to develop more normally and to meet whatever demands society places on them. But there appear to be no cures for the emotional, mental, psychiatric, and neurological problems of childhood.

I can again quote Herrick by saying that success in treatment like "Success in life depends very largely on our ability to recognize and evaluate native capacities and limitations, to make the most of the former and compensate in every particular way for the latter [1956, p. 6]."

The nature of childhood is a state of becoming, while at any one point in time each child exists as a complete and unique individual. This is the trend of evolution. Childhood psychiatric, emotional, and mental problems interfere with this state of becoming or evolution. Research in child psychiatry, too, is in a state of becoming; it is open-ended. Each study only suggests further investigations. This is a characteristic of all the work that I have done in this field, a portion of which I have discussed here.

References

BANKS, B. G., & LARROCHE, J. C. Periventricular leukomalacia of infancy. *Archives of Neurology*, 1962, **7**, 386–410.

BENDER, L. The cerebellar control of the vocal organs. *Archives of Neurology and Psychiatry*, 1928, **19**, 319–329.

BENDER, L. Emotional problems in children. *Proceedings of the Second Institute on the Exceptional Child*. Langhorne, Penn., 1935, **2**, 49–64.

BENDER, L. Behaviour problems in children of psychotic and criminal parents. *Genetic Psychology Monograph*, 1937, **19**, 229–338.

BENDER, L. *A visual motor gestalt test and its clinical use*. Research Monograph #3. New York: American Orthopsychiatric Association, 1938.

BENDER, L. Art and therapy in mental disturbances in children. *Journal of Nervous and Mental Diseases,* 1939, **86,** 249–263.

BENDER, L. The Goodenough Test (Drawing of a Man) in chronic encephalitis in children. *Journal of Nervous and Mental Diseases,* 1940, **91,** 277–286.

BENDER, L. Cerebral sequelae and behavior disorders following pyogenic meningoencephalites in children. *Archives of Pediatrics,* 1942, **59,** 772–783. (a)

BENDER, L. Childhood schizophrenia. *The Nervous Child,* 1942, **1,** 138–141. (b)

BENDER, L. Postencephalitic behavior disorders in childhood. In J. B. Neal (Ed.), *Encephalitis: A clinical study.* New York: Grune & Stratton, 1942. (c)

BENDER, L. Burn encephalopathies in children. *Archives of Pediatrics,* 1943, **60,** 75–87.

BENDER, L. Organic brain condition producing behavior disturbances. In Nolan D. C. Lewis and B. L. Pacella, (Eds.), *Modern Trends in Child Psychiatry.* New York: International University Press, 1946. (a)

BENDER, L. There is no substitute for family life. *Child Study,* 1946. (b)

BENDER, L. Childhood schizophrenia: A clinical study of 100 schizophrenic children. *American Journal of Orthopsychiatry,* 1947, **17,** 40–56. (a)

BENDER, L. Psychopathic behaviors disorder in children. In R. M. Lindner and R. V. Seliger (Eds.), *Handbook of Correctional Psychology.* New York; Philosophical Library, 1947. (b)

BENDER, L. Genesis of hostility in children. *American Journal of Psychiatry,* 1948, **105,** 241–245. Also in *Psychoanalytic Review,* 1963, **50,** 95.

BENDER, L. Anxiety in disturbed children. In Paul H. Hoch and Joseph Zubin (Eds.), *Anxiety.* New York: Grune & Stratton, 1950.

BENDER, L. *Child psychiatric techniques: diagnostic and therapeutic approach to normal and abnormal development through patterned, expressive, and group behavior.* Springfield, Ill.: Charles C Thomas, 1952.

BENDER, L. *Aggression, hostility and anxiety in children.* Springfield, Ill.: Charles C Thomas, 1953.

BENDER, L. *A dynamic psychopathology of childhood.* Springfield, Ill.: Charles C Thomas, 1954.

BENDER, L. Specific reading disabilities as a maturational lag. *Bulletin of the Orton Society,* 1957, **7,** 9–18. (a)

BENDER, L. What are the influential factors that predispose the youth of our society to delinquency and crime? In Frank J. Cohen (Ed.), *Youth and crime.* New York: International Universities Press, 1957. (b)

BENDER, L. Problems of conceptualization and communication in children with developmental alexia. In Paul H. Hoch and Joseph Zubin (Eds.), *Psychopathology of communication.* New York: Grune & Stratton, 1958.

BENDER, L. Autism in children with mental deficiency. *American Journal of Mental Deficiencies,* 1959, **64,** 81–86. (a)

BENDER, L. Children and adolescents who have killed. *American Journal of Psychiatry,* 1959, **116,** 510–513. (b)

BENDER, L. Concept of congenital aphasia: psychiatric aspects. In Spencer Brown (Ed.), *Concept of congenital aphasia from the standpoint of dynamic differential diagnoses.* Thirty-fourth Annual Convention American Speech and Hearing Association, Washington, D.C., 1959. (c)

BENDER, L. The concept of pseudopsychopathic schizophrenia in adolescence. *American Journal of Orthpsychiatry,* 1959, **29,** 491–512. (d)

BENDER, L. Diagnostic and therapeutic aspects of childhood schizophrenia. In P. W. Bowman (Ed.), *Mental retardation.* Proceedings of the First International Medical Conference. New York: Grune & Stratton, 1960. (a)

BENDER, L. Emotional deprivation in infancy and its implication in child psychiatry. *A Crianca Portuguesa,* 1960, **19,** 83–107. (b)

BENDER, L. Mental illness in childhood and heredity. *Eugenics Quarterly,* 1963, **10,** 1–11.

BENDER, L. Offender and offended children. In R. Slosenko (Ed.), *Sexual behavior and the law.* Springfield, Ill.: Charles C Thomas, 1964.

BENDER, L. The concept of plasticity in childhood schizophrenia. In P. Hoch and J. Zubin (Eds.), *Psychopathology of schizophrenia.* New York: Grune & Stratton, 1966.

BENDER L. A psychiatrist looks at deviancy as a factor in juvenile delinquency. *Federal Probation,* 1968, **32,** 35–41.

BENDER L. Hostile aggression in children. In S. Garattini and S. B. Sigg, (Eds.), *Biology of aggressive behavior.* Amsterdam: Excerpta Medica, 1969. (a)

BENDER, L. The nature of chilhood psychosis. In John G. Howard (Ed.), *Modern perspectives in international child psychiatry* Edinburgh: Oliver & Boyd, 1969. (b)

BENDER, L. The life course of schizophrenic children. *Biological Psychiatry,* 1970, **2,** 165–172. (a)

BENDER, L. The maturation process and hallucinations. In Wolfram Keup, (Ed.), *Origin and mechanisms of hallucinations.* New York: Plenum Press, 1970. (b)

BENDER, L. The use of the Visual Motor Gestalt Test in the diagnosis of learning disabilities. *Journal of Special Education,* 1970, **4,** 29–39. (c)

BENDER, L. Psychopathic personality or schizophrenia in adolescence. *Biological Psychiatry,* 1971, **3,** 197–204. (a)

BENDER, L. Remission rate and long term results of convulsive therapy of schizophrenic children. Read at the American Society of Biological Psychiatry, 1971. In press. (b)

BENDER, L. Aggression in children. *Proceedings of the Research Association of Nervous and Mental Diseases,* 1974, **52,** 201–208.

BENDER, L. The life course of children with schizophrenia. *American Journal of Psychiatry,* 1973, **30,** 783–786. (b)

BENDER, L. Schizophrenic spectrum disorders in the families of schizophrenic children. Read at the American Psychopathological Association. New York, 1973. In Press. (c)

BENDER, L. Prescription for treatment of children. In Daniel X. Freedman and Jarl E. Dyrud (Eds.). *The American Handbook of Psychiatry,* 1975. In Press.

BENDER, L. & ANDERMAN, C. Brain damage in blind children with retrolental fibroplasia. *Archives of Neurology and Psychiatry,* 1965, **12,** 644–649.

BENDER, L., & CURRAN, F. J. Children and adolescents who kill. *Journal of Criminal Psychopathology,* 1940, **1,** 296–322.

BENDER, L., & DEWITT, L. M. Hematological studies on experimental tuberculosis of the guinea pig. *American Review of Tuberculosis,* 1923, I-**8,** 138–162; 1924, II-**9,** 65–71; 1924, III-**9,** 477–486.

BENDER, L., & FARETRA, G. Pregnancy and birth histories in children with psychiatric problems. *Proceedings of the Third World Congress of Psychiatry,* 1962, **2,** 1329–1333.

BENDER, L., & FARETRA, G. Body image problems in children. In H. I. Lief, V. F. Lief, and N. R. Lief. (Eds.), *The psychological basis of medical practise.* New York: Harper & Row, 1963.

BENDER, L., & FARETRA, G. Relationship between childhood schizophrenia and adult schizophrenia. In Arnold R. Kaplan (Ed.), *Genetic factors in schizophrenia.* Springfield, Ill.: Charles C Thomas, 1972.

BENDER, L., & FREEDMAN, A. M. A study of the first three years in the maturation of schizophrenic children. *Quarterly Journal of Child Behavior,* 1952, **4,** 245–270.

BENDER, L., FREEDMAN, A., GRUGETT, A. E., & HELME, W. Schizophrenia in childhood: A confirmation of the diagnosis. *Transactions of the American Neurological Association,* 1952, **77,** 67–73.

BENDER, L., & HELME, W. A quanitative test of theory and diagnostic indicators of childhood schizophrenia. *Archives of Neurology and Psychiatry,* 1953, **70,** 413–427.

BENDER, L., & HITCHMAN, I. L. A longitudinal study of ninety schizophrenic women. *Journal of Nervous and Mental Diseases,* 1956, **124,** 337–345.

BENDER, L., & PASTER, S. Homosexual trends in children. *American Journal of Orthopsychiatry,* 1941, **11,** 730–740.

BENDER, L., & RAPOPORT, J. Animal drawings of children. *American Journal of Orthopsychiatry,* 1944, **14,** 521–527.

BENDER, L., & SCHILDER, P. Encephelopathia alcoholica. *Archives of Neurology and Psychiatry,* 1933. **29,** 990–1053.

BENDER, L., & SCHILDER, P. Impulsions: A specific disorder of the behavior of children. *Archives of Neurology and Psychiatry,* 1940, **44,** 990–1008.

BENDER, L., & SCHILDER, P. Mannerisms as organic motility syndrome. *Confinia Neurology,* 1941, **3,** 321–330.

BENDER, L., & SCHILDER, P. Graphic art as a special ability in children with reading disability. *Journal of Clinical and Experiment Psychopathology,* 1951, **12,** 147–156.

BENDER, L., & YARNELL, H. An observation nursery: A report of 250 children on the psychiatric division of bellevue hospital. *American Journal of Psychiatry,* 1941, **97,** 1158–1172.

BLAU, A., Mental changes following head trauma in children. *Archives in Neurology and Psychiatry*, 1936, **35**, 723–766.

BOWLBY, J. Forty-four juvenile theives. *International Journal of Psychoanalysis*, 1944, **25**, 19–52 & 107–128.

BOWLBY, J. *Maternal care and mental health*, Geneva: World Health Organization, Monograph #3, 1951.

BOWMAN, K. M., & BLAU, A. Psychiatric states following head and brain injuries in adults and children. In S. Brock (Ed.), *Injuries of the skull, brain and spinal cord*, 2nd ed. Baltimore: Williams & Wilkins, 1943.

CAPLAN, H. The role of deviant maturation in pathogenesis of anxiety. *American Journal of Orthopsychiatry*, 1956, **26**, 94–98.

CHESS, S. Developmental language disability as a factor in personality distortion in childhood. *American Journal of Orthopsychiatry*, 1944, **14**, 483–490.

COLBERT, E. G., KOEGLER, R. I., & MARKHAM, C. H. Vestibular dysfunction in childhood schizophrenia. *American Archives of General Psychiatry*, 1959, **1**, 600–617.

COTTINGTON, F. The treatment of schizophrenia of childhood. *The Nervous Child*, 1942, **1**, 171–187.

DE HIRSCH, K., JANSKY, J. J., & LANGFORD, W. S. *Predicting reading failure*. New York: Harper & Row, 1966.

FABIAN, A. A. Vertical rotation in visual motor performance in relationship to reading reversals. *Educational Psychology*, 1945, **36**, 129–135.

FABIAN, A. A., & BENDER, L. Head injuries in children: Predisposing factors. *American Journal of Orthopsychiatry*, 1947, **17**, 68–79.

FISH, B. Longitudinal observations of biological deviations in a schizophrenic infant. *American Journal of Psychiatry*, 1959, **116**, 25–33.

FISH, B. Contributions of development research to a theory of schizophrenia. In J. Helmuth (Ed.), *Exceptional infant*. Vol. 2: *Studies in abnormalities*. New York: Brunner-Mazel, 1971.

FISH, B., & ALPERT, M. Patterns of neurological development in infants born of schizophrenic mothers. *Recent Advances in Biological Psychiatry*, 1963, **5**, 34–37.

FISH, B., WILE, R., SHAPIRO, T., & HALPERN, F. Prediction of schizophrenia in childhood II: A ten year follow-up. In P. Hoch and J. Zubin (Eds.), *Psychopathology of schizophrenia*. New York: Grune & Stratton, 1966.

FREEDMAN, A. M. Maturation and its relation to the dynamics of childhood schizophrenia. *American Journal of Orthopsychiatry*, 1954, **24**, 487–491.

GESELL, A. *Embryology of behavior*. New York: Harper & Bros., 1945.

GESELL, A., & AMATRUDA, C. S. *Developmental diagnosis*, 2nd ed. New York: Hoeber, 1947.

GIBBS, C. E. Behavior disorders in chronic epidemic encephalites. *American Journal of Psychiatry*, 1930, **9**, 619–625.

GOLDBERG, I. Use of remedial reading tutoring as a method of psychotherapy for schizophrenic children with reading disabilities. *Quarterly Journal of Child Behavior*, 1952, **4**, 273–280.

GOLDFARB, W. Infantile rearing and problem behavior, *American Journal of Orthopsychiatry*, 1943, **13**, 249–265.

GOLDFARB, W. Effects of psychological deprivation in infancy and subsequent stimulation. *American Journal of Psychiatry*, 1945, **13**, 249–265.

GOLDFARB, W. Emotional and intellectual consequences of psychologic deprivation in infancy: A revaluation. In Paul H. Hoch and Joseph Zubin (Eds.), *Psychopathology of Childhood*. New York: Grune & Stratton, 1955.

GREENACRE, P. Predisposition to anxiety. *Psychoanalytic Quarterly*, 1941, **10**, 66–95, 610–639. Also in *Trauma growth and personality*, New York: Norton, 1952.

HERRICK, C. J. *The evolution of human nature*. Austin: University of Texas Press, 1956.

HESTON, L. L. The genetics of schizophrenia and schizoid disease. *Science*, 1970, **167**, 249–255.

KANNER, L. *Childhood psychosis: Initial studies and new insights*. Washington, D.C.: V. H. Winston & Sons, 1973.

KEELER, W. R., & BENDER, L. A follow-up study of children with behavior disorders and sydenham's chorea. *American Journal of Psychiatry*, 1952, **109**, 421–428.

KETTY, S. S. Genetic environment interaction in the schizophrenic syndrome. In R. Cencro (Ed.), *The schizophrenic reaction*. New York: Brunner-Mazel, 1970.

KNOBLOCH, H., & PASAMANICK, B. Complications of pregnancy and mental deficiency. In P. W.

Bowman and H. V. Mautner (Eds.), *Mental Retardation*. New York: Grune & Stratton, 1960. See bibliography for more references.

LORENTE DE NO, R. Vestibular-ocular reflex arc. *Archives of Neurology and Psychiatry*, 1933, **30**, 245–253.

MAHLER, M. *On human symbiosis and the vicissitudes of individuation*. Vol. 1: *Childhood psychosis*. New York: International Universities Press, 1968.

ORTON, S. T. "Word blindness" in children. *Archives of Neurology and Psychiatry*, 1928, **14**, 581–652.

ORTON, S. T. *Reading, writing and speech problems in children*. New York: W. W. Norton, 1937.

PEEKE, J. Incidence of reading disabilities on the Bellevue Psychiatric Children's Service. Thesis for candidate of graduate degree at New York School of Social Work (unpublished), 1945.

POLLACK, M., & KRIEGER, H. P. Oculomotor and postural patterns in schizophrenic children. *Archives of Neurology and Psychiatry*, 1958, **79**, 720–726.

RABINOVITCH, R. Observation on the differential study of severely disturbed children. *American Journal of Orthopsychiatry*, 1951, **22**, 230–236.

RACHMAN, S., & BERGER, M. Whirling and postural control in schizophrenic children. *Journal of Child Psychology and Psychiatry*, 1963, **4**, 137–155.

RAPOPORT, J. The psychopathology of childhood schizophrenia. *The Nervous Child*, 1942, **1**, 188–195.

RAPOPORT, J. Fantasy objects in children. *Psychoanalytic Review*, 1944, **31**, 1–6.

ROBERTS, L. Functional plasticity in cortical speech areas and the integration of speech, *Associated Research in Nervous and Mental Disease*, 1958, **36**, 449–466.

ROSENTHAL, D. Genetic research in the schizophrenic syndrome, In H. Cancro (Ed.), *The schizophrenic reaction*. New York: Brunner-Mazel, 1970.

SCHILDER, P. *Brain and personality*. Nervous and Mental Disease Monograph, #53, 1931. Also New York: International Universities Press, 1951.

SCHILDER, P. *Image and appearance of the human body*. London: Kegan Paul, Trench, Trubner, 1935. Also, New York: International University Press, 1950.

SCHILDER, P. The psychology of schizophrenia. *Psychoanalytic Review*, 1936, **26**, 380–385.

SCHILDER, P. Vita and bibliography. *Journal of Criminal Psychopathology*, 1940, **2**, 225–230.

SCHILDER, P. *Mind, perception and thought in their constructive aspects*. New York: Columbia University Press, 1942.

SCHILDER, P. *Contributions to developmental neuropsychiatry*. New York: International Universities Press, 1964.

SCHILDER, P., & CURRAN, F. J. A constructive approach to the problems of childhood and adolescence. *Journal of Criminal Psychopathology*, 1940, **2**, 120–129.

SILVER, A. A. Postural and righting responses in children. *Journal of Pediatrics*, 1952, **41**, 493–498.

SILVER, A. A., & HAGIN, R. Specific reading disability: A delineation of the syndrome and relationship to cortical dominance. *Comprehensive Psychiatry*, 1960, **1**, 126–134.

SPITZ, R. A. Hospitalism, an inquiry into the genesis of psychiatric conditions of early childhood. *The Psychoanalytic Study of the Child*, 1945, **1**, 53–74.

SZENTAGOTHAI, J. Specificity and plasticity of neural structures and functions. In M. H. Brazier (Ed.), *Brain and behavior*, American Institute of Biological Sciences, 1961.

TEICHER, J. D. Preliminary survey of motility in children. *Journal of Nervous and Mental Diseases*, 1941, **94**, 277–304.

TOLOR, A., & SCHULBERG, H. C. *An evaluation of the Bender Gestalt Test*, Springfield, Ill.: Charles C Thomas, 1963.

TOWBIN, A. Central nervous system damage in human fetus and newborn infant. *Diseases of Childhood*, 1970, **119**, 529–542.

VON ECONOMO, C. *Encephalitis lethargica*. English translation, New York: Oxford University Press, 1931.

WENDER, P. *Minimal brain dysfunction in children*. New York: Wiley Interscience, 1971.

WERTHEIMER, M. Untersuchuchungen zur Lehre von der Gestalt. *Psychologiste Forschung*, 1923, **4**, 332–337. Translated in W. D. Ellis (Ed.), *A source book of gestalt psychology*, New York: Harcourt, Brace & Co. 1938, 71–88.

THE ANATOMY OF A PERIPATETIC CHILD PSYCHIATRY RESEARCHER

REGINALD S. LOURIE

As I understand my assignment, it is to answer two questions: (1) How did you get to be a researcher in child psychiatry? (2) What was behind the actual research studies? I accepted it because it offered the rare opportunity to look back and see how I got here and to give credits where they belong, particularly as there have been so many important influences along the way. It is a process that creates humility and a debt of gratitude, payable only by passing on what I have learned.

The answer to the first question is a long one. It must begin with my physician father. I cannot, like Tristram Shandy, report precisely what happened before my conception. But I can summarize the kind of model my father was in stimulating curiosity by telling how he came to the United States. He ran away from home in Russia at 12 to follow his inspiring teacher to America and gave himself a new name, Inte. *I* stood for *intelligence, N* for *knowledge, T* for *truth,* and *E for eternity.*

Another lasting influence was my best friend, Abraham Maslow. We were inseparable through grammar school, high school, and even into the second year of college, before he got married. Abe later became the founder of the field of humanistic psychology, the basis on which the Esalen and other innovative concepts began.

The beginning stimulus for actual research came in my college years at Cornell, where there was the opportunity to work under Emerson, a pioneer

REGINALD S. LOURIE, Director Emeritus, Department of Psychiatry, Children's Hospital National Medical Center, Washington; Medical Director, Hillcrest Children's Center; Professor Emeritus of Child Health and Development, Psychiatry and Behavioral Sciences, George Washington University School of Medicine, Washington.

in genetics (sharing laboratories with graduate students, including Beadle, who later became a Nobelist).

One experience that should have warned me away from the frustrations of research happened when, in a year-long experiment in collaboration with Dunn at Columbia on breeding mice for coat color, a custodian allowed the heat to go over 110° for a weekend and all my more-than-500 mice died.

There were also Rahn in bacteriology and Sharp in cytology, who provided me the opportunity to do small independent research projects in which methodology was stressed. Another model was a graduate student with whose family I lived, A. Leon Winsor, who was a contributor in physiological psychology and whose techniques were the basis for my own later doctoral research. It was also made possible for me to spend time in the New York City Health Department, before and after graduation, with William H. Park, whose leadership eliminated diphtheria as a dread disease in this country and who was working with a vaccine for gonorrhea when he died. I was labeled a bacteriologist, but it was Park who persuaded me that the only way to be a bacteriologist was to study medicine.

My medical school in Brooklyn prided itself in turning out family doctors, but I had the opportunity there to do research with a new machine (which took up most of a large room) called the electrocardiograph. My first published paper—which I did in collaboration with a fellow student, Sidney Margolin, and a young physiology instructor, David Abramson, both of whom became noted research contributors—was on experimental extrasystoles in the cat (Abramson et al., 1936). Because of my laboratory background I was an assistant in clinical microscopy under a research-oriented professor, Louis Johnson, who was also a book reviewer for the *New York Times*.

The logical place to intern for a laboratory man in the mid 1930s was in pediatrics, which was then heavily rooted in biochemistry and bacteriology. A place was available at the medical-school hospital pediatric service, where, with residency training, there was a rare opportunity to combine clinical information with the clinical and laboratory research taking place in the use of prontosil, the first of the now-familiar antibiotics that have changed the practice of pediatrics. The valuable part of these years was that I learned to think both like a pediatrician and like a child. However, the questions that intrigued me and for which there were only fragmentary answers available were about what to do for the children whose thinking provided answers that led to behavioral, adjustment, and psychosomatic problems. Especially troublesome were those seen in their own poverty-stricken and often strife-ridden homes in the Red Hook section of Brooklyn.

Ambulance duty took us not only into every other Red Hook home but also onto ships, where we saw sick sailors with exotic diseases. In addition, it forced us to learn about the reactions of humans in misery and under stress, such as when one is delivering a pregnant nun in a hideout at gunpoint.

It became clear that my next step in training should be to get a background in child psychiatry to try to find answers to the questions that were most challenging. My chief of pediatrics, Charles Weymuller, arranged for me to spend some time with Bronson Crothers at the Boston Children's Hospital and with Leo Kanner at the Harriet Lane Home of the Johns Hopkins Hospital. Crothers as a model provided an insatiable interest in combining what he was learning about the developing nervous system with the development of behavior. It was no surprise when he later wrote the book *A Pediatrician in Search of Mental Hygiene* (1937). He liked my plan to concentrate on child psychiatry but warned me that "It's a fascinating and important emerging field, but you can't make a living in it." Kanner, on the other hand, was an encyclopedia of information about the manifestations of childhood disorders and the common-sense approach to applying what was known to clinical pediatrics. As an available and interested model of the inquiring mind, he remained as a sort of godfather for a young man with an open mind in search of child psychiatry.

There were two other lasting influences during my pediatric training years. When on a rotation for contagious disease experience at the Chapin Hospital in Providence, Rhode Island, I had the opportunity to spend considerable time at the Emma Pendleton Bradley Home, where the first work with the electroencephalogram in the United States was being carried out on children by Jasper and his group, and where Charles Bradley was beginning to explore the use of stimulants in childhood schizophrenia and hyperactivity. During this period I had a most important meeting with Arnold Gesell, in which he clarified for me what my future research involvement would be. When I persistently asked him the reasons for the developmental stages he was describing, he finally said, "I am interested in finding out and detailing what happens. I am leaving it to you to find out *why* it happens."

In spite of Gesell's admonition my first research venture in child-psychiatric-related studies was spent in finding out what happens. My old friend and college roommate, Edward Strongin, persuaded me to take my psychiatric residency at his base of operations, the New York State Psychiatric Institute and Hospital at the Columbia Presbyterian Medical Center, where he was a research and clinical psychologist. He was working with the parotid secretory rate as a diagnostic technique, using Lashley's techniques as modified by Winsor. I began to test the rate in children, seeing it as a potential bridge to measure the function of the autonomic nervous system as related to developing behavior. Later, during the early days of World War II, I was fortunate to be close to Strongin's work on newer physiological techniques for pilot selection centering on measuring function under stress. These techniques later became part of the selection process for astronauts. They impressed me with what later became the basis for my current studies in the developmental aspects of the synthetic functions of the ego.

The Psychiatric Institute was alive with psychiatric research. Kalinowski had brought over the first electric shock machine from Italy; Kallman was studying the genetics of schizophrenia; Barrera and Ferrera were carrying out a variety of neuropathological research with psychiatric patients; Piotrowski and Kelly were developing standards for the new Rorschach test; Landis and Zubin were carrying out statistical and clinical psychological investigations in a range of psychiatric syndromes; and Jervis was doing neurochemical studies in mental retardation. Clinically I had my first exposure to leading psychoanalytic thinking and fortunate contacts with Howard Potter, a pioneer in studies of childhood psychosis and initiator of modern concepts in mental retardation, and with William Langford, who introduced me to pediatric psychiatry and clinical research in child psychiatry at Babies Hospital.

My second year of psychiatric residency was at Bellevue Psychiatric Hospital, where my assignment was to work with Lauretta Bender on the children's ward. This ward was a museum of psychological and organic pathology and a center for research. In addition to Bender's wide-ranging, prodigious research output, Wechsler, Halperin, and Mackover were perfecting the WISC and a group of projective tests with children. Most important was my being selected a Paul Schilder's "secretary" and note taker, which meant accompanying this genius on his rounds and participating in his therapeutic innovation, which later became known as group therapy. Most of the notes became the basis for additions to his extensive publications. Penetrating insights on mental functioning as related to organicity became available as well as a research philosophy that was later both to be productive for me and to lead to blind alleys. This philosophy was based on one that Schilder had learned from his teacher, Warner-Juaregg, and was summed up as, "If an idea sounds good, it has a good chance of being right." Once, after he had published a brilliant paper based on some rounds notes, I mentioned to Schilder that he had not been sure of these formulations. He replied, with a twinkle in his eye, that if the paper stimulated someone to prove that he was wrong it had served an important purpose.

The director of the Psychiatric Institute, Nolan D.C. Lewis, had been sufficiently impressed with my beginning work on the function of the autonomic nervous system and the parotid secretory rate to arrange a Markle Foundation fellowship for me to complete these studies and become a candidate for a doctoral degree in medical science at the medical school at Columbia. Although I had a laboratory at the Psychiatric Institute, it was also arranged for me to continue studies begun at Bellevue with Bender and Schilder, who had opened the way for personal contact at their home and with their family.

It was also arranged through Bill Langford for me to have as basic project research subjects the study population of Myrtle McGraw's Normal

Child Development Laboratory at Babies Hospital. This introduced me to still another research dimension, child development studies, with a superbly trained but unorthodox and innovative research team. At the same time I could continue training in clinical child psychiatry with Langford and Katherine Wickman. The Babies Hospital experience made it possible for me to share the thinking of fine research minds such as Hattie Alexander, John Coffey, and Ashley Weech, as well as Rustin McIntosh and Frederick Bartlett, who wrote the "baby book" by which children were reared between Holt's and Spock's baby books. A consultantship was also arranged in which I collaborated with Benjamin Spock in training well-baby clinic pediatricians in preventive pediatric psychiatry for the New York City Health Department. This three-year combined research and clinical training fellowship ended with my joining the Navy until the end of World War II.

In naval hospitals there was the opportunity to do studies with combat neuroses and combat fatigue, using both the hypnosis techniques learned from Schilder and what could be called behavior modification. One such behavior-modification approach was a time saver. When as officer of the day I had the duty to catheterize all postoperative patients who hadn't voided by the time of evening rounds, I sent a corpsman around to find those patients and tell them that if they didn't void, a psychiatrist was going to catheterize them. I never had to do a catheterization.

Following the Navy were two clinical and teaching years in Rochester before I came to Children's Hospital in Washington, D.C., and the George Washington University School of Medicine, where I have been since, combining clinical research and teaching in pediatric psychiatry and completing my own psychoanalytic training. However, becoming an independent researcher happily did not end my opportunities to work with great thinkers and innovators. I have had such interchanges on programmatic research with fine minds from many disciplines on the President's Panel on Mental Retardation; the National Mental Health Advisory Council; White House task forces, which developed the Head Start and the national Parent and Child Center programs; the Joint Commission on Mental Health of Children; and seven of the Delos Symposions on Human Settlements. In the latter I have had rare opportunities to exchange research ideas with such students as Arnold Toynbee, Buckminster Fuller, Margaret Mead, Baron de Juvenal, Constantinos Doxiadis, and many others. More recently, there have been the meetings of the International Study Group of the International Association of Child Psychiatry and Allied Professions.

In answer to the second question: looking back, I find two qualities that have been useful in whatever research contributions have emerged from my background: an ability to translate the principles from one field to others and a touch of a polymorphous perverse tendency leading to a widespread range of interests and involvements. The end result has been a research generalist rather than a research specialist. There are also two periods involved, before and after psychoanalytic training.

The studies of the autonomic nervous system (1943) when my independent research studies began, involved simplifying the techniques for use with children to measure the parotid secretory rate with what came to be called "the spitometer." Normal values for early-to-late age levels were established, demonstrating that parasympathic controls do not become mature until five to six years of age, at which time the rates begin to approach adult levels. When these standards were applied to clinical problems, it appeared that in children with impulse-control problems, including hyperactivity, the parotid secretory rates continue at the high early levels, while in neurotic manifestations the rates are at normal levels. This finding has implications for the still incompletely clear problem of symptom choice. What impressed me lastingly from these studies was the role of individual constitutional differences in determining solutions to the stages of personality development. Although interest in the use of the easily measured parotid secretory rate in child psychiatry has not continued, the techniques and normal values have found a useful place in the work of investigators at the National Institute for Dental Research and other dental study groups. These techniques and values are also being used in studies of cystic fibrosis at the National Institute of Child Health and Human Development.

Another set of base-line studies involved the natural history of rhythmic patterns in childhood, their use and their distortions (Lourie, 1949). I was first stimulated to do these studies by trying to understand the repetition compulsion and Bender and Schilder's concepts of early childhood repetitive patterns, which they called "impulsions" while at Bellevue. This interest was furthered by Kubie's work on the repetitive core of the neuroses. My interest was crystallized while I was working as pediatric–psychiatric liaison at Strong Memorial Hospital in Rochester, when I was challenged by the practical problems posed by bed rockers and head bangers. It was possible to define when and how a variety of rhythmic patterns were used in normal development, became "partialized," continued to serve tension-relieving purposes, and in some children persisted in more primitive form as anxiety manifestations.

One amusing situation I encountered during the study involved a two-year-old who rocked her crib violently for two to three hours every night. The noise could be heard by the neighbors in the apartment house in which she lived. When we had found a variety of daily rhythmic patterns to substitute so that the troublesome rocking could be given up, the father met the man whose bedroom was directly under the child's. "The child's rocking must have been annoying," the father said. The neighbor, startled, said, "So that's what it was! You have no idea what a reputation you have in this neighborhood. Every night for two or three hours! You are known as 'What-a-Man Smith.'"

Mittleman later told me that these studies were the basis for his own series of reports on the psychodynamic meanings of movement. In addition to their use in clinical practice, I am told that these original studies are being used in the theories of dance therapy. Howard Hansen consulted me about using them in teaching music theory at the Eastman School. If I had written the paper on rhythmic patterns after my psychoanalytic training, it would have had a few additional dimensions. In addition to the use of rhythmic patterns as a method of maintaining homeostasis and therefore as a part ego function, the relationship of rhythmic patterns to the expression of libidinal and aggressive drives would be useful to annotate as a constitutionally based, readily available expression that can be easily cathected and offers a readily available source of drive sublimation.

Another type of base-line study was the investigation of the use of comic books and their effect on children (Bender & Lourie, 1941). I did this study as a research fellow in collaboration with Bender at Bellevue at a time when there was great concern about the deleterious effects of the then-new and eagerly consumed comic books. There had been similar concerns earlier about the harmful effects of movies and radio serials on children, just as there is still concern about the effects of violence on television. In fact, there were, and still are, reports of children having nightmares or acting out violent themes or copying delinquent activities of the villains after exposure to all these media. Our findings were that the themes in the comic book stories were age-old basic themes, handed down in children's literature from generation to generation but brought up-to-date to include modern-day or futuristic technology, such as rockets, ray guns, and interplanetary transportation and communication systems, with a touch of the supernatural and magic. In terms of upsetting children, this form of literature acted like the pulling of a gun's trigger: only if the gun was loaded was there a reaction. Hearing about these studies, the man who wrote Superman stories for the radio came to discuss his worries about harming children because he was receiving indignant letters from mothers of acting-out children and children with sleep disturbances. In spite of my reassurance he decided to undo the supposed harm by putting on radio, in a series called "Adventure Parade," the classic stories that children were supposed to be reading instead of reading comic books or listening to radio serials. To his amazement and chagrin he found that these classics contained so much blood and gore and villainy that they had to be "cleaned up" to fit the radio code!

My research involvements in my first 10 years in the Department of Psychiatry of Children's Hospital of D.C. were closely linked to the clinical problems we were in some ways forced to investigate. A prime example was our

studies on pica. Sam Bessman (now a renowned pharmacologist), in his work
as the pediatric biochemist at Children's Hospital, developed the first chelating
agent for deleading children with clinical lead poisoning. He stopped me in a
corridor one day and said, "Reg, you've got to find out why these children eat
the lead paint in the first place. I delead them, but many come back again and
again, and each time with more evidence of brain damage." With Frances
Millican and Emma Layman I began studies (1963) that only in the last few
years have been experimented with in official circles as a logical basis for the
prevention of lead poisoning. It appeared that young children turn to the
ingestion of nonfood substances most often when meaningful, protective
mothering is unavailable. There were many reasons why mothers were
unavailable to their one- and two-year-old children, but if the reasons were
successfully dealt with, the symptom of pica was readily given up. Fortunately
we were dealing with conflict areas not yet internalized. It also appeared that
lead paint from peeling plaster was only one source of the ingested lead, so
that redoing the walls of old houses could not be the only method of preventing
lead poisoning. There are eaters of dirt, newspapers, pencils, broken dishes,
etc., many of which involve a source of lead. Besides, since pica is not confined
to the children of the poor, it is important to see it as an indicator that some
distortion is taking place in the quality of mothering. When we looked more
closely, we found depressed mothers, mentally ill mothers, hopeless, helpless,
passive, apathetic mothers, alcoholic and drug-addicted mothers, and pleasure-
loving teen-age mothers. There is some pica that is culturally determined,
which later focused our research attention on cross-cultural differences
(Layman *et al.*, 1965). Because so many authorities felt that pica was a young
child's attempt to correct a nutritional deficiency, an independent nutritional
study was developed under Gutelius (Gutelius *et al.*, 1962), which showed no
connection between any food or metabolic deficiency and pica. The South Af-
rican studies (Lanskowsky, 1949) that showed that pica cleared up with iron
injections were repeated, and all our pica patients given intramuscular iron
stopped their pica. However, all the controls who were given saline injections
also gave up their pica.

Probably the most gratifying investigations and those that shaped my
later research directions have been the clinical and developmental studies of
the problems of the first years of life. These began with attention to the psychosomatic problems of infants, including such manifestations as functional
diarrheas, nonorganic failures to thrive, ruminations, and other problems that
were life threatening (Lourie, 1959). It appeared that the babies involved often
had some constitutionally based predisposing factor that made them vulnerable
to handling that did not take into account these individual differences. The
challenge was to define these individual vulnerabilities, such as sensory
hypersensitivities, vegetative imbalances, etc., and build a program of care

around them. Then an individualized program had to be built to "sell the human race" back to these babies, who had often give up on people and turned to their own bodies for the few satisfactions were available to them. The results were gratifying. Rumination, for example, in which there was an expectable 75 percent mortality, was overcome in 100 percent of our cases so handled. These studies formed a base line, added to as will be described further, for an approach in training to the most neglected area in child psychiatry, the first years of life. We have the beginnings of the subspecialty of infant psychiatry.

It was when I was a member of John Kennedy's President's Panel on Mental Retardation that our more comprehensive applied research approach was conceptualized. The broad perspective made available by the outstanding thinkers in this formidable group showed that 75 percent of the retardation in this country was functionally determined. Most of it resulted from child rearing in the most deprived parts of our populations, inner city and rural, whose emphasis was on the development of survival intelligence at the cost of development of the skills that are necessary in formal learning. Much of this was known,—for example, from Pavenstedt and Malone's reports (1971), which we confirmed, symbolized by the three-year-old who could go shopping at the corner store for bread and milk, get the right change, and get it all safely home across busy streets. This most impressive, precocious survival task was achieved at considerable cost. If you asked the child what else was in the store, he didn't know. If you turned him around, he lost his direction.

As we pulled pictures such as this together from over the country, it became apparent that the roots of functional mental retardation were in the first years of life. Our studies of pica and the psychosomatic problems of infants had provided a more detailed look at many of the constitutional and experiential factors involved, as well as evidence that they were both preventable and available to remedial programs. This hopeful outlook was reinforced by my participation in a mission to the Soviet Union, where there were active infant-rearing and early-childhood-rearing programs and where the incidence of mental retardation at least appeared to be confined to the organic, genetic, and metabolic problems. Thus, as in Sweden and a few other countries, the incidence was .5 percent in contrast to our 3–5 percent of the population. When the facts were pointed out to a Congressional committee recently, I was accused publicly and personally by our then Vice President as advocating the Sovietization of American children.

Based on a resolve to apply what we knew to the solution of the problem, an applied research program was developed in our Department of Psychiatry, ambitiously titled the "Prevention of Culturally Determined Retardation." An outstanding early-child-development research staff was slowly formed. With Allen Marans, our basic hypotheses on the disadvantaged child were formulated and published (Marans & Lourie, 1961). Dorothy Huntington was brought in to lead the group. Lois Murphy joined it later as a half-time senior research consultant and, in the spirit of the project, produced one of the most valuable of the staff's contributions, a vulnerability inventory and index for both clinical and research application (Murphy, 1968). We had a population of "boarder babies" in the hospital. They were wards of the D.C. Department of Welfare for whom it was possible to develop individually determined care programs, under Dr. Huntington's perceptive leadership, as a demonstration of what could be accomplished preventively. When "our" babies, who had learned to trust relationships and whose explorations were encouraged, were transferred to other child-care facilities, they were not liked, because if their needs were not met, they became irritable and demanding instead of apathetic or depressed.

Because there appeared to be culturally determined factors underlying developmental distortions of some children in the deprived segments of our inner-city population, we felt it would be useful to compare this aspect of the problem with other cultures. Through colleagues, former staff members, and trainees a personal survey was made in three countries: Italy, Israel, and Greece. In Israel the health and educational authorities knew they had culturally deprived populations and problems similar to ours and were ready to collaborate in cross-cultural infant-rearing studies, but they couldn't decide who should carry them out. In Italy they had the same problems, were unwilling to acknowledge them, and therefore were in no position to do anything about them. In Greece they had the problems and were ready and eager to do something about them in a collaborative cross-cultural research and training program. Our collaborator was Spyros Doxiadis, who is an international pediatric authority, chief of the Children's Hospital Aghia Sophia in Athens, and president of the Metera, a model infant-rearing institution. We began a still-ongoing, productive, comparative infant-development study with our Children's Hospital child-development research team, which included exchanges of staff for periods of time.

This Greek liaison led to my later fortunate involvement with Dr. Doxiadis's brother, Constantinos, the world planner and founder of the science of human settlements (ekistics). This liaison resulted in my becoming part of the series of Delos Symposions he sponsored and was a result of being in the right place at the right time. The cross-disciplinary as well as cross-cultural contributions involved in "The Delos" provided an irreplaceable opportunity for me to develop a much-broadened perspective on the range of factors involved. Putting together the information from child psychiatry and child development with the problems faced by planners, city developers, architects, and a variety of other educators, historians, legal minds, and political and business leaders, as well as scientists, has resulted in a new type of research for me to be involved in: how to build cities for human development. It turns out that many of the leaders concerned with planning or redoing human habitations, from houses to cities, are challenged by the fact that there is a body of information about the developmental needs of children that has implications for their designs. My own involvement follows a familiar pattern in research: a combination of serendipity and one thing's leading to another.

The field of infant-rearing research and programming was expanding, but a major unsolved problem was what to do with the babies in the new preventive "stimulation" approaches. To attempt to define where the deficits in ego functions are that should be addressed in these programs, Dale Meers came to our research team from the Hampstead Clinic. He decided to analyze ghetto children who at the beginning of their school careers were labeled as educational failures. His findings have made a unique contribution as a collaborative project between a psychoanalytic institute and a department of child psychiatry.

Even though the necessary information is far from complete, there has been pressure for the application of at least what we do know. This pressure has resulted in a type of applied mental health research programming on a national scale. A small group was called together by Robert Cooke for Sargent Shriver and the Office of Economic Opportunity and asked if there wasn't something that could be done for the four- and five-year-old disadvantaged children before they got to schools, where so many of them were not learning. Some of us said that there was a great deal known about programming for that age group but that for many of those children it was already too late. Others said that there should be small pilot projects first. We ended by defining a program called Head Start with seven priorities, of which learning was well down on the list. Then began an experiment that demonstrated that we can take giant steps as well as the small, careful ones we are usually committed to as researchers. We learned a great deal from the successful Head Start programs. We learned also that as we learn from the failures we must at the same time stand by to pick them up. At our Hillcreat Children's Center we had a part of the therapeutic nursery devoted to dropouts from Head Start.

Subsequently President Johnson set up a White House task force on programs for the first years of life chaired by J. McVicker Hunt, in which we defined a program for the enhancement of the family and the earliest life experience of babies in their first two years of life. This program, on a much more modest level than Head Start, was established as the Parent and Child Center program. These demonstrations of what could be accomplished for deprived children became one of the major forces behind the pressures for universally available, quality day care.

The move from bench research to clinical research to program research can take the child psychiatric researcher increasingly far from his beginnings if he doesn't watch out. I didn't watch out and was named President and Chairman of the Joint Commission on the Mental Health of Children. The work of the Joint Commission was done by close to 600 of the people in this country most knowledgeable about every aspect of childhood. After they finished six volumes of reports, there remained, as is true in every form of research, the job of integrating their findings and recommendations. This was accomplished by a small group: Julius Richmond, Nicholas Hobbs, and Norman Lourie, along with our executive director, Joseph Bobbitt (*Crisis in Child Mental Health: Challenge for the 1970's,* 1970). Each of them had demonstrated, and still is demonstrating, impressive synthetic capacities in research. The child advocacy concept, which evolved as a major recommendation of the Joint Commission, is an example of teaming such capacities.

One of the unfulfilled needs I felt strongly about was explored by a distinguished group made possible by the Stern Family Fund. This was the need for a research group to function as a strategy and planning body in the child health and mental health field. The concept became one of the recommendations of the Joint Commission. It is gratifying after many vicissitudes to see it now a fledgeling reality as the Human Services Institute for Families and Children. Hopefully there can now be a more thorough structure to allow the thinking through of comprehensive, coordinated programs for children instead of so many decisions made to meet crises, adding to our current fragmented, overlapping, uncoordinated programs for children in this country.

Unfortunately not all one's good research projects come to fruition. Many die aborning. For example, there is our action research project for dealing with the developmental roots of racism. Since racism has been identified as a major problem in this country and since we have information about how and when racist attitudes can begin, it seems timely to test a program to attempt preventive approaches. We know that it is between two and four years of age that a child looks at himself and others and asks the question; Is black or white or yellow or red good or bad, clean or dirty, beautiful or ugly? We know that first answer can provide a foundation for later attitudes toward others who are different. Helping parents to help young children find good answers as early as possible seems feasible, although we recognize at the same time the difficulties involved in such an oversimplification and the hazards to be expected. However, it should be recognized that one important and usually unspoken characteristic of the successful child psychiatric researcher is salesmanship. With this project, as with others before it, after the sales pitch, when the hat was passed around, it returned empty. It helps in this aspect of the field to be an optimist.

In all this my real wish is to return to bench research, where the most fundamental answers to our problems in child psychiatry will be found. If there can be an integrated approach to understanding the range of ways that cells and groups of cells defend themselves or fail to in the presence of stress or danger, and what chemical mediators are involved, do we have clues to the nature of the defenses of the mind? And in all this, with this mandate to look back, what I am proudest of are the young people who have gone on from our programs to establish themselves as contributors to child psychiatric research.

References

ABRAMSON, D., MARGOLIN, S., & LOURIE, R. Experimental extrasytoles in the cat. *Heart,* 1936, **110,** 76–81.

BENDER, L., & LOURIE, R. Effect of comic books on the ideology of children. *Am. J. Orthopsychiatry,* 1941, **11,** 54–65.

Crisis in child mental health: challenge for the 1970's. Report of the Joint Commission on the Mental Health of Children. New York: Harper and Row, 1970.

CROTHERS, B. A. *The pediatrician in search of mental hygiene.* New York: Commonwealth Fund, 1937.

GUTELIUS, M., MILLICAN, F. K., LAYMAN, E. M., COHEN, G., & DUBLIN, C. C. Nutritional studies of children with pica. *Pediatrics,* 1962, **29,** 1012–23.

LANSKOWSKY, P. Investigation into the etiology and treatment of pica. *Arch. Dis. Child.,* 1959, **34,** 140–148.

LAYMAN, E. M., MILLICAN, F. K., LOURIE, R. S., & TAKAHASHI, L. Y. Cultural influence and symptom choice: Etiology of pica. *Psychol. Rev.,* 1965, **13,** 249–257.

LOURIE, R. Autonomic nervous system function in children. *AMA J. Dis. Child.,* 1943, **65,** 455–470.

LOURIE, R., The role of rhythmic patterns in childhood. *Am. J. Psychiatry,* 1949, **105,** 653–661.

LOURIE, R. Psychosomatic problems in infants, in *Problems of communication.* New York: Grune and Stratton, 1955.

LOURIE, R., LAYMAN, E. M., & MILLICAN, F. K. Why children eat things that are not food. *Children,* 1963, **10,** 143–146.

MARANS, A., & LOURIE, R. Hypotheses regarding the effects of child rearing patterns on the disadvantaged child. In J. Hellmuth (ed.), *The disadvantaged child* (Vol. 1). Seattle: Special Child Publications, 1961.

MURPHY, L. A vulnerability inventory. In: C. Chandler, R. Lourie, & A. Peters (eds.), *Early child care: the new perspectives.* New York: Atherton Press, 1968.

PAVENSTEDT, E., & MALONE, C. *The drifters.* New York: International University Press, 1971.

EPILOGUE

THE STATE OF THE ART AND SCIENCE IN CHILD PSYCHIATRY[1]

E. James Anthony

A review of the changes in child psychiatry over the past two decades would suggest that although some minor shifts in attitude and orientation have occurred, putting an emphasis on different issues, the practice has remained relatively unaffected, apart from the trial of different therapeutic maneuvers. The minimal research that has emerged in this period has had little impact on the establishment of a scientifically based body of knowledge.

Child psychiatry remains as service-oriented as ever, and its training programs are designed to produce new service-oriented child psychiatrists to carry on the tradition. The therapeutic skills developed with experience are impressive, although their efficacy remains to be rigorously evaluated. In fact, the art has flourished, but the science has stood still. I presumptuously offer here a tentative blueprint for future development, although there is ground for skepticism, based on past performance, that this will bridge the chasm between the science and the art. Efforts of this nature, nevertheless, must be made if this fragile discipline is to be salvaged from its present predicament.

There are certain challenging moments in the history of science that when first encountered have something of a shock value in reordering one's conception of things. A good example of this is the French mathematician-philosopher Poincaré's (1952) consideration of the relativity of space:

> Suppose that in one night all the dimensions of the universe became a thousand times larger. . . . When I awake in the morning, what will be my feeling in face of such an astonishing transformation? Well, I shall not notice anything at all. The most exact measures will be incapable of revealing anything of this tremendous change, since the yard-measures I shall use will have varied in exactly the same

[1] Read before the annual meeting of the Society of Professors of Child Psychiatry, Los Angeles, March 2, 1973, and published in the *Archives of General Psychiatry*, Volume 29, September 1973

E. JAMES ANTHONY, The Harry Edison Child Development Research Center, Washington University School of Medicine, St. Louis.

proportions as the objects I shall attempt to measure. In reality the change only
exists for those who argue as if space were absolute [page 94].

Suppose (we could ask) that all textbooks, annual reviews, journals, and
research papers (miniscule though these are) were collectively destroyed
overnight. What would we notice the next morning, the next year, or the next
decade in the day-to-day practice of child psychiatry? As things are now, we
would probably notice nothing, because very little appears to feed into the art
from the science. This is in part because the science is undeniably still embryonic, in part because research and application are not currently regarded as
mutually related, and in part, sad to report, because the busy and service-com-
mitted practitioner does not, in general, keep up with the psychiatric and
psychological literature pertaining even to his own specialty once he has
passed his board examination.

Having focused on the gloomiest element in the picture, I think it is
equally important to mention the assets that have combined to keep the
profession alive although not altogether well. A growing population of child
psychiatrists is gradually distributing itself across the country and helping to
give direction, leadership, and psychiatric impetus to a large number of clinics
that previously had functioned nondescriptively as guidance and counseling
agencies. The individual child psychiatrist seems less confused than previously
about his identity and seems more self-assured about his overall responsibilities
within the clinic. He is entering the larger world of the community with a confidence based on technical skills rather than on status. Within a comparatively
short time textbooks have been written and specialty examinations instituted,
an academy has been founded, and a journal, documenting the scientific
growth of the membership, has made its appearance. Although we are
probably in much better shape than our enemies think we are, let us admit, at
least to ourselves, that we are suffering from certain defects and disabilities
that are becoming chronically ingrained and are very liable to impede our
future progress as an art–science.

We can discuss the diagnosis in the context of two well-known parables.
The first is the story of Buridan's ass, who died from indecision when exposed
to two equal lots of hay. He succumbed from having too much to consider. The
second parable (a favorite of Freud's) tells of another ass, who was doing a
good job until the skinflint directors of the organization began to wonder
whether he could not do what he did on less. So they cut his food ration in
half, and the hard-working little ass continued to function just as well. He
made no complaints at all, or perhaps no one heard him if he did, because he
was constitutionally endowed with quite a soft voice. Each day the organization reduced his ration of hay until they got him down to a single straw, and
then they took even that away. The next day the poor little ass died, and no
one was more surprised than the directors of the organization.

As diagnosticians we must ask very candidly which sort of ass is child psychiatry. On the surface, and in the context of the severe federal cuts, it would seem to be suffering from the same problem as the second ass, who continued to work with characteristic diligence and masochism in the face of dwindling resources. In a profounder and different sense, however, child psychiatry can be equated with the first ass. Child psychiatrists invariably get themselves overcommitted to a multitude of attractions—running clinics, consulting with schools, working with the community, training students and residents, and attempting to treat every "fascinating" patient who appears on the doorstep. How can they possibly find time for scholarship and research?

In spite of these dire forebodings and in spite of the financial threats hanging over our heads at the present time, enough organizational work has been done to ensure the survival of child psychiatry as a profession. For one thing, schools of medicine have grown accustomed to having us around, even though they may sometimes wonder vaguely who we are and what on earth we are doing on the campus. Being where we want to be, within a school of medicine, is not enough; we must do what we ought to be doing toward making our specialty more of a science. Our need is to project an image of ourselves that compares not too unfavorably with the images of neighboring disciplines and to make significant contributions to both the medical and the behavioral sciences. This is not to deny that they may already have gained from us something of our intrinsic humanism, which could help to moderate a little of the "coldness" of pure science. In order to achieve our completest identity and make our fullest offering, we should cultivate both the art and the science of our specialty. It is always impressive to observe how artistically the therapy is carried out in many centers, but if one asks about clinical investigation, there is generally an embarrassed mumble about time and service pressures. There can be no concern, therefore, about the survival of child psychiatry as a diagnostic and therapeutic art, and a marvelously transmittable art at that, but there should be real anxiety about its continuance as a science.

Up to the present its deceptive health and identity have been largely based on borrowings from medical and behavioral disciplines and attempts "to make them our own" by a process of synthesis and integration; but will such products ever be quintessentially "child psychiatric"? As Goethe said, long ago, only what we have struggled to bring into being ourselves is ever really our own. We cannot survive predominantly on transplants.

Following up on this line of thought, our interests should be gravitating toward building our own scientific house from the foundation upward, and if we have to borrow (which, admittedly, at the present stage we have to do), we should limit our plagiarism to method rather than content. This limit should enable us to produce a body of knowledge relevant to our own specific needs and situations. We must manufacture and garnish our own frames of reference in our own inimitable styles. We can do this not by passively reading what others have written for us but by writing for ourselves and our own advancement. In this sense we should not identify with our patients and assume postures of dependency. There is nothing in these suggestions that could be construed as foolishly advocating a policy of self-sufficiency and self-containment. An important part of our scientific activity is to penetrate and explore the sciences around us that are much farther ahead in their development and can provide us with necessary models for generating, storing, and using relevant data. Nevertheless, we must be aware of the hazards entailed in doing even this, since imported scientific attitudes and methods may not prove very useful, and unless we have done a great deal of preparatory work for ourselves, we may be more bewildered than benefited by what we try to assimilate.

In 1724 the author of *Gulliver's Travels* (1971) warned us of this possible danger when discussing the relationship between the world of science, as represented by the Flying Island of Laputa hovering in the air, and the solid, earth-based country of Balnibarbi, with all its pretensions and aspirations. On some occasion a few inhabitants of Balnibarbi paid a visit to Laputa and returned "with a very little Smattering in Mathematics" but "full of Volatile Spirits acquired in the Airy Region." (Have we not all returned elated at some time from visits in the rarified atmospheres of National Institutes and Centers for Advanced Study!) Swift proceeds with this comment (which we should take very much to heart):

> These Persons upon their Return, began to dislike the Management of every Thing below; and fell into Schemes of putting all Arts, Sciences, Languages, and Mechanics upon a new Foot. To this end they procured a Royal Patent for erecting an Academy . . . !

Here we must part company from these aspiring Balnibarbians. When your science is in trouble, the solution does not lie in erecting an Academy or Society or Association; too often all this does is to organize, institutionalize, and ritualize the nonscientific trends in the making. Nor does the solution consist in thrusting a hastily acquired Smattering in Mathematics upon resistant colleagues and inviting them to exchange psychoanalysis for statistical analysis. They will often inform you, in no uncertain terms, what you can do with the latter! Nor is there any remedy in that well-known panacea for all earthly ills: the appointment of a committee, with a subcommittee and a chairman for each portion of the problem. The only workable answer is in a change of heart and a change of head. We must become thinking as well as feeling people and focus on cognition as much as we focus on affect. We must school ourselves to dedicate our interests as much to projects as to patients and to write science into our working lives. All this requires a redistribution of cathexis, an expansion of our professional curiosity, and a new numerical consciousness that makes findings in two patients twice as interesting as the same findings in one patient. However, as every physician knows, prescriptions are easily written but less easily followed. When the patient is a professional discipline, its body of members is not always able or ready to recognize the diagnostic implications that indicate a need for change in functioning. Institutions are notoriously hypochondriacal in this respect and are constantly complaining about real or imaginary maladjustments in the organization. For this reason an ailing society or association can become chronically dispirited and disabled without anyone's taking the matter too seriously. One reason for this *laissez-faire* is the fads and fashions that transiently engage the interest and then vanish. Diagnoses and prescriptions are undoubtedly a reflection of particular times, and the significance of either diminishes with the passage of time. We can appreciate this by turning to history.

Diagnosis, Prescription, and Prediction 20 Years Ago

Twenty years ago, David Levy (1952) gave the academic address to the American Psychiatric Association, the subject being "The Critical Evaluation of the Present State of Child Psychiatry." Seen from the perspective of today, his title is intriguing and raises a number of questions. Would his concerns now seem outdated, his suggested regimes outmoded, and his conjectures about future developments falsified by time?

Since this was still within the golden era of the child guidance movement, he was, as one might have expected, preoccupied with the "team approach" in terms of its advantages and disadvantages. On the positive side he allowed that the team had been instrumental in alerting clinics to the total situation of the child and to the multiple factors involved in etiology, thus laying the groundwork for a genuine social psychiatry, which was never, unfortunately, followed to its logical conclusion. On the negative side he regarded the team approach as putting "a checkmate on scientific values" and consequently as detrimental to the further development of child psychiatry. Among other debits he enumerated the overlapping and blurring of professional functions, leading to a blunting of specific skills, the almost exclusive focus on therapy to the comparative neglect of diagnosis and prognosis, and the loss of professional identity that reduced the child psychiatrist, for all practical purposes, to a "lay psychiatrist." Yet he was unready to recommend the eviction of the psychological and social members of the team. They should remain, he thought, if their roles were clarified and subordinated and their functions defined within the general context of the medical tradition.

Where did he suppose child psychiatry was going? It is intriguing to note that his prophesies, like the prophesies of all prophets, both scientific and lay, follow on the projections of his own work. He felt that the observational studies that he had pioneered would multiply and provide a body of empirical data; that the processes and materials involved in treatment would be subject to systematic investigation along the lines that he had laid down; and that psychopharmacology would not only grow in importance but render the child psychiatrist increasingly conscious of his medical origins.

In a discussion of this paper at the time, Kanner (1952), whatever misgivings he had about the interchangeability of roles and functions, was driven to admit that the "holy trinity" had indeed become indispensable to the practice of clinical child psychiatry. In the course of our evolution we had grown these appendages and could not shed them without endangering our survival. His personal diagnosis of the profession was that it suffered from narrowness. The Freudian viewpoint was paramount, and giants like Meyer, Kraeplin, Kretschmer, Bleuler, and Janet were all dismissed as dismal "old fogies." Extremists, whether geneticists, organicists, intrapsychic determinists, or transactionists, maintained their respective positions rigidly and exclusively, so that nobody learned or was prepared to learn from anybody else. His prescription, like Levy's, was dictated largely by his own eclectic interests. According to him, there were two basic movements in child psychiatry: the centripetal one concerned with knowing more about the inner structure of the developing individual (as evident in the work of Binet, Piaget, Stern, Buhler, and Freud), and the centrifugal one dealing with the external milieu and its interface with the internal environment of the growing child. This latter was largely based on American effort. Kanner saw the two movements as complementary and felt sure that their convergence would eventually lead to "a new and fruitful step forward in the rapid advance of child psychiatry." He recognized, however, that some preliminary unfreezing of doctrinaire positions would be necessary before this pluralistic and relativistic viewpoint could be generally adopted.

The second discussant of Levy's address was the redoubtable Frederick Allen (1952), whose main consideration, predictably, was helping children and their parents psychotherapeutically to live more comfortably with one another. The team was not only indispensable for this purpose but also "one of the far-reaching and unique contributions of child psychiatry," since each member was able to grow and develop *vis-à-vis* the other. This was the mystique of the "holy trinity" in its most developed form—one in three and three in one. Allen was not concerned with the families as such but with children and their parents, and he was concerned with both. He hoped that the child psychiatrists of the future would feel better disposed toward parents, who were having a rough time in the literature around that period. The guilt stemming from parental abuse was beginning to set in. Winnicott (1956), for example, was reminding analytic psychotherapists that they should always be grateful for the hard work done by parents in the first five years of life because it made their own work in transference years later so much easier. One could imagine the bedtime prayer of the psychotherapist: "Thank you, Lord, for the average, good-enough parents who have helped to make my work tolerable!"

Levy, Kanner, and Allen, looking at the state of child psychiatry 20 years ago, appear to have come to somewhat different conclusions about diagnosis, treatment, and prognosis. Levy undoubtedly scored highest in his forecasts of further empirical development, but it is Kanner's theoretical comments on the convergence of inner and outer knowledge that appear most pertinent to the current trend in conceptualization, although, sad to say, Mayer, Kraeplin, Kretschmer, Bleuler, and Janet would be still regarded in child psychiatric circles as "old fogies." (This is probably another indication of *memento mori*, and along the lines of Mark Twain's thoughts about his father that the closer one gets to becoming an "old fogey," the more strongly one feels that there is a great deal to be learned from them; it has been referred to as presenile *folie à deux*.) Allen had least to predict except more of the same thing—more team-work, more casework, and more nondirective guidance. It seems from this one discussion that he had a fairly limited notion of child psychiatry as merely one other therapeutic agency working toward the growth and differentiation of the child.

The State of the Art–Science Today

Where then are we today? On the face of it we still seem to be struggling with the same dilemmas as in the past: between doing child guidance or child psychiatry, between being a community agency or a medical facility, and between having a psychoanalytic orientation or a biopsychosocial one. In spite of our community interests and contacts we are not regarded as a social or community psychiatry, although many of us are heavily involved in mental health centers. We continue to pursue the psychiatric and psychosocial investigation of our cases in collaboration with our colleagues, but we would be far more hesitant to acknowledge that this represented the "unique contribution" that child psychiatry had to make to psychological medicine. This is not to say that any general conclusion has been reached by this subdiscipline as to what its unique contribution could or should be, and part of the problem is that we remain befuddled about our identities and allegiances. Isolation, and a certain amount of persecution, has at times caused us to react like any minority faction. We occasionally seem to see ourselves as chosen people with an inherent empathic capacity not only to understand children but to act as "superconsultants" in the role of communicators, integrators, and transmitters for interprofessional groups. Behind this grandiosity, as always, are feelings of insecurity and inadequacy, which we can only thinly disguise by sheltering within our academies, associations, and societies.

The diagnosis we would make today is different from 20 years ago, and if we are honest with ourselves, we would be more inclined to emphasize our "character" disorder. There is no doubt that child psychiatry is regarded by hard-nosed medical and behavioral scientists as a "soft" profession and child psychiatrists as essentially soft-hearted individuals with a curious and somewhat puzzling affinity for children. With a scientifically unbecoming subjectivity we display a credulity about evidence, an often-passionate dogmatism about our intuitive hunches, and an overinvolvement with our patients and their families. In this respect we stand at the opposite pole from most of our colleagues. We are the humanists of the "two-culture" system described by Snow (1959), and there are many diagnostic pointers to indicate this. Bennis (1969), for example, has suggested that the process of learning is radically different within the two cultures: in a scientific culture the learner scans the content of the material regardless of who produces it, rarely recalling the author and tending to depersonalize the information that he retains; the humanistic trainee, on the other hand, learns through identification, sets up influential models, and is extremely aware of the personalities that have guided him. He is, in fact, the typical child psychiatrist in the making. In child psychiatry, training is carried out through a system of supervised apprenticeship, and the trainee picks up procedures in the way children assimilate the practice of parenthood from their parents, first by acting as children, then by becoming surrogate parents, and finally by becoming parents. The contact with the patient is likewise humane, tender, and personalized. We do mainly "soft" things with them, such as talking to them empathically, playing with them nondirectively, and providing them with an understanding of their predicament in a harsh world. For many of us it may have been some time since we examined a child medically or pricked him with a needle, and some of our more tender-hearted colleagues shudder at the thought of inflicting even minimal pain on the small patient.

Can we afford to remain so "soft?" True, the cultivation of "softness" may have enhanced our considerable therapeutic skills in psychological treatment, and we may be understandably reluctant to sacrifice a characteristic that pays off so well in practice. However, if we follow our own proclivity and analyze the origin and meaning of our "softness," we may develop some doubt about its lasting value for our own professional advancement. We must work rather at becoming useful both to ourselves and to our patients and refrain from making "sacrifices" for the sake of treatment. It does not take much analysis of unconscious factors to unearth a massive identification with both mother and child in the original dyadic state and thereby to compensate for any deficiencies in parenting that once existed and from which the child must be rescued. In the identification with the child we strive to recapture, vicariously, the lost narcissism of childhood, together with some of the omnipotence and omniscience that had so little realistic basis. We can use this interpretation to explain, in part, why we are such saviors as a group and why our slender hunches seem to carry so much conviction, irrespective of the realistic criticism to which we are subjected.

There is no question that in the next two decades the pressure will be on us. Can we afford not to change? Can we afford not to develop a much wider range of approach? Can we afford not to consider a broader spectrum of theories and theorists, even including some of the "old fogies"? Can we afford not to abandon points of view that have served their purpose and become outdated with the accretion of new evidence? Can we afford not to test our clinical hunches systematically and attempt to disprove them? Can we afford not to have laboratories in our buildings in addition to playrooms? Gut knowledge is all very well and may even be true, but it can only be transmitted from person to person within the shaping process of supervision, and gut knowledge dies with the gut.

If we wish to enter the brotherhood of scientific professions, we must have more solid and verifiable underpinnings of knowledge than we currently possess. We owe much too much to psychoanalysis and with good reason. It helped to get us off the ground, to sustain us during our development, and to make us into sensitive therapists but inept scientists. It has consolidated our suspicion of experiment. In this context one can recall Freud's famous postcard to Rosenzweig (1962) in 1934, in which he commented on the latter's attempt to study repression experimentally: "I cannot put much value on these confirmations because the wealth of reliable observations on which these assertions rest makes them independent of experimental verification." However, he added graciously, "Still, it can do no harm." This attitude is completely suitable for psychoanalysis, which is largely a self-contained and self-sufficient discipline, but it simply cannot provide a model for child psychiatry, which is hemmed in on all sides by medical and behavioral sciences, with which it must transact in order to survive. Psychoanalysis has helped us to become good therapists; we must now look to other sciences to help us become good scientists. We must provide settings in which empirical explorations are given free scope, and we must give equal time to both art and science. This point brings us to consider the crucial problem of time and the way in which we clutter up the entire day with a plethora of competing interests: supervision, teaching, administration, treatment, consultation, video taping, staff meetings, group sessions, etc., representing one bundle of hay, and quiet reflection, creative jottings, the sketching out of research projects, the reading of pertinent articles, the writing of reviews summarizing knowledge in an area, etc., representing the other bundle of hay. What is the poor ass going to do? If he is a shrewd and not a stupid and self-destructive ass, he will marshal his resources and deploy them within the limits of time as strategically as he is able. We do not want to see him paralyzed between art and science; we do not want to see him the complete artist and certainly not the nothing-but scientist. We want him to learn to pursue this art–science to the furthest and fullest, but in order to do so he must learn to master the problem of time in his professional life. Piaget, in bidding farewell to the author 20 years ago, gave him one parting word of advice that he himself rigorously followed: every day, for three hours in the afternoon, he should walk beside a river or over the hills meditating on his work and hatching new ideas. Otherwise there was a danger of his becoming just another professional in the field.

Being given a gift of time, the next problem is to discover what to do with it. Free time for anyone, including the busy clinician, may represent nothing but the unguarded exposure to exotic or erotic daydreaming, unless we begin to develop scientific free associations akin to the ones we already use in therapy. We can, in time, become as curious about a project as about a patient and cultivate a "floating" attention to suit both circumstances.

As a second prelude to the development of a scientific attitude, we need to become accustomed to the process of conjecture and thereby to establish predictive skills, that is, in more rigorous terms, to distribute probabilities among different possible futures. To do this we require an adequate knowledge of past and present contingencies.

We will not begin in a state of complete naïveté: we are already excellent historians with a sound developmental sense of the past, and we are in the process of becoming good observers of the present scene. We need, however, to become reliable predictors of the future, and to do this we must acquire a comprehensive system of knowledge of the developing child and, based on this knowledge, practice in short-term and long-term forecasting. As a matter of fact, we can write this small scientific exercise into our everyday work by formulating prognoses specifically and systematically with every history and diagnosis that we construct.

The importance of this procedure cannot be overstated. Comte (1966), who specialized in integrating scientific fields, had this to say:

> The aim of every science is foresight [*prévoyance*]. For the laws established by observation of phenomena are generally employed to foresee their succession. All men, however little advanced [and we may take comfort from this], make true predictions, which are always based on the same principle, the knowledge of the future from the past. For example, all men predict the general effects of terrestrial gravity [for example, when we jump off the earth we come back to it, or at least some of us do!] and a multitude of other phenomena sufficiently simple and usual for the least capable and attentive spectator to be aware of their order of succession. The faculty of foresight in each person is measured by his science.

What Comte was saying here so reassuringly is that everyone is a bit of a scientist, and some are more so than others. Every time we diagnose and treat a child, we are laying odds on the future outcome, and although we may express it in fairly simple terms, such as "getting better," "losing his symptoms," or "becoming better adjusted," we are, in fact, carrying out a scientific project that time will prove or disprove. We can restrict ourselves to such diffuse statements or become more specific. We can refer to general trends with a larger prospect of turning out to be right—the child will be better, worse, or stay the same—or we can make a more critical forecast, predicting, for example, that the child will have a schizophrenic breakdown early in adult life. In making forecasts we are also making selections, and since nobody is so omniscient as to forecast all possible outcomes, the best we can often do is to choose certain elements from the past and present that we can project into the future.

Although we can make predictions within the framework of everyday practice, we need something more when we undertake scientific research into the future. As already indicated, we must have a certain minimal reservoir of knowledge, and this, unfortunately, we still lack in child psychiatry. Furthermore, what we have is mostly borrowed knowledge. There are two kinds of knowledge that can come together to form a consolidated body of knowledge and a basis for scientific prediction: knowledge accumulating within the child psychiatrist about the child and knowledge about the growth of knowledge in the child.

Knowledge about the child includes knowledge of his development within a complicated milieu of persons and things. It includes a knowledge of processes, of environments, and of the relationship of body to mind. There already exist several developmental maps with which we have reason to be fairly satisfied. They trace the course of psychosexual, psychosocial, and psychocognitive developments according to Freud, Mahler, Erikson, and Piaget. We are also accumulating direct observational knowledge about critical and optimal phases of development and the impact of phase-specific stresses on the further course of development. To these we have added sporadic facts stemming from the work of the academic developmental psychologists subscribing to learning theories.

The knowledge of processes has added an important dimension to our total understanding, since it employs a micro- and macro-analytic approach across time, which gives a more vivid and experiential grasp of knowledge. One of the major shifts in the training of residents, for example, takes place when they develop an understanding of the temporal processes that underlie the content of diagnostic or therapeutic interviews. The GAP Committee on Child Psychiatry (in press) has pioneered this avenue over the past two decades and has opened up the conventional areas of child psychiatry—diagnosis, classification, treatment planning, and treatment—to the investigation of process. Treatment planning, for instance, is no longer regarded as an *ad hoc*, intuitively made decision to institute a certain therapeutic program; instead, the process approach enlarges and elaborates the whole area between diagnosis and treatment, throwing into relief the team discussions of discomforts, the interactions between the clinicians and the family, the mode of communicating diagnostic findings to parents and children, the mutual discussions concerning the needs of the patient and the facilities for meeting them, etc. In its analysis of the therapeutic process the GAP committee is concentrating on the similarities and the dissimilarities of process in dyadic, familial, or group situations and the way in which transference and transaction are affected by age, sex, and sociocultural factors present in both patient and therapist. The therapeutic process can also be looked at in terms of the flow of affect, which can be followed through the series of cycles that run through the session. For example, sexual or aggressive impulses may elicit guilt; remorse; a wish to make amends; the development of inhibitions, regressions, or passivity; responses of shame to ensuing feelings of inferiority; and the need to overcompensate for all of these. The process of play has been subjected to micro- and macroanalysis by Erikson (1940) through a sequence comprising a common-sense description of a unit of play; the morphoanalysis of affects, spatial relationships, and behavioral modes; a subjective impression of latent possibilities based on past experience; an interpretation of symbols and metaphors following the analysis of defenses; a developmental reconstruction and analysis of configurations; and finally, a confirmation of the conclusions reached in the outcome of further events.

The knowledge of environments has also recently enlarged its scope and represents a more sophisticated development of the home visits carried out by social workers in the early days of child psychiatry. Today we are no longer content simply to describe the different environments; we wish also to understand why they evolved in a particular form. Brutalizing environments in which children are exposed to battering and sadistic attacks have been shown to emerge predictably from the environments experienced by the parents as children, and the environment of psychosis, with its peculiar inconsistency and incoherence, can be predictably linked to the eventual symptomatic behavior of the children, anxiously puzzled and searching for ways to make sense of the irrationality. Conflictual environments are essentially predivorce settings that may or may not culminate in divorce and that may or may not extend into bitter postdivorce resentments and recriminations. It is often the lot of children to be caught up as volunteers or conscripts in the marital struggle and sometimes to have to struggle with both parties or even to change sides under conditions of threat or seduction. To survive in such an environment sometimes demands huge capacities for denial, distancing, and distraction, but to understand the choice of defense or offense, we must study the conflictual process as it evolves in the family. Environments of psychosocial isolation and impoverishment create their own curiosities of psychopathology, often demonstrating that the mind is as susceptible to undernourishment as the body and even less liable to recover from its effects. In time the researching child psychiatrist will be able to correlate these several environments with both the child's behavior and his inner representation of the circumstance. To understand the child's reaction, it is not sufficient to assess the world he lives in as the investigating adult perceives it; the child may not see it at all in this fashion and may even paradoxically reconstruct it inwardly in an opposite form, causing his responses to appear paradoxical unless one becomes aware of this "psychic" reality. Nevertheless, it is equally important (if only to gauge the extent of the paradox) to evaluate the real environment psychosocially, epidemiologically, and ecologically and to examine the "behavior day" of the child within this larger context.

The knowledge of the body in relation to the child's mind, and the impact of physical illness and physical discomfort on his emotional life have already become a specialized interest for a number of researching child psychiatrists who are currently reconstructing the "natural history" of certain chronic diseases, to include the psychological adaptation of the child and his family. What he feels about the privacy of his body can be most vividly inferred from his reactions to medical intrusions, and it is therefore of importance for the child psychiatrist to be around when the child is being subjected to these inevitable stresses, which are natural experiments that need to be understood in their entirety.

This rewarding preoccupation with the microanalysis of human attitudes and feelings in the process of formation should not blind us to the macroscopy of environments—the gross conditions of inner cities, ghettos, and slums— which can also be correlated with developing psychopathology. We should bear in mind that big things can be as harmful as little things, and outside things as harmful as inside things—facts that are often overlooked by the microanalyst. To formulate an overview, it should become the essence of our observational training to look bifocally at the child's environment, not only as we see it but also as he sees it, and we will then begin to understand how he fits himself into it.

We come finally to the way in which we get to know the child as a knower, as the constructor of a knowledge bank that will render him a competent human being for the remainder of his life. The philosophical term for this is *epistemology*, and after many years of study Piaget (1950) saw fit to bring his accumulation of development facts together and to establish a new discipline of genetic epistemology at his center in Geneva, which every child psychiatrist should visit at least once in his lifetime. In genetic epistemology the inquiry can take both cognitive and affective directions: we can learn how the outer world is conceived of by the child in terms of cognitive appreciation, and we can also learn how the most important chunk of this world, namely, the group of people with whom he becomes emotionally related, is represented within him, as well as to what extent the two inner worlds are clearly differentiated within themselves and between themselves. The better this inner representation, the more skillfully does he learn to manage his everyday life, and the more likely is he to become increasingly self-reliant and self-confident. This new and vital theory of personal, interpersonal, and organizational competence will undoubtedly dominate research in child psychiatry over the next two decades. Competence has two parts to it: a representation competence that provides the child with a working model of the outside world and an executive competence that has to do with his organizational abilities within his particular environment. The more completely competent the child is, the less vulnerable he should prove in relation to the many risks—genetic, reproductive, constitutional, environmental, and traumatic—that seem ready to overpower him. Competence can also be related to other good ego qualities, such as resilience and maturity of defenses, excellence of coping skills, and the power to synthesize experience.

This is some, but by no means all, of the knowledge that we need to carry out our predictive work reliably, and if we add to it the knowledge of developmental psychobiology, we should certainly have enough at our scientific disposal for the next 20 years. An inquisitive speaker at the meeting of the Society of Professors of Child Psychiatry in 1993 may well ferret out this presentation and, we can hope, find that in these dim and dismal times, plagued by financial crises that undermine the growing programs of training and research, child psychiatry was at least beginning to deal with some of the right and rewarding issues.

References

ALLEN, F. Discussion of: Critical evaluation of the present state of child psychiatry. *American Journal of Psychiatry*, 1952, **108**, 492–494.

BENNIS, W. A psychoanalytic inquiry into the "two cultures" dilemma. *Psychoanalytic Forum*, 1969, **3**, 161–183.

COMTE, A. *A system of positive polity*. New York: Franklin, 1966, Vol. 4.

ERIKSON, E. Studies in the interpretation of plays. I: Clinical observation of play disruption in young children. *Genetic Psychology Monographs*, 1940, **22**, 557–671.

GAP COMMITTEE ON CHILD PSYCHIATRY. *From diagnosis to treatment: An approach to treatment planning for the emotionally disturbed child*. Group for the Advancement of Psychiatry. In press.

KANNER, L. Discussion of: Critical evaluation of the present state of child psychiatry. *American Journal of Psychiatry*, 1952, **108**, 490–492.

LEVY, D. The critical evaluation of the present state of child psychiatry. *American Journal of Psychiatry*, 1952, **108**, 481–490.

PIAGET, J. *Introduction to genetic epistemology*. Paris: PUF, 1950.

POINCARÉ, H. *Science and method.* New York: Dover, 1952.

ROSENZWEIG, S. Postcard from S. Freud. In L. Postman (Ed.), *Psychology in the making.* New York: Knopf, 1962.

SNOW, C. *The two cultures and the scientific revolution.* Cambridge: Cambridge University Press, 1959.

SWIFT, J. *Gulliver's travels.* New York: Oxford University Press, 1971.

WINNICOTT, D. W. Clinical varieties of transference. *Int. J. Psycho-Anal.,* **37,** 386, 1956.

INDEX

495